T0263824

Implantable Devices: Design, Manufacturing, and Malfunction

Editors

KENNETH A. ELLENBOGEN
CHARLES J. LOVE

CARDIAC ELECTROPHYSIOLOGY CLINICS

www.cardiacEP.theclinics.com

Consulting Editors
RANJAN K. THAKUR
ANDREA NATALE

June 2014 • Volume 6 • Number 2

ELSEVIER

1600 John F. Kennedy Boulevard • Suite 1800 • Philadelphia, Pennsylvania, 19103-2899

http://www.theclinics.com

CARDIAC ELECTROPHYSIOLOGY CLINICS Volume 6, Number 2
June 2014 ISSN 1877-9182, ISBN-13: 978-0-323-32315-4

Editor: Adrianne Brigido
Developmental Editor: Barbara Cohen-Kligerman

Cardiac Electrophysiology Clinics (ISSN 1877-9182) is published quarterly by Elsevier Inc., 360 Park Avenue South, New York, NY 10010-1710. Months of issue are March, June, September, and December. Subscription prices are $200.00 per year for US individuals, $293.00 per year for US institutions, $105.00 per year for US students and residents, $225.00 per year for Canadian individuals, $331.00 per year for Canadian institutions, $285.00 per year for international individuals, $354.00 per year for international institutions and $150.00 per year for Canadian and foreign students/residents. To receive student/resident rate, orders must be accompanied by name of affiliated institution, date of term, and the signature of program/residency coordinator on institution letterhead. Orders will be billed at individual rate until proof of status is received. Foreign air speed delivery is included in all Clinics subscription prices. All prices are subject to change without notice. **POSTMASTER:** Send address changes to Cardiac Electrophysiology Clinics, Elsevier Health Sciences Division, Subscription Customer Service, 3251 Riverport Lane, Maryland Heights, MO 63043. **Customer Service: 1-800-654-2452 (US and Canada). From outside of the US and Canada, call 314-477-8871. Fax: 314-447-8029. E-mail: JournalsCustomerService-usa@elsevier.com (for print support); JournalsOnlineSupport-usa@elsevier.com (for online support).**

Reprints. For copies of 100 or more of articles in this publication, please contact the Commercial Reprints Department, Elsevier Inc., 360 Park Avenue South, New York, NY 10010-1710. Tel.: 212-633-3874; Fax: 212-633-3820; E-mail: reprints@elsevier.com.

Contributors

CONSULTING EDITORS

RANJAN K. THAKUR, MD, MPH, MBA, FHRS
Professor of Medicine and Director, Arrhythmia Service, Thoracic and Cardiovascular Institute, Sparrow Health System, Michigan State University, Lansing, Michigan

ANDREA NATALE, MD, FACC, FHRS
Executive Medical Director, Texas Cardiac Arrhythmia Institute, St. David's Medical Center, Austin, Texas; Consulting Professor, Division of Cardiology, Stanford University, Palo Alto, California; Adjunct Professor of Medicine, Heart and Vascular Center, Case Western Reserve University, Cleveland, Ohio; Director, Interventional Electrophysiology, Scripps Clinic, San Diego, California; Senior Clinical Director, EP Services, California Pacific Medical Center, San Francisco, California

EDITORS

KENNETH A. ELLENBOGEN, MD, FAHA, FACC, FHRS
Kontos Professor of Cardiology, VCU School of Medicine, Pauley Heart Center, Richmond, Virginia

CHARLES J. LOVE, MD, FACC, FAHA, FHRS, CCDS
Professor of Clinical Medicine, Division of Cardiology, Heart Rhythm Center, New York University Langone Medical Center, New York, New York; President, International Board of Heart Rhythm Examiners, Washington, DC

AUTHORS

CARINA BLOMSTRÖM-LUNDQVIST, MD, PhD
Professor of Cardiology, Department of Cardiology, Institution of Medical Science, Uppsala University, Uppsala, Sweden

MARIA GRAZIA BONGIORNI, MD
Cardiology Department, University Hospital of Pisa, Pisa, Italy

PIERRE BORDACHAR, MD, PhD
Medical Doctor, Hôpital Cardiologique du Haut-Lévêque, CHU Bordeaux, IHU LIRYC, Université Bordeaux, Bordeaux, France

MARTIN C. BURKE, DO
Director, Section of Cardiology; Professor, Department of Medicine, Heart Rhythm Center, University of Chicago, Chicago, Illinois

YONG-MEI CHA, MD
Professor of Medicine, Division of Cardiovascular Diseases, Department of Internal Medicine, Mayo Clinic, Rochester, Minnesota

JANE CHEN, MD, FACC, FHRS
Associate Professor, Cardiovascular Division, Department of Medicine, Washington University School of Medicine, St Louis, Missouri

GEORGE H. CROSSLEY, MD, FACC, FHRS, CCDS
Associate Professor, Vanderbilt Heart Institute, Vanderbilt University, Nashville, Tennessee

IAN CROZIER, MD
Department of Cardiology, Christchurch Hospital, Christchurch, New Zealand

MATTHEW DALY, MBChB
Department of Cardiology, Christchurch Hospital, Christchurch, New Zealand

CHRISTOPHER R. ELLIS, MD, FACC
Assistant Professor, Cardiac Electrophysiology, Vanderbilt Heart and Vascular Institute, Nashville, Tennessee

LAURENCE M. EPSTEIN, MD
Brigham & Women's Hospital, Boston, Massachusetts

ROMAIN ESCHALIER, MD, PhD
Medical Doctor, Hôpital Cardiologique du Haut-Lévêque, CHU Bordeaux, IHU LIRYC, Université Bordeaux, Bordeaux; Cardiology Department, ISIT-CaVITI, CHU Clermont-Ferrand, Clermont Université, Clermont-Ferrand, France

MIKAEL HANNINEN, MD
Division of Cardiology, University of Western Ontario, London, Ontario, Canada

BENGT HERWEG, MD, FACC, FHRS
Associate Professor of Medicine, Director, Electrophysiology and Arrhythmia Services, Department of Cardiovascular Disease, Tampa General Hospital, University of South Florida Morsani College of Medicine, Tampa, Florida

DARREN HOOKS, PhD, MBChB
Department of Cardiology, Christchurch Hospital, Christchurch, New Zealand

KAROLY KASZALA, MD, PhD, FHRS
Director, Cardiac Electrophysiology Laboratory, Hunter Holmes McGuire Veterans Affairs Medical Center; Associate Professor of Medicine, Virginia Commonwealth University, Richmond, Virginia

CHARLES KENNERGREN, MD, PhD, FETCS, FHRS
Senior Consultant, Associate Professor, Department of Cardiothoracic Surgery, Sahlgrenska University Hospital, Gothenburg, Sweden

AMMAR M. KILLU, MBBS
Fellow, Division of Cardiovascular Diseases, Department of Internal Medicine, Mayo Clinic, Rochester, Minnesota

GEORGE J. KLEIN, MD
Professor of Medicine, Division of Cardiology, University of Western Ontario, London, Ontario, Canada

MATTHEW J. KOLEK, MD
Vanderbilt Heart and Vascular Institute, Nashville, Tennessee

ANDREW D. KRAHN, MD, FRCPC, FHRS
Division of Cardiology, Diamond Health Care Centre, University of British Columbia, Vancouver, British Columbia, Canada

ERNEST W. LAU, MD
Department of Cardiology, Royal Victoria Hospital, Belfast, United Kingdom

TAYLOR LEBEIS, MD
Division of Clinical Cardiac Electrophysiology, Emory University Hospital, Atlanta, Georgia

MICHAEL S. LLOYD, MD, FACC, FHRS
Division of Clinical Cardiac Electrophysiology, Emory University Hospital, Atlanta, Georgia

CHARLES J. LOVE, MD, FACC, FAHA, FHRS, CCDS
Professor of Clinical Medicine, Division of Cardiology, Heart Rhythm Center, New York University Langone Medical Center, New York, New York; President, International Board of Heart Rhythm Examiners, Washington, DC

CIORSTI J. MACINTYRE, MD, FRCPC
Division of Cardiology, QE II Health Sciences Centre, Halifax, Nova Scotia, Canada

JAIMIE MANLUCU, MD
Assistant Professor of Medicine, Division
of Cardiology, University of Western
Ontario, London, Ontario, Canada

JOSEPH E. MARINE, MD
Associate Professor of Medicine, Johns
Hopkins University, Baltimore, Maryland

MELANIE MAYTIN, MD
Brigham & Women's Hospital, Boston,
Massachusetts

IAIN MELTON, MBChB
Department of Cardiology, Christchurch
Hospital, Christchurch, New Zealand

SAMAN NAZARIAN, MD, PhD
Assistant Professor of Medicine, Johns
Hopkins University, Baltimore, Maryland

RATIKA PARKASH, MD, MS, FRCPC, FHRS
QE II Health Sciences Centre, Halifax, Nova
Scotia, Canada

SYLVAIN PLOUX, MD
Medical Doctor, Hôpital Cardiologique
du Haut-Lévêque, CHU Bordeaux, IHU
LIRYC, Université Bordeaux, Bordeaux,
France

PHILIPPE RITTER, MD
Medical Doctor, Hôpital Cardiologique du
Haut-Lévêque, CHU Bordeaux, IHU LIRYC,
Université Bordeaux, Bordeaux, France

SIMONE L. ROMANO, MD
Cardiology Department, University Hospital
of Pisa, Pisa, Italy

DAVID WILSON, MD
Assistant Professor of Medicine, Staff
Electrophysiologist, James A. Haley VA
Medical Center, University of South Florida
Morsani College of Medicine, Tampa, Florida

OMAIR YOUSUF, MD
Chief Cardiology Fellow, Johns Hopkins
University, Baltimore, Maryland

Contents

specialized functions are helpful, many have not been shown to benefit patients in randomized trials. Automated and programmable features have dramatically increased in number and complexity.

The use of cardiac implantable electronic devices (CIEDs) has increased rapidly over the past 2 decades due to landmark clinical trials and expanding indications for use. As devices are implanted in increasingly complex patients with multiple comorbidities, the incidence of CIED infections has outpaced the growth in new CIED systems and presents a major and preventable complication. Careful antimicrobial stewardship at the time of implantation is the cornerstone of preventing CIED infections. Specific strategies to prevent infections have been evaluated, and evidence-based methods are reviewed here.

The first-generation subcutaneous implantable cardioverter defibrillator (S-ICD) effectively detects and terminates induced and spontaneous malignant ventricular arrhythmias with an inappropriate shock rate comparable with that of transvenous defibrillators. The S-ICD is an option for implantable defibrillator candidates who do not require pacing for bradycardia, cardiac resynchronization, or antitachycardia pacing indications. It is recommended for patients with compromised vascular or cardiac access and should be considered in younger patients and those needing a shock-only device. Wider implementation is dependent on randomized clinical trial data showing noninferiority to the transvenous ICD, together with the results of long-term registries.

The entirely subcutaneous implantable cardioverter defibrillator (S-ICD) is a new implant intended to prevent sudden cardiac death. The S-ICD detects and treats ventricular tachyarrhythmias and presents both common and unique mechanisms of malfunction and complication in comparison to the traditional transvenous ICD implant procedure. This article endeavors to specifically detail the function and possible malfunctions, as well as complications related to patient selection, the implant procedure, and programing of the device for follow-up.

A lead is an insulated conductor cord. The conductors fail by fracture caused by fatigue from cyclic stresses superimposed on background stresses. High amplitude low frequency cyclic stresses shorten the fatigue life more than low amplitude high frequency cyclic stresses. High background stresses shorten the fatigue life for the same cyclic stresses. The insulations fail by abrasion, creep, environmental stress cracking, metal ion–induced oxidation and chain scission. The body's immune and inflammatory responses and bacteria participate in the lead's degradation. Implantation techniques may help reduce lead malfunction. Lead design evolves to meet clinical demands, which should include extractability alongside reliability.

Cardiac implantable electrical devices (CIEDs) have undergone revolutionary changes in the last decade, linked to growth in both indications and capability. These changes have led to an increase in the use of both pacemakers and implantable cardioverter defibrillators (ICDs), collectively known as CIEDs. It is projected that the population with heart failure will double by the year 2025, and the absolute number of patients eligible to receive an ICD for primary prevention or cardiac resynchronization therapy will likely increase accordingly. These epidemiologic observations will translate into a significantly increased burden on the health care system, with fiscal pressures that will be hard pressed to cope with this projected demand.

In recent years, the number of centers performing transvenous lead extraction (TLE) in Europe has increased. Recently, the European Heart Rhythm Association (EHRA) conducted 2 surveys on TLE to characterize the clinical practice of extracting centers in Europe. These surveys highlighted the need for a prospective registry to achieve better analysis of TLE among European countries. In 2012, EHRA carried out the ELECTRa (European Lead Extraction Controlled) Registry, the first large prospective, multicenter registry of patients undergoing TLE in Europe.

 Video of overcoming an engaged active fixation mechanism accompanies this article

Millions of patients are currently living with implanted leads. Lead management mandates premeditated hardware selection with design features that balance implantability and extractability. The implanter should consider the hardware choices that might result in decreased need for extraction and, if extraction is needed, the hardware choices that will make it safer and easier, keeping in mind the concepts of lead control and tensile strength. The future may mitigate or even obviate these considerations as leadless systems and systems that avoid the vasculature entirely are developed.

Lead extraction has become a common and highly successful procedure. However, complications are possible and errors can be made. This article presents an overview of these issues.

Cardiac resynchronization therapy (CRT) has been shown to be highly efficacious in the treatment of congestive heart failure in patients with a wide QRS. Achieving successful left ventricular lead placement is the key step in achieving successful CRT. Leads have been developed that reduce the possibility of lead dislodgement after implantation. Lead technology has been developed that allows for the reprogramming of the stimulation vector so that phrenic nerve stimulation can be avoided while successful resynchronization therapy is maintained. Implantation tools have been developed that help achieve successful CRT implantation.

CARDIAC ELECTROPHYSIOLOGY CLINICS

NOW AVAILABLE FOR YOUR iPhone and iPad

Foreword
TED of Implantable Devices

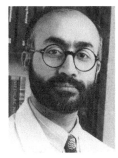
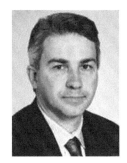

Ranjan K. Thakur, MD, MPH, MBA, FHRS   Andrea Natale, MD, FACC, FHRS
Consulting Editors

The modern era of cardiac pacing began with the development of the cardiac pacemaker in the late1950s. TED forces (Technology, Engineering, and Design) have shaped the development of cardiac rhythm devices over the last half-century. Now patients have access to pacemakers, implantable cardioverter-defibrillators, implantable loop recorders, subcutaneous defibrillators, leadless pacemakers, and so forth, and new innovations are on the way.

These advances were made possible by an interplay of ideas, concepts, and developments in technology, engineering, and design. As a result, these devices have become very complex. Tremendous technological sophistication is required in the manufacture of these devices, leads, and implantation tools. Not surprisingly, unanticipated problems have also arisen, as exemplified by the recent Riata™ (St. Jude Medical, St. Paul, Minnesota) issues. The externalization problem could not have been anticipated during the design phase.

TED forces will also ultimately solve many of the current clinical problems and improve the care of patients with cardiac arrhythmias.

We thank Drs Ellenbogen and Love for focusing on issues related to design, manufacture, and malfunction of cardiac implantable electronic devices (CIED). They cover lead-related issues (lead design, lead selection and extraction, and new left ventricular lead design), advances in CIED hardware and software seen in the "newer" CIEDs, and analysis and troubleshooting of these complex devices.

Electrophysiologists, cardiologists, and all those involved in the care and follow-up of patients with CIEDs will find this volume of the *Cardiac Electrophysiology Clinics* useful as a review of contemporary issues.

Ranjan K. Thakur, MD, MPH, MBA, FHRS
Sparrow Thoracic and Cardiovascular Institute
Michigan State University
1200 East Michigan Avenue, Suite 580
Lansing, MI 48912, USA

Andrea Natale, MD, FACC, FHRS
Texas Cardiac Arrhythmia Institute
Center for Atrial Fibrillation at
St. David's Medical Center
1015 East 32nd Street, Suite 516
Austin, TX 78705, USA

E-mail addresses:
thakur@msu.edu (R.K. Thakur)
andrea.natale@stdavids.com (A. Natale)

http://dx.doi.org/10.1016/j.ccep.2014.04.002
1877-9182/14/$ – see front matter

cardiacEP.theclinics.com

Preface

Implantable Devices: Design, Manufacturing, and Malfunction

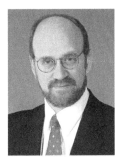

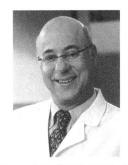

Kenneth A. Ellenbogen, MD, FAHA, FACC, FHRS   Charles J. Love, MD, FACC, FAHA, FHRS, CCDS

Editors

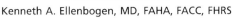

We are pleased to introduce to you this issue of *Cardiac Electrophysiology Clinics*. We have gathered a group of international experts to provide insight into some of the most important and evolving issues in cardiac implantable electronic devices (CIEDs) and the patients that rely on them.

Management of pacing and implantable cardioverter defibrillator (ICD) leads is a concern of many of our colleagues. Recent "recalls" and reliability concerns have created a great deal of interest in these critical components of CIED systems. Thus, we have particularly sought to focus on issues regarding lead selection, lead design, and lead extraction. A number of the contributions to this work focus on these aspects of device therapy, including experiences from our colleagues in Europe and Canada. We discuss new left ventricular lead technology as well as analyze design and construction issues with ICD leads that have failed. An important aspect of lead management is preventing the need to extract leads. Therefore, the prevention of device infections and the role of new technology in this area are reviewed as well.

The level of sophistication present in current device hardware and software has increased exponentially in recent years. In that regard, we highlight the subcutaneous ICD, the implantable loop recorder, remote monitoring, and new technology for ICDs. In addition, the evolving role of MRI and CIEDs is addressed, as well as new design and technology considerations.

Finally, analyzing and troubleshooting the electrocardiogram of patients with ICDs and cardiac resynchronization devices are a challenging yet critical part of device management. With all of the new algorithms in devices, interpretation of these strips has become a nearly impossible task without the advanced diagnostic features and annotated rhythm printouts that the programmers provide. In this context, we provide a discussion of pseudo-device malfunction and review a number of the more common (and troublesome) new algorithms that have been and are being incorporated into CIEDs.

We are deeply indebted to our colleagues and appreciate their time, effort, and enthusiasm to finish their articles in a timely fashion. We also thank Barbara Cohen-Kligerman for her help and professionalism in editing this volume. We are certain that the readers of this work will appreciate the

Card Electrophysiol Clin 6 (2014) xv–xvi
http://dx.doi.org/10.1016/j.ccep.2014.04.001

cardiacEP.theclinics.com

content and learn much useful clinical information from this volume.

Kenneth A. Ellenbogen, MD, FAHA, FACC, FHRS
VCU School of Medicine
Pauley Heart Center
Gateway Building, 12th and Marshall Street
Third Floor, Room 3-223
Richmond, VA 23219, USA

Charles J. Love, MD, FACC, FAHA, FHRS, CCDS
New York University Langone Medical Center
Heart Rhythm Center
403 East 34th Street
RIV-4th Floor
New York, NY 10016, USA

E-mail addresses:
kellenbogen@mcvh-vcu.edu (K.A. Ellenbogen)
Charles.love@nyumc.org (C.J. Love)

Troubleshooting the Malfunctioning Pacemaker: A Systematic Approach

Karoly Kaszala, MD, PhD, FHRS

KEYWORDS

- Pacemaker • Troubleshooting • Capture • Sensing • Noise • Lead fracture • Pacemaker algorithm

KEY POINTS

- Pacemaker troubleshooting requires an integrated approach with special emphasis on clinical history, physical examination, and device interrogation.
- Successful patient management requires an in-depth understanding of the basics of pacing and device features.
- If an abnormal device function is suspected, a wide differential diagnosis should be established and a didactic approach used to uncover the final diagnosis.

INTRODUCTION

Expectations for a pacing system are high. Pacemaker leads should withstand the hostile intravascular environment for decades, characterized by excessive chemical and mechanical stress. Pacemaker generators are expected to operate on a single battery without a flaw for 10+ years and appropriately react to cardiac signals without being affected by noise from the neighboring environment. Over the 60-year history of cardiac pacing, as technology continued to evolve, many lessons have been learned and, as a result, the reliability of modern pacemaker systems has reached an exceptional level.[1] In spite of these achievements, an occasional problem with device components continues to occur.[2] More frequently, abnormalities or pseudoabnormalities may be encountered, caused by complexities in device programming and algorithms. Differentiation between these is important in order to ensure proper management and safe patient care. An approach to pacemaker troubleshooting is discussed here.

PATIENT EVALUATION (CLINICAL HISTORY, PHYSICAL EXAMINATION, STUDIES/TESTING)

In all aspects of medicine, a systematic approach for evaluation of a clinical problem minimizes the chance of overlooking the correct diagnosis, and this is also true during pacemaker troubleshooting. Although a complete evaluation is the goal, the extent of initial investigations should be determined by the urgency of the problem. A focused clinical history, physical examination, and ancillary testing should be performed in most cases. The troubleshooting process is significantly enhanced with meticulous record keeping during the implantation procedure and routine device follow-up visits.

Clinical History

The first step is to identify the presence and circumstances of symptoms that may direct attention to specific problems (**Table 1**). Focused questions should also be directed to screen for specific abnormalities in select patient groups (such as

The author has nothing to disclose.
Cardiac Electrophysiology Laboratory, Hunter Holmes McGuire Veterans Affairs Medical Center and Virginia Commonwealth University, 1201 Broad Rock Boulevard, Room 111(J3), Richmond, VA 23249, USA
E-mail address: karoly.kaszala@va.gov

Card Electrophysiol Clin 6 (2014) 187–205
http://dx.doi.org/10.1016/j.ccep.2014.02.004
1877-9182/14/$ – see front matter Published by Elsevier Inc.

Table 1
Differential diagnosis of symptoms related to pacemaker system malfunction

Clinical Event or Symptom	Possible Abnormality	Causes
Fatigue, dizziness, chest pain, palpitation, syncope	Pacemaker syndrome	Loss of atrial pacing or capture; nontracking pacing mode; VVI pacing caused by ERI; inadequate AV delay, RV pacing Inadequate rate support
Chest pain (pleuritic)	Lead perforation; pneumothorax, pulmonary embolization	RA or RV lead perforation, perioperative lung injury, DVT
Palpitations	Failed mode switching, inappropriate mode switching, PMT, RNRVAS Upper rate behavior, loss of capture or sensing, intermittent operation of special algorithms Inaccurate sensor rate pacing New arrhythmia	Failed mode switch algorithm caused by undersensing Mode switch is turned off; suboptimal programming of refractory periods or mechanical complication Suboptimal programming of rate sensor or special algorithms
Hiccup/ diaphragmatic stimulation	Lead dislodgement, positional change in phrenic nerve and pacer lead proximity	Atrial lead dislodgement or lateral lead positioning LV lead dislodgement/movement
Muscle twitching	Pectoral stimulation	Insulation defect, loose lead pin, unipolar pacing and pocket stimulation
Chest wall stimulation	Perforation, thin body habitus	Lead perforation, far-field capture of skeletal muscle
Heart failure	New heart failure symptoms	Switched A and V lead pin, high % RV pacing, suboptimal AV or VV delay, frequent rapid pacing
Cardiac surgery	Heart manipulation, electrocautery	Lead dislodgement, EMI, device compromise
Other surgery	Electrocautery	EMI
Cardioversion	High electric current	EMI, device compromise, threshold change
Radiofrequency ablation	Local heat production Electric current	EMI, threshold change, lead dislodgement
Therapeutic radiation	Radiation injury	Device reset, circuitry damage

Abbreviations: A, atrial; AV, atrioventricular; DVT, deep vein thrombosis; EMI, electromagnetic interference; ERI, elective replacement indicator; PMT, pacemaker-mediated tachycardia; RA, right atrial; RNRVAS, repetitive nonreentrant ventriculoatrial synchrony; RV, right ventricular; V, ventricular; VVI, ventricular pacing and sensing with inhibition.

pacemaker-dependent patients, patients with biventricular devices). Certain symptoms may be intermittent or the patient may not relate those to the pacemaker. Indications for device therapy and symptoms before device implantation should be queried. In the medical history, recent interventions such as surgeries (EMI [electromagnetic interference] noise, circuitry damage), cardioversions (increased threshold, circuitry damage), ablation procedures (lead dislodgement, increased threshold), or therapeutic radiation (device reset and memory problems; rarely damage to the circuitry and decreased battery life) should be noted. New diagnoses such as renal failure, heart failure, myocardial infarction, or new medication prescriptions should be recorded.

Implant and device clinic data should be reviewed with special attention to the implant report. Lead and device type and serial numbers, access site, pacemaker pocket location, any procedural difficulties, or problems during follow-up should be noted. The timeline in relation to device implantation and symptoms may also provide clues for specific causes. Examples are listed in **Box 1**.

Physical Examination

Focused physical examination is an important part of device troubleshooting and follow-up. The device site should be inspected and palpated to ensure proper healing and to rule out erosion or impending erosion. Presence of muscle twitching

---

Box 1
Possible causes of failure to capture related to timing of device implantation

Early (<3 months) abnormalities

- Lead dislodgement
- Loose lead connector
- Acute/subacute perforation
- Tissue reaction during lead maturation (change in sensing/threshold)

Late (>3 months) abnormalities

- Local fibrosis
- Myocardial infarction
- Lead fracture
- Lead insulation defect
- Battery depletion
- Delayed perforation

---

may suggest mechanical malfunction or lead dislodgement (see **Table 1**). Abnormal characteristics of the jugular venous pulsation may suggest loss of atrioventricular (AV) synchrony (Cannon A waves) or, in the case of increased jugular venous pressure, to heart failure or pericardial effusion. Lung examination should evaluate for wheezing (contraindication to certain medications), rales (congestive heart failure), or pneumothorax (complication in postimplantation period). In the right clinical settings, the presence of cardiac rub, murmur, or gallop provides additional guidance to further diagnostic tests. Other signs and symptoms of heart failure, such as orthopnea, paroxysmal nocturnal dyspnea, and peripheral edema should also be assessed.

Diagnostic Studies and Tests

Several ancillary tests may add valuable information to clarify the cause of a pacemaker abnormality.

Electrocardiogram

A 12-lead electrocardiogram (ECG) is part of routine evaluation. Besides diagnosing the base rhythm, analysis of the tracing should identify whether pacing is present and whether there is adequate sensing and capture. Paced ECG morphology helps to identify the site of pacing (**Fig. 1**).[3] In most cases, magnet application over the pacemaker causes asynchronous pacing at the magnet rate. The magnet rate provides information on pacemaker battery status and proper capture even without a programmer at hand.[4]

Holter or event monitor

If symptoms cannot be reproduced and are rare, long-term ECG monitoring may be helpful to correlate the symptoms with any abnormal pacer behavior. For complex cases, some companies provide a specific Holter monitor feature that also records the device marker channel.

Chest radiograph

A chest radiograph in anteroposterior and lateral projections should be performed after device implantation to document lead position and rule out procedural complications. The following acute complications may be identified: pneumothorax, pleural effusion/hemothorax, pericardial effusion, inadvertent lead placement in the arterial system or via an intracardiac shunt (ie, patent foramen ovale), lead dislodgement, and improper lead pin connection. During follow-up, a delayed perforation, lead dislodgement, or radiographic evidence of lead failure may be identified (**Fig. 2**).

Echocardiogram

Echocardiogram serves an important tool in management of a pacing system. It provides a noninvasive means to assess ventricular hemodynamic parameters, screen for structural heart disease, or screen for the presence of pericardial effusion. Hemodynamic effects of iterations of pacing intervals in a biventricular pacing system (AV delay, right ventricle to left ventricle pacing delay) may be evaluated and followed. Echocardiogram is also useful to identify the pacer lead position (ie, to rule out lead placement in the left ventricle) and occasionally identify a lead perforation.

Laboratory evaluation

Laboratory evaluation is rarely helpful in troubleshooting but, in certain situations, the results may explain an apparent pacemaker malfunction. Sensing and capture parameters may change in the setting of severe metabolic and electrolyte abnormalities. Certain medications (such as class I and III antiarrhythmics), or toxic medication levels (such as digoxin, lithium) may also contribute to changes in pacing parameters or clinical symptoms.

Device interrogation

The most important part of testing is device interrogation. Each company provides a proprietary programmer that allows 2-way communication with the device using induction-based or radiofrequency technology. The incorporation of microprocessors and increasing random access memory (RAM) in current state-of-the-art models allows storage of a wealth of information beyond

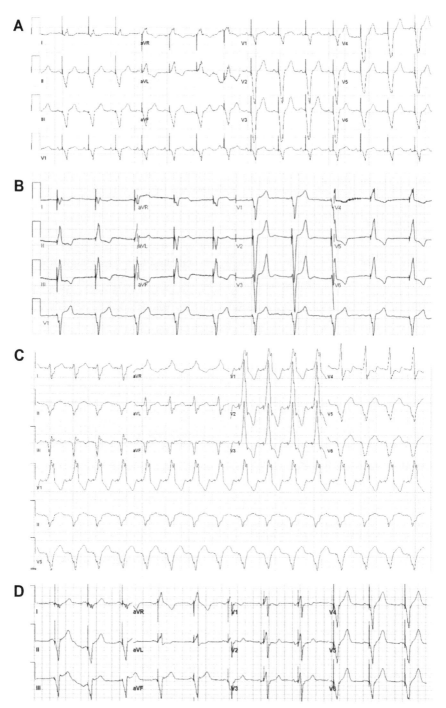

Fig. 1. Typical ECG configurations of ventricular pacing. (*A*) Right ventricular (RV) apical pacing. QRS axis is typically left superior, and left bundle branch block–type morphology is present in lead V_1 with negative concordance. (*B*) RV pacing from the high septum. QRS is narrow and there is an inferior axis. (*C*) Left ventricular (LV) pacing in a patient with a biventricular device and RV pacing turned off because of lead fracture. The axis is right superior with monophasic R wave present in lead V_1 and R-wave transition in V_5. (*D*) Biventricular pacing. In typical lateral lead position, there is a QS wave in lead I and an R wave in V_1.

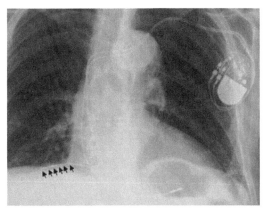

Fig. 2. Lead perforation. A chest radiograph in a patient 2 weeks after placement of a dual chamber pacemaker for sinus node disease. The patient complained of occasional diaphragmatic stimulation. The atrial lead impedance was markedly increased and there was loss of sensing and capture. The chest radiograph shows atrial lead perforation into the pleural space (*arrows*). The main risk factor for perforation was chronic high-dose oral prednisone use. (*Adapted from* Kaszala K. Evaluation, troubleshooting and management of pacing system malfunctions. In: Ellenbogen K, Kaszala K, editors. Cardiac pacing and ICDs. 6th edition. New York: Wiley-Blackwell; 2014. p. 272–322.)

basic pacing parameters, including longitudinal lead and threshold parameters, pacing statistics, arrhythmias with stored electrograms (EGM), arrhythmia burden, and histograms, all of which may be helpful in clinical management or troubleshooting (**Fig. 3**).

Intraoperative evaluation

In cases in which proper diagnosis of a malfunction cannot be established, intraoperative evaluation may, rarely, be required to clarify a particular problem. An intraoperative test may confirm a loose lead pin connection, visualize an insulation breach in the pacemaker pocket, and allow testing of the leads using a programmer to differentiate between device and lead abnormalities. This type of testing is usually performed when invasive system revision is necessary anyway.

PRESENTATION

There are 3 main reasons (and the combination of these) that may lead to suspicion of a pacemaker problem.

1. Presence of a symptom. Although certain symptoms are commonly attributed to pacemaker malfunction (ie, syncope), others may be subtle or nonspecific (ie, hiccups) and may not be readily attributed to a pacemaker malfunction.

With an aging population and frequent presence of multiple comorbidities, significant time and experience is sometimes required to sort through unrelated, nonspecific complaints.

2. Routine ECG or telemetry recording. Although many of these abnormalities are explained by filtering of pacing stimulus artifact, low-amplitude signals, noise on the tracing, or operation of a special pacemaker algorithm (**Fig. 4**), a true pacemaker abnormality may also be identified (**Fig. 5**).

3. Routine device check. The importance of routine device check is to periodically reassess the clinical status of the patient and evaluate the system components to ensure proper function. Device interrogation allows a comparison of current and long-term data, such as impedance, sensing, and threshold measurement. Review of real-time marker channel events and comparison with stored electrograms and interpretation of histograms may allow correlation of symptoms with specific events or reproduction of an abnormal device behavior.

DIFFERENTIAL DIAGNOSIS
Pacing Problems: Loss of Capture, Loss of Pacing

Pacing rate in a simple single-chamber device is determined by the lower rate (or sensor rate) settings. If dual chamber devices are programmed in tracking mode (such as in DDD mode [dual chamber pacing and sensing with inhibition and tracking]), atrial pacing is at the lower rate limit, but ventricular pacing is accelerated to the atrial rate (up to the upper tracking rate) as long as intrinsic conduction is slower than the programmed AV delay. Lack of pacing in general may simply mean that the intrinsic rate and AV conduction are faster than the programmed settings. If there is no pacing artifact at the expected time point, certain special algorithms should be considered (ie, MVP mode [managed ventricular pacing]). Next, oversensing of an electric event or structural abnormalities such as lead fracture and battery depletion should be considered.

Capture of the myocardium requires a minimum current density in the myocardium that surrounds the electrode tip to allow initiation and propagation of an action potential. Because capture threshold may fluctuate for various reasons, including diurnal changes, it is generally accepted to program chronic pacing output at twice the voltage threshold (measured at pulse width slightly more than chronaxie) for clinical safety. Any abnormalities in the pacemaker system components (pacemaker circuit and battery, header, lead pin, lead

A

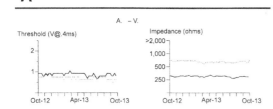

Threshold (V@.4ms) — A. – V. — Impedance (ohms)

Oct-12 Apr-13 Oct-13

Arrhythmia Summary: 10/11/12 to 10/30/13			
Mode Switch Count	2,270 (1.2 hrs/day - 5.2%)	VHR Episodes	9
AHR Episode Trigger	Mode Switch > 30 sec	VHR Detection	150 ppm for 5 beats
AHR Episode	44	VHR Termination	150 ppm for 5 beats
AHR Detection	150 bpm - No Delay	SVT Filter	On

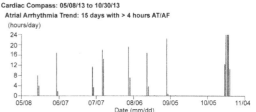

Type	Date/Time	Duration hh:mm:ss	Rates (bpm): Max A	Max V	Avg V	Sensor	EGM
VHR							
First	03/11/13 12:03 PM	:37	150	226	150	84	No
Fastest	07/12/13 5:51 PM	:06:26	>400	274	166	75	No
Longest	07/13/13 6:45 AM	:06:34	>400	240	165	88	No
	10/17/13 5:12 AM	:04	111	175	150	91	Yes
Last	10/19/13 7:37 PM	:04	178	226	150	89	Yes
AHR							
First	11/07/12 4:51 AM	9:01:46	>400	256	93	87	No
Longest	03/30/13 2:35 PM	>96:00:00	>400	226	92	63	No
	10/19/13 9:11 PM	44:29:53	>400	248	108	76	Yes
	10/21/13 5:41 PM	23:30:59	>400	202	93	60	Yes
Last	10/22/13 5:12 PM	27:00:05	>400	240	107	81	Yes

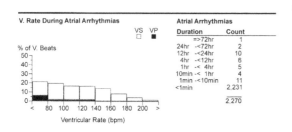

V. Rate During Atrial Arrhythmias

VS VP

% of V. Beats

< 80 100 120 140 160 180 200 >
Ventricular Rate (bpm)

Atrial Arrhythmias

Duration	Count
=>72hr	1
24hr -<72hr	2
12hr -<24hr	10
4hr -<12hr	6
1hr -< 4hr	5
10min -< 1hr	4
1min -<10min	11
<1min	2,231
	2,270

Cardiac Compass: 05/08/13 to 10/30/13

Atrial Arrhythmia Trend: 15 days with > 4 hours AT/AF

(hours/day)

05/08 06/07 07/07 08/06 09/05 10/05 11/04
Date (mm/dd)

B

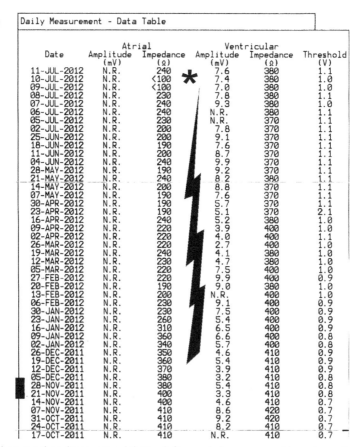

Daily Measurement - Data Table

Date	Atrial Amplitude (mV)	Atrial Impedance (Ω)	Ventricular Amplitude (mV)	Ventricular Impedance (Ω)	Threshold (V)
11-JUL-2012	N.R.	240	7.6	380	1.1
10-JUL-2012	N.R.	<100	7.4	380	1.0
09-JUL-2012	N.R.	<100	7.0	380	1.0
08-JUL-2012	N.R.	230	7.8	380	1.1
07-JUL-2012	N.R.	240	9.3	380	1.0
06-JUL-2012	N.R.	240	N.R.	380	1.1
05-JUL-2012	N.R.	230	N.R.	370	1.1
02-JUL-2012	N.R.	200	7.8	370	1.1
25-JUN-2012	N.R.	200	9.1	370	1.1
18-JUN-2012	N.R.	190	7.6	370	1.1
11-JUN-2012	N.R.	200	8.7	370	1.1
04-JUN-2012	N.R.	240	9.9	370	1.1
28-MAY-2012	N.R.	190	9.2	370	1.1
21-MAY-2012	N.R.	240	8.2	380	1.1
14-MAY-2012	N.R.	200	8.8	370	1.1
07-MAY-2012	N.R.	190	7.6	370	1.1
30-APR-2012	N.R.	190	5.7	370	1.1
23-APR-2012	N.R.	190	5.1	370	2.1
16-APR-2012	N.R.	240	5.2	380	1.0
09-APR-2012	N.R.	220	3.9	400	1.0
02-APR-2012	N.R.	220	4.0	400	1.1
26-MAR-2012	N.R.	220	2.7	400	1.0
19-MAR-2012	N.R.	240	4.1	380	1.0
12-MAR-2012	N.R.	230	4.7	380	1.0
05-MAR-2012	N.R.	220	7.5	400	1.0
27-FEB-2012	N.R.	220	9.9	400	0.9
20-FEB-2012	N.R.	190	9.0	380	1.0
13-FEB-2012	N.R.	200	N.R.	400	1.0
06-FEB-2012	N.R.	230	9.1	400	0.9
30-JAN-2012	N.R.	230	7.5	400	0.9
23-JAN-2012	N.R.	260	5.4	400	0.9
16-JAN-2012	N.R.	310	6.5	400	0.9
09-JAN-2012	N.R.	360	6.6	400	0.8
02-JAN-2012	N.R.	340	5.7	400	0.8
26-DEC-2011	N.R.	350	4.6	410	0.9
19-DEC-2011	N.R.	360	5.4	410	0.9
12-DEC-2011	N.R.	370	3.9	410	0.9
05-DEC-2011	N.R.	380	3.2	410	0.8
28-NOV-2011	N.R.	380	5.4	410	0.8
21-NOV-2011	N.R.	400	3.3	410	0.8
14-NOV-2011	N.R.	400	4.6	410	0.7
07-NOV-2011	N.R.	410	8.6	420	0.7
31-OCT-2011	N.R.	410	9.2	420	0.7
24-OCT-2011	N.R.	410	8.2	410	0.7
17-OCT-2011	N.R.	410	N.R.	410	0.7

Fig. 3. Selected pacemaker diagnostics. (*A*) Top left panel shows normal long-term threshold and impedance trends in the atrial and ventricular lead. The arrhythmia summary helps to estimate the arrhythmia burden. In this case, the mode switch burden was 5.2%. The ventricular rate control was suboptimal during atrial arrhythmias. (*B*) Long-term tabular data of amplitude, impedance, and threshold. Gradual decline and variability in atrial lead impedance (lightning sign and *asterisk*) are seen, consistent with insulation failure. ([*B*] *Adapted from* Kaszala K. Evaluation, troubleshooting and management of pacing system malfunctions. In: Ellenbogen K, Kaszala K, editors. Cardiac pacing and ICDs. 6th edition. New York: Wiley-Blackwell; 2014. p. 272–322.)

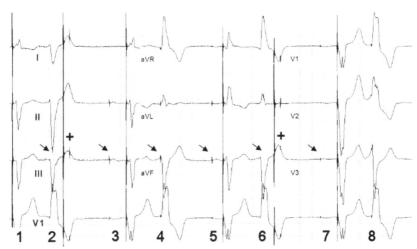

Fig. 4. Complex pacemaker ECG. The patient was referred to the clinic because of suspected pacemaker abnormality. The ECG shows dual chamber pacing and ventricular bigeminy. The second and sixth beats were the main concerns for undersensing. Careful examination of the tracing shows atrial pacing artifacts (*arrows*) buried in the premature ventricular contraction (PVC) beats (beats 2, 4, 6). Because the PVC originates from the left ventricle (right bundle branch block [RBBB]–like morphology), it is sensed late at the RV pacing lead. In beats 2 and 6, postatrial ventricular blanking resulted in functional undersensing and RV pacing (first pacing artifact over the T wave). There was no capture because of functional myocardial refractoriness. Because this device has a beat-to-beat autocapture feature, a second ventricular stimulus is delivered (marked as +) at an increased output, 80 milliseconds following the initial ventricular pacing stimulus.

conductor(s), tip-to-myocardium coupling) or change in myocardium properties (medication effect, electrolyte abnormalities, myocardial infarction) may result in abnormality in capture. Loss of capture is identified by the lack of electrical depolarization in the chamber that is being paced (ie, pacing artifact is present but not associated with a P wave or R wave). Capture only occurs if the myocardium is excitable at the time of pacing (see **Fig. 5**). Once non–pacer-related myocardial causes are excluded, it is best to stratify a capture abnormality according to timing relative to the device implantation. In the acute phase (<3 months),

the most common reasons include excessive tissue reaction at the lead tip, lead dislodgement, lead perforation, or loose lead pin connection. The diagnosis is based on changes in pacing parameters; chest radiograph result; and, if needed, intraoperative evaluation. It is important to remember that severe, temporary tissue reaction may still occur following acute lead implant despite the universal use of steroid eluting tips in intravenous pacemaker leads. In these cases, the threshold may improve after several weeks following the original implantation. It is therefore important to program a higher pacing output for

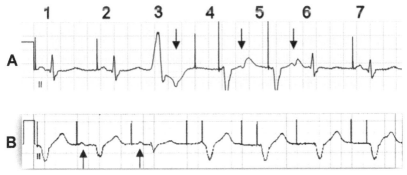

Fig. 5. Loss of capture. (*A*) Dual chamber pacing. The first 2 beats are atrial pacing; the third beat is a PVC with retrograde conduction (*arrow*). This falls in the postventricular atrial refractory period (PVARP) and is not tracked. The next atrial pacing stimulus fails to capture because of functional atrial refractoriness. Beats 4 and 5 are pacemaker-mediated tachycardia (PMT) (arrows point to retrograde p wave), which terminates when beat 6 conducts and atrial pacing resumes. (*B*) Loss of atrial capture. Atrial pacing stimulus is not followed by atrial depolarization (arrows point to P waves).

the first several months to cover the lead matura-tion process. In the chronic phase (>3 months but usually years after implantation), investigations should be directed more toward structural device or lead abnormalities. Adequate device battery status should be confirmed during device interro-gation. Battery depletion (normal or early) should be considered. Other possible causes include lead integrity failure (fracture, insulation damage), change in lead-tissue interface (fibrosis, myocar-dial infarction), or inadequate programming.

Sensing Problems: Undersensing/Oversensing

Proper sensing depends of integrity of the pace-maker system components (pacemaker circuit and battery, header, lead pin, lead conductor(s), tip-to-myocardium coupling). Sensing of a myocardial signal means acknowledgment of an electrical signal by the timing cycle algorithm following acquisition, filtering, and signal process-ing. If a signal amplitude falls to less than a set sensing threshold, the signal is not registered (undersensing; see **Fig. 5**). In addition, signals that fall into traditional blanking periods are not sensed (functional undersensing; see **Fig. 5**; **Fig. 6**). Thus, when sensing is evaluated, it is important to understand the programmed device parameters and timing cycles. Sensing threshold in traditional pacemakers is fixed, as opposed to implantable defibrillators (ICDs), in which beat-to-beat variability and increased sensitivity level are used in order to properly identify ventricular fibrilla-tion and also atrial arrhythmias. These algorithms with higher sensitivity predispose to oversensing. In newer pacemakers, ICD-type sensing algo-rithms are increasingly being used.

Under most circumstances, undersensing is manifested by pacing at earlier than the expected interval. The most common reason for this abnor-mality is a programming mistake or a change in sensing parameters (ie, lead dislodgement, local fibrotic changes), but a secondary change in myocardium properties (ie, medication effect, electrolyte abnormalities) should also be consid-ered. It is important to remember that sensing is derived from activation at the myocardium adja-cent to the pacing lead. On occasion, the signifi-cant delay from the initial ECG deflection to local activation (ie, to right ventricular [RV] lead tip in right bundle branch block [RBBB]) may result in pacing with the appearance of undersensing (**Fig. 7**).

Oversensing results in delay in pacing (**Fig. 8A–C**). Atrial oversensing may result in increased ventricu-lar pacing rate caused by tracking (if tracking mode is programmed), recording of spurious atrial ar-rhythmias, inappropriate mode switching, and acti-vation of atrial antitachycardia pacing therapy (**Fig. 9**). In ICDs, ventricular oversensing may result in inappropriate therapy and inhibition of pacing. In pacemakers, oversensing of low-frequency events (such as T waves) results in delay in pacing. If high-frequency events, such as EMI, fall repeatedly

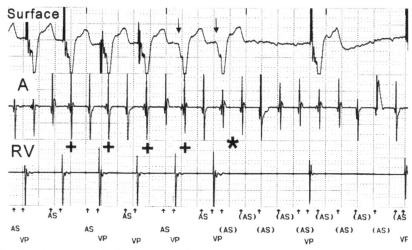

Fig. 6. Functional undersensing. The beginning of the tracing shows atrial flutter and functional undersensing. Every other flutter wave falls in the postventricular atrial blanking period (PVAB) (+) and is not sensed; therefore, mode switching is not initiated and 2:1 tracking is present. In the middle segment, atrial flutter response algo-rithm is activated with uncovering of the blanked atrial events and proper mode switching (*). Note the sudden change in pacing rate. Two arrows on the surface QRS indicate the lack of pacing artifact likely caused by filtering. A, atrial signal; RV, right ventricular signal. (*Adapted from* Kaszala K. Evaluation, troubleshooting and management of pacing system malfunctions. In: Ellenbogen K, Kaszala K, editors. Cardiac pacing and ICDs. 6th edition. New York: Wiley-Blackwell; 2014. p. 272–322.)

in the retriggerable noise reversion window (commonly 40–50 milliseconds after the blanking period) or in the ventricular refractory period, most pacemakers initiate temporarily asynchronous pacing in order to avoid possible asystole during external noise oversensing. Crosstalk is another common form of oversensing. AV crosstalk may occur if atrial pacing stimulus or polarization artifact is sensed by the ventricular channel, which may have severe consequences in the pacemaker-dependent patient because ventricular oversensing may result in asystole (see **Fig. 8**). Blanking periods are used following a pacing stimulus to eliminate oversensing (postatrial ventricular blanking or post-ventricular atrial blanking period). Asystole caused

by AV crosstalk is also mitigated by the introduction of safety pacing algorithms (see **Fig. 7**). Ventriculo-atrial (VA) crosstalk is the result of oversensing of a paced or sensed far-field R-wave signal in the atrial channel, which is the most common type of over-sensing. It results in spurious mode switching, spurious recording of atrial arrhythmias, and potential loss of AV synchrony (see **Fig. 9**; **Fig. 10**).

Sensing problems may be identified on a rhythm strip, showing earlier than expected stimulus or a delayed pacing stimulus. Review of stored or real-time electrograms with mismatch between cardiac signals of interest and device markers serve as the ultimate proofs of the particular abnormality. Undersensing is managed by increasing sensitivity or, rarely, with lead revision. Oversensing of cardiac signals or myopotentials may be managed by decreasing sensitivity or increasing blanking periods or refractory periods. Lead fracture or perforation usually requires lead revision. EMI is best managed by avoidance of trigger or in-hospital settings with asynchronous pacing (if indicated).

Unexpected Pacing Rate or Sudden Change in Pacing Rate or Intervals

Faster-than-expected pacing
The pacing rate is determined by the lower rate limit, tracking rate, or sensor rate, depending on the clinical situation. An abnormally high pacing rate is often explained by one of these features. A lower rate limit may be programmed unusually high following an AV node ablation procedure to minimize risk of torsades de pointes or following a systemic illness if a higher base rate is desired to improve cardiac output. A new atrial arrhythmia may result in increased pacing rate because of an increased lower rate limit during mode switching or tracking (if arrhythmia is slower than the mode switch rate, if mode switching fails, or if mode switch is turned off). A special situation is 2:1 flutter lockout, in which every other flutter wave falls in the postventricular atrial blanking period (PVAB) and results in 2:1 tracking. Special flutter response algorithms are helpful to correct this problem (see **Fig. 6**). These algorithms uncover the blanked flutter wave by temporarily extending the postventricular atrial refractory period (PVARP). Inappropriate sensor activation (for example, interaction between a minute ventilation rate sensor and a respiratory rate intensive care unit monitor) or an overly sensitive sensor algorithm may also cause accelerated pacing (**Box 2**).

Runaway pacemaker is a dangerous but largely extinct problem. It is a serious medical emergency with accelerated pacing beyond the programmed

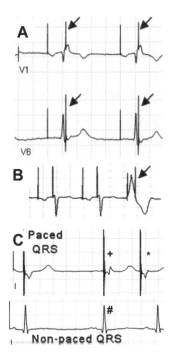

Fig. 7. Examples of fusion on surface ECG. (*A*) An example of pseudofusion. A pacing artifact appears late in the QRS (*arrows*) without change in the QRS morphology. This artifact is commonly seen in RBBB (as in this example) caused by late activation of the right ventricle. This phenomenon is often confused with undersensing. (*B*) An example of pseudo-pseudo fusion. AV pacing takes place but a PVC coincides with the atrial stimulus (third beat), giving an appearance of ventricular capture by atrial pacing. The ventricular pacing occurs at shortened AV interval caused by safety pacing (*arrow*), and signifies that the PVC was sensed in the safety pacing window. A ventricular stimulus is released to avoid asystole, because sensing in this window may also be the result of AV crosstalk (sensing atrial polarization artifact). (*C*) True fusion (+) with QRS morphology appearing as the sum of fully paced QRS (*) and intrinsic QRS (#).

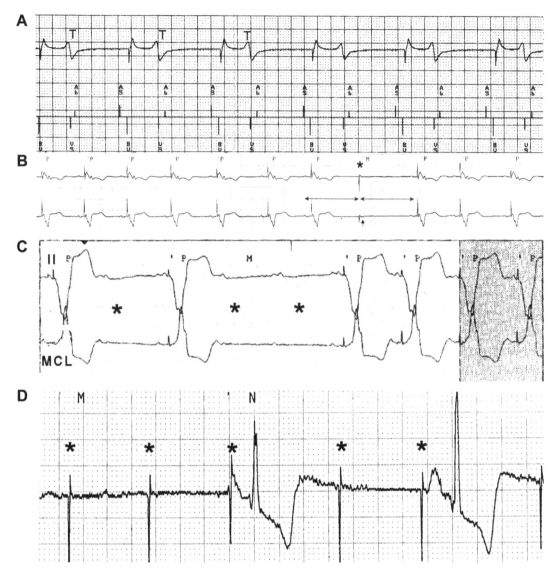

Fig. 8. Examples of ventricular pacing and sensing abnormalities. (A) T-wave oversensing in a biventricular device. VS (ventricular sense) events correlate with T wave (the first T waves are marked with T). The following sinus beat falls in the PVAB period (Ab) and is not tracked. This pacemaker-dependent patient presented with increased dyspnea. The effective ventricular rate was 42 beats per minute (bpm). (B) AV crosstalk with inhibition in a pacemaker-dependent patient. Atrial pacing (*) results in capture (*single arrow*), but ventricular pacing is inhibited (no ventricular pacing artifact). Double arrows from A to pacing spike are shorter than pacing spike to next V (AA time vs AA+AVD), confirming that the pacing spike (*) has an atrial origin. (C) Intermittent loss of pacing caused by oversensing (*). Because there is no atrial pacing, AV crosstalk is ruled out. This loss of pacing is an example of RV lead fracture with intermittent noise and inhibition. Note the large R wave in the MCL lead (modified chest lead). This patient has a biventricular device and there is capture from the LV lead. Because of noise, LV output was intermittently inhibited. This example underscores that asystole may develop in a patient with a biventricular device with RV lead fracture even if there is a functioning left ventricle lead. (D) Loss of capture (*) in a single-chamber ventricular pacemaker. Sensing is preserved because the fourth pacing output is reset by the intrinsic beat.

upper rate caused by mechanical device malfunction. Often, there is no response to magnet application or to commands from the programmer. Treatment of this problem requires immediate pulse generator replacement.[5]

Pacemaker-mediated tachycardia is an iatrogenic reentrant tachycardia in patients with multichamber devices. The circuit is established by ventricular pacing and retrograde atrial conduction (**Fig. 11**). The retrograde P wave is then tracked

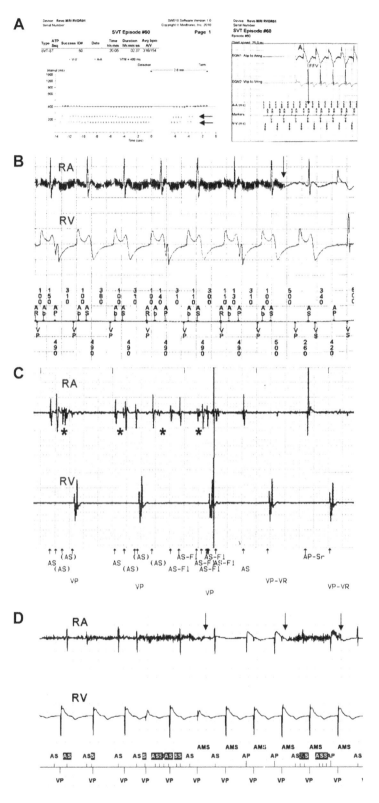

Fig. 9. Atrial oversensing. (*A*) Far-field R-wave oversensing. The plot on the left shows a typical train-track appearance in the atrial signals (*arrows*). Atrial electromyogram in the plot on the right is followed by a signal that correlates with the R wave (FFV [far-field ventricular signal], *down arrow*) marked as AR (A refractory). There is typical atrial group-beating appearance. This problem is best mitigated by careful lead placement during implantation. Atrial sensitivity or PVAB may be modified in the postimplantation period. (*B*) EMI with atrial oversensing and tracking at maximum upper rate. EMI is typically a high-frequency, low-amplitude signal with sudden onset and termination (*arrow*). (*C*) Atrial oversensing caused by insulation abnormality. Nonphysiologic, high-frequency, and unpredictable signals are seen in the atrial channel (*). (*D*) Myopotential oversensing with sudden onset and termination (*arrows*) and tracking. These signals have low amplitude and high frequency and are often reproducible with specific isometric exercise.

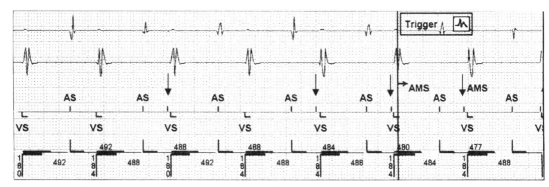

Fig. 10. Far-field R-wave oversensing. A special type of far-field R-wave oversensing is shown here with mode switching (AMS, horizontal arrow). Far-field R-wave sensing precedes R-wave sensing (sensing signal is marked with vertical arrows before the VS marker). In this case, changing PVAB does not help; atrial sensitivity has to be adjusted. AMS, auto mode switch; AS, atrial sense; VS, ventricular sense.

(ventricular pacing) and the arrhythmia continues. PVARP is designed to minimize this problem. If an atrial signal falls within the PVARP, it is not tracked and the arrhythmia cannot be maintained. Because PVARP is part of the total atrial refractory period (TARP = AV delay + PVARP; TARP

Box 2
Possible causes of unexpected pacing rate

Accelerated pacing rate
- Atrial tracking
- Mode switch failed or turned off
- Sensor rate pacing
- Rate hysteresis
- Safety pacing
- Automatic capture test
- Rate regularization algorithm
- Sinus overdrive pacing algorithm
- Sense response in biventricular pacemaker
- Rate reduction response
- Pacemaker-mediated tachycardia
- Runaway pacemaker (rare)

Decreased pacing rate or pause
- Sleep rate
- Rate hysteresis
- Hybrid pacing mode (see text)
- Change in atrial rate and tracking
- Flutter response algorithm
- Upper rate behavior
- Oversensing
- Battery depletion

determines highest programmable upper rate), the upper tracking rate may be limited if long PVARP is programmed. By extending the PVARP, another problem sometimes arises, called repetitive nonreentrant ventriculoatrial synchrony.[6] In this case PVARP covers the retrograde P wave but, if the next V-AP interval (ventricular sense or pace to atrial pace interval) is short enough, the atrium may not be captured because of refractoriness. AP and atrial noncapture is followed by VP (ventricular paced) with retrograde conduction and the abnormality continues (**Fig. 12**). Symptoms are similar to VVI (ventricular pacing and sensing with inhibition) pacing. To fix this problem, it may be necessary to decrease the atrial pacing rate and shorten the AV delay.

Accelerated pacing rate may also be seen during operation of special algorithms. Automatic capture algorithms are increasingly used in pacemakers to optimize safety and enhance follow-up. During the test, these algorithms usually initiate temporary pacing at greater than the intrinsic rate or shorten the AV delay.

A variety of algorithms have been designed to minimize bradycardia and pause-dependent arrhythmias (see **Box 2**). These algorithms provide overdrive suppression of premature atrial complexes (PACs), premature ventricular contractions (PVCs), or regularize ventricular rate during atrial fibrillation. These algorithms remain in use only in select patients because clinical benefits are increasingly being questioned.[7,8] Ventricular sensed response or triggered pacing is commonly used in biventricular devices when there is intrinsic, nonpaced ventricular activity (because of PVCs or nontracked atrial arrhythmias). To promote at least some resynchronization, the algorithm provides (usually left ventricular) triggered pacing following a sensed (RV) event. In these cases the pacer

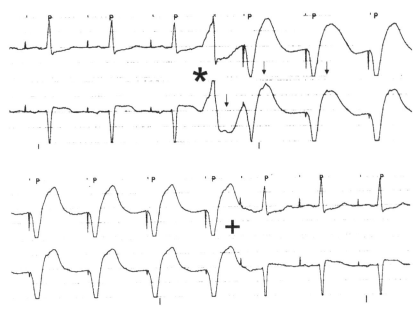

Fig. 11. PMT. Illustrative telemetry strip showing the initiation and termination of a PMT. This arrhythmia may only develop if tracking mode is programmed on. Following a PVC (*), the retrograde P wave (the first examples are marked with vertical arrows) is tracked. RV pacing in turn causes another retrograde P wave and the circuit continues. Once the device activates the PMT algorithm, the last p wave is not tracked (+) and the arrhythmia terminates. Increasing PVARP is the usual first step to eliminate the problem.

artifact is commonly localized in the middle of the QRS complex even at a rapid rate (**Fig. 13**).

Sudden rate increase may be seen if rate hysteresis is programmed on. In this case, pacing is withheld until a lower rate (hysteresis rate) is reached, but then pacing is initiated at a (higher) lower rate limit. If intrinsic rate overtakes pacing, the algorithm allows heart rate to decrease again to less than the lower rate limit. A specialized temporary hysteresis response is used to treat cardioinhibitory vasovagal syncope (ie, rate reduction response; sudden brady response). If sudden bradycardia is detected, the algorithm allows temporary rapid dual chamber pacing to minimize symptoms and risk of syncope (**Fig. 14**).

Lower-than-expected pacing rate
A lower rate may be seen when sleep rate or rate hysteresis algorithm is active (discussed earlier). Newer algorithms are designed to minimize RV pacing (MVP, Medtronic, RythmIQ, Boston Scientific, SafeR, Sorin). These hybrid pacing modes (practically AAI [atrial pacing and sensing with inhibition] mode with some form of ventricular safety

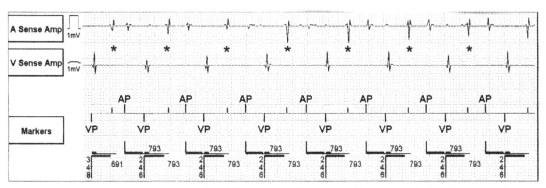

Fig. 12. Repetitive nonreentrant ventriculoatrial synchrony (RNRVAS). This arrhythmia is initiated by the same mechanism as PMT (see **Fig. 11**). The difference is that the P wave falls in the PVARP and is not tracked. The subsequent atrial pacing stimulus does not capture because of the functional refractoriness of the atrial tissue (functional loss of capture). The following RV pacing conducts to cause retrograde P wave (*) and the arrhythmia perpetuates.

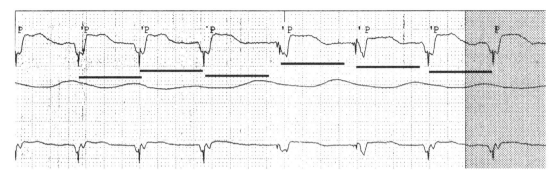

Fig. 13. Triggered LV pacing. The telemetry tracing shows atrial fibrillation and ventricular pacing. Many pacing artifacts are seen in the middle of the QRS complex. The timings of pacing artifacts are different (horizontal lines are the same length), which is consistent with left ventricle–triggered pacing in a biventricular device in order to improve resynchronization. See text for details.

backup) may produce findings of unusual pacing behaviors such as PR interval prolongation, occasional AV block and pauses, and sudden change in AV delay (**Fig. 15**). Sudden slowing of heart rate may be seen when mode switch is activated following initial tracking of an atrial arrhythmia (see **Fig. 6**). In the setting of AV block or short programmed AV delays, upper rate behavior may be seen if sinus rate exceeds upper tracking rate (**Fig. 16**). If sinus cycle length is less than TARP, 2:1 AV block may occur.

Oversensing of a noise (commonly T wave, electric artifact from lead fracture, or EMI), intermittent loss of capture, or device battery depletion are other causes of slowed pacing rate (see **Fig. 8**).

Abnormalities Identified During Device Interrogation

Although diagnostic information provided by different pacemaker models is not uniform, some key components are generally present. Basic information includes data on battery status, lead status, pacing mode, and programmable timing intervals. For a thorough evaluation, it is best to perform device testing with a systematic approach.

The battery status should be checked first. Although there are iterations on how different companies provide battery information (measured voltage or impedance or fuel gauge–type meter), in general the 3 main battery states are good, elective replacement indicator (ERI; device needs to be replaced within 1–3 months), or end-of-life (EOL; unreliable device function). If a pacemaker cannot be interrogated, the battery may be exhausted. As an alternative, the wrong programmer may be used or there is a logic controller problem in the device. If there is a suspected near depletion of a battery in a pacemaker-dependent patient (for example, there is evidence of noncaptured beats), it is safer to insert a temporary pacemaker before the device is interrogated because a telemetry connection may deplete the battery enough to cause asystole.

Impedance, a measure of opposition against electrical current in a circuit, is a key parameter of lead integrity. In general, a breach in lead insulation results in lower impedance (increased path for current flow). In contrast, conductor fracture causes increased impedance (reduced path for current flow). Subtle decline in lead impedance after an active fixation lead implant is common and part of the normal lead maturation process. Significant peri-implant impedance change may indicate dislodgement or perforation. In chronic follow-up, abnormal impedance values may be

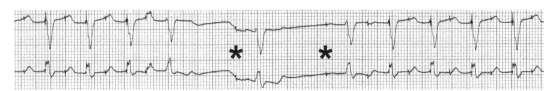

Fig. 14. Rate drop response. The patient presented to the emergency room with palpitations. He had incessant rapid pacing at 110 bpm with termination only for a few beats. AV pacing was present, thus PMT was ruled out. He was paced for 2 minutes as part of a rate drop response algorithm, but, because of subsequent bradycardia (*), another rate drop therapy was initiated. The tracing shows termination and reinitiation of the algorithm, which was easily eliminated with reprogramming.

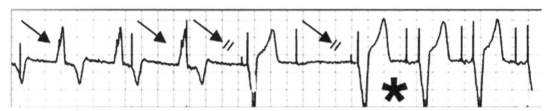

Fig. 15. Managed ventricular pacing algorithm. The telemetry tracing shows atrial pacing with long AV conduction (*arrows*). Blocked AV conduction (*double lines*) results in pause and AV pacing with short AV delay. After 2 of 4 atrial beats are blocked, the device switches to DDD mode (*). This device behavior is typical during the operation of the algorithm.

intermittent and are not always reproducible even at device check, potentially because of a make-or-break–type lead integrity failure (lead fracture). High-frequency, sudden-onset signal with occasional saturation of the amplifier is common in this case. In contrast, gradual increase in impedance is not characteristic of lead fracture. Myopotential oversensing and EMI are characterized by sudden-onset, high-frequency, low-amplitude signals (see **Fig. 9**). During real-time EGM monitoring, provocative measures may bring out an otherwise intermittent system abnormality. Repeat impedance testing during pocket manipulation and arm movement may reproduce noise from a lead fracture. Testing and comparing lead impedance in bipolar and unipolar configuration (tip to ring, tip to can, ring to can) may reveal which conductor connection is defective (should not be tested in

pacemaker-dependent patients but polarity switch may be tried in an emergency). Isometric arm exercise, deep breathing, or change in position (leaning forward, laying on the back or sides) may bring out oversensing of pectoral muscle or diaphragmatic myopotentials or reproduce phrenic nerve capture. Lead impedance fluctuations are not expected if noise is the result of EMI or myopotential oversensing. Impedance changes and noise may also be seen with loose lead pin connections. Pocket manipulation may provoke electrical abnormality in this case.

Testing of sensing and capture threshold with real-time EGM monitoring is the key component of the examination. Although these measurements are simple in most cases, different pacing modes may need to be used to confirm the test results. It is helpful to look at a simultaneous surface

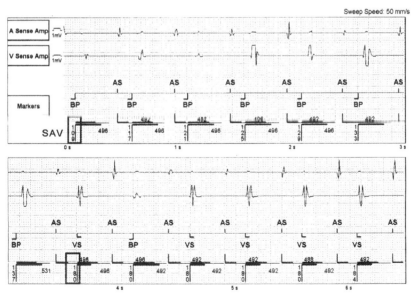

Fig. 16. Upper rate behavior. A biventricular device tracing with sensed AV delay (SAV) of 110 milliseconds at the beginning of the top panel. As the heart rate accelerates, AV delay is progressively prolonged in order to conform with the upper tracking rate limit. In this case, intrinsic conduction takes over (*bottom panel*). In a pacemaker-dependent patient, AV delay progressively prolongs until a following P wave falls in the PVARP and is no longer tracked. Note increased sweep speed at 50 mm/s.

ECG tracing. Based on measured thresholds, sensing level and pacing output may be programmed. In general, sensitivity is programmed between 30% and 60% of the measured sensed parameter but sensitivity should be adjusted in special clinical situations (such as unipolar lead, pacemaker-dependent patients, problems with sensing low-amplitude extrasystoles). In the atrial channel, sensitivity is often programmed at a high level to optimize sensing of low-amplitude arrhythmias, such as atrial fibrillation. It is important to make sure that far-field R-wave oversensing is avoided (see **Figs. 9** and **10**).[9] Details of capture abnormalities are discussed earlier.

Analysis of pacing statistics data and stored EGMs adds another layer of information to troubleshooting. Careful review of the data may suggest an impending clinical abnormality. Heart rate trend and histogram may help to assess the activity level of patients and provides a simple measure to screen for chronotropic incompetence. If clinically indicated, rate-modulated pacing may be programmed on. The histogram pattern may also assist with long-term monitoring of heart rate control in permanent or persistent atrial fibrillation (see **Fig. 3**). Specific heart rate distribution (ie, double hump) may suggest the presence of frequent ectopic beats, which may be the cause of symptoms or cardiomyopathy in some patients. Current data from the literature suggest that frequent RV pacing (>40%) may be associated with heart failure and cardiomyopathy and therefore it should be avoided, if possible. If AV nodal conduction is largely intact, programming efforts should be

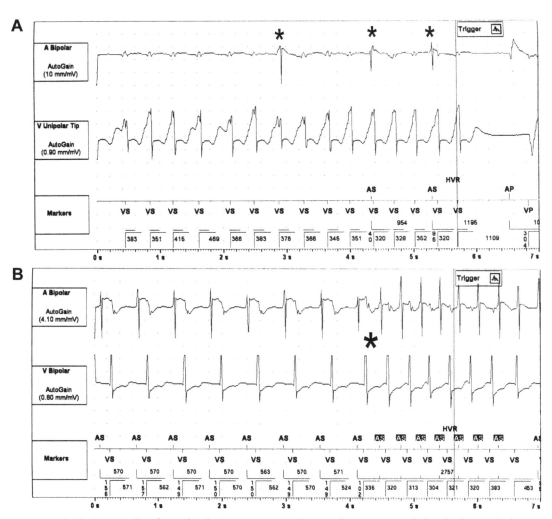

Fig. 17. Arrhythmia recording from the device memory. Both episodes were recorded as high ventricular rate events. (A) Ventricular tachycardia with VA dissociation (atrial electrogram in the A channel, marked with an asterisk). (B) Sudden-onset tachycardia (*), initiated in the A channel. Bipolar ventricular signal is similar to sinus. This recording is most consistent with an atrial tachycardia and not a ventricular tachycardia.

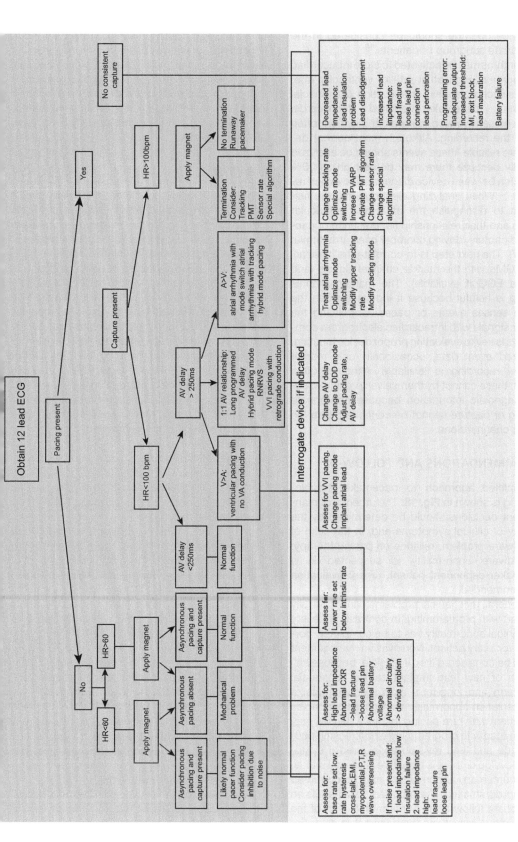

Fig. 18. A simplified approach for pacemaker troubleshooting. The initial work-up and differential diagnosis (*red area*) is derived from the baseline ECG findings and magnet response. The blue area highlights further work-up with additional ancillary tests and device interrogation. (*Adapted from* Kaszala K. Evaluation, troubleshooting and management of pacing system malfunctions. In: Ellenbogen K, Kaszala K, editors. Cardiac pacing and ICDs. 6th edition. New York: Wiley-Blackwell; 2014. p. 272–322.)

directed toward minimizing RV pacing. Biventricular device upgrade should be considered in the appropriate subgroup of patients.[10]

Algorithms may be activated to store intracardiac electrograms. High atrial rate or ventricular rate, mode switch episodes, or activation of a special algorithm (pacemaker-mediated tachycardia [PMT], noise reversion, magnet application) often trigger the recording. Although most current devices are reliable, these events should be analyzed carefully because there may be as high as 30% mismatch between device diagnosis and expert review.[11,12] When analyzing electrograms, the first step is to distinguish the atrial and ventricular signals and their relationship (ie, presence of pacing and capture, driving chamber of an arrhythmia; **Fig. 17**). The next step is to correlate the intracardiac EGMs with the marker channel signals (and surface ECG if available). The marker channel reading is helpful because it indicates when the device senses events or paces. Correlating the marker signals with intracardiac electrogram components is key to evaluating proper device function. In stored event data, occasionally only marker channel recording is available. Although often helpful, these cannot by themselves provide absolute diagnostic information because appropriate sensing or capture cannot be confirmed from the marker channel alone.

RECOMMENDATIONS AND FOLLOW-UP

A simplified approach to pacemaker troubleshooting is shown in **Fig. 18**. The urgency of management decisions should be determined by the severity of clinical symptoms and, in the case of a hardware problem, reliance on pacing therapy. If hardware abnormality is suspected in a pacemaker-dependent patient, urgent evaluation is recommended.

In general, mechanical problems cannot be fully resolved with programming. In contrast, not every mechanical abnormality has to be completely corrected for every patient. Noninvasive management should be considered first, if feasible, because any revision or new lead implant carries substantial short-term and long-term risks. For example, a lead insulation abnormality with occasional noise in a patient with rare pacing for sinus pauses may be managed with programming a nontracking pacing mode and lead revision considered if symptoms develop or there is a change in clinical status.

Although many abnormalities may be corrected with reprogramming, it is important to schedule an appropriate follow-up to confirm resolution of the symptoms or reevaluate the pacemaker data. For example, enhanced surveillance is recommended following reprogramming when borderline sensing or increasing capture threshold is observed. Additional tests should be considered on occasion; for example, a repeat hall-walk test or exercise test when fine tuning of a rate-modulating sensor is required in an active patient with chronotropic incompetence. Device surveillance is markedly eased with the advent of remote, Internet-based device monitoring.

SUMMARY

Although the basic principles of cardiac pacing have not changed over recent decades, providers taking care of complex modern pacemakers continue to be challenged with system problems and device interactions. They are required to master not only basic principles of pacing but also to develop a thorough knowledge of device features. Troubleshooting may be aided by knowledgeable technical support staff from the device companies and they are especially helpful to clarify certain device idiosyncrasies. However, the final decision on clinical care should be made by the medical providers, who must integrate the clinical information, patient characteristics, and device data and weigh the risks and benefits with each available option. If any of these three pillars of care fails, patient outcomes may become compromised.

REFERENCES

1. Maisel WH. Pacemaker and ICD generator reliability: meta-analysis of device registries. JAMA 2006; 295(16):1929–34.
2. Hauser RG, Hayes DL, Kallinen LM, et al. Clinical experience with pacemaker pulse generators and transvenous leads: an 8-year prospective multicenter study. Heart Rhythm 2007;4(2):154–60.
3. Coman JA, Trohman RG. Incidence and electrocardiographic localization of safe right bundle branch block configurations during permanent ventricular pacing. Am J Cardiol 1995;76(11):781–4.
4. Jacob S, Panaich SS, Maheshwari R, et al. Clinical applications of magnets on cardiac rhythm management devices. Europace 2011; 13(9):1222–30.
5. Raitt MH, Stelzer KJ, Laramore GE, et al. Runaway pacemaker during high-energy neutron radiation therapy. Chest 1994;106(3):955–7.
6. Serge Barold S. Repetitive reentrant and non-reentrant ventriculoatrial synchrony in dual chamber pacing. Clin Cardiol 1991;14(9):754–63.
7. Lian J, Mussig D, Lang V. Ventricular rate smoothing for atrial fibrillation: a quantitative comparison study [Comparative Study]. Europace 2007;9(7): 506–13.

8. Tse HF, Newman D, Ellenbogen KA, et al. Effects of ventricular rate regularization pacing on quality of life and symptoms in patients with atrial fibrillation (Atrial fibrillation symptoms mediated by pacing to mean rates [AF SYMPTOMS Study]). Am J Cardiol 2004;94(7):938–41.

9. Kolb C, Wille B, Maurer D, et al. Management of far-field R wave sensing for the avoidance of inappropriate mode switch in dual chamber pacemakers: results of the FFS-test study. J Cardiovasc Electrophysiol 2006;17(9):992–7.

10. Witte KK, Pipes RR, Nanthakumar K, et al. Biventricular pacemaker upgrade in previously paced heart failure patients—improvements in ventricular dyssynchrony. J Card Fail 2006; 12(3):199–204.

11. de Voogt WG, van Hemel NM, van de Bos AA, et al. Verification of pacemaker automatic mode switching for the detection of atrial fibrillation and atrial tachycardia with Holter recording. Europace 2006;8(11): 950–61.

12. Defaye P, Leclercq JF, Guilleman D, et al. Contributions of high resolution electrograms memorized by DDDR pacemakers in the interpretation of arrhythmic events. Pacing Clin Electrophysiol 2003; 26(1 Pt 2):214–20.

Troubleshooting the Malfunctioning Implantable Cardiac Defibrillator: A Systematic Approach

Pierre Bordachar, MD, PhD[a],[*], Romain Eschalier, MD, PhD[a],[b], Sylvain Ploux, MD[a], Philippe Ritter, MD[a]

KEYWORDS

- Implantable cardiac defibrillator • Troubleshooting • Management • Oversensing • Lead fracture
- Ventricular arrhythmias

KEY POINTS

- Implantable cardiac defibrillators (ICDs) have evolved prominently since their introduction, with broader indications as primary prevention.
- ICDs have become extremely complex and offer many programmable parameters.
- A physician should be thoroughly familiar with the nuances of each model to confirm or dispute the diagnosis made by the ICD as well as reprogram the parameters with a view to adapting them specifically to the characteristics of individual device recipients.
- A systematic stepwise approach (clinical history, physical examination, radiographic techniques, and an analysis of the stored electrograms) is essential for correctly identifying the cause of suspected defibrillator malfunction.

INTRODUCTION

Implantable cardiac defibrillators (ICDs) have evolved prominently since their introduction in clinical practice in 1980. The indications for implant of the original shock boxes were limited to secondary prevention after the survival of at least 2 episodes of sudden cardiac death. The devices delivered only high-energy monophasic shocks between pericardial patches implanted by cardiac surgeons.[1–3] Practice guidelines, based on large international clinical trials, include primary prevention as an indication for implantation of ICD, and the devices are most commonly implanted by cardiologists, using endocardial leads. Antitachycardia pacing (ATP) therapy limits the need to deliver shocks, and the programmable shock polarity and waveforms have increased the efficacy of the system.[4–6]

ICDs have become complex and offer many programmable parameters, whether for cardiac pacing, the memory functions, or the various therapies.[7–10] Because of this technological evolution and the characteristics of devices available from a single manufacturer or among various manufacturers, the acquisition of knowledge is constantly changing. A physician should probably take advantage of every possible source of assistance,

Funding Support: None.
Financial Disclosures or Conflicts of Interest: The authors have nothing to disclose.
[a] Hôpital Cardiologique du Haut-Lévêque, CHU Bordeaux, IHU LIRYC, Université Bordeaux, 1 Avenue Magellan, Bordeaux 33604 Pessac Cedex, France; [b] Cardiology Department, ISIT-CaVITI, CHU Clermont-Ferrand, Clermont Université, BP 10448, Clermont-Ferrand F-63003, France
[*] Corresponding author.
E-mail address: bordacharp@hotmail.com

including review of the technical manual of the device and contacting the manufacturer for help. It is, nevertheless, indispensable for them to be thoroughly familiar with the nuances of each model to confirm or dispute the diagnosis made by the ICD regarding a stored event, as well as, perhaps, reprogram the parameters with a view to adapting them specifically to the characteristics of individual device recipients. A systematic approach is essential for correctly identifying the cause of suspected defibrillator malfunction. Patients may present with excessive or inadequate device therapy or in contrast with insufficient therapy, with a single or multiple ICD discharges, syncope with no perceived ICD therapy, ICD therapies without previous symptoms. By a careful evaluation of the clinical history, physical examination, and radiographic techniques and then a comprehensive analysis of the stored electrograms (EGMs) and of the information obtained by telemetry (including battery voltage, charge time, function and appearance of the lead system, pacing parameters assessment), the cause of malfunction can often be determined.

In this article, a stepwise approach is presented to the most common troubleshooting cases encountered in an ICD clinic, focusing on the several multiple stages that lead to the final diagnosis, with a solution to the problem posed.

SYSTEMATIC OVERSENSING OF A PHYSIOLOGIC CARDIAC SIGNAL

The systematic oversensing of a physiologic cardiac signal at each cycle (oversensing of the T-wave, oversensing of the P-wave, and double counting of the R-wave) results in 2 signals with different morphologies alternating between 2 intervals (1 short, 1 long).

Patient 1: T-Wave Oversensing and Shock

A 41-year-old man suffering from hypertrophic cardiomyopathy received an Atlas (St. Jude Medical) single-chamber ICD for management of sustained ventricular tachycardia (VT). He was seen after having received an electrical shock while exercising without previous symptoms or sensation of tachycardia.

Clinical history and physical examination
Clinical assessment should systematically include the indication for implantation, activity preceding the episode, symptoms experienced during the episode, duration of the episode, and information from the family or any bystander.

This episode highlights a characteristic commonly found in presence of T-wave oversensing.

Inappropriate therapies often occur during exercise; effort is associated with a decrease in the R-wave and an increase in the T-wave amplitudes. The speed of the signal is also increased, which modifies the slew rate, bringing the T-wave into a bandwidth at which it is sensed as an R-wave, causing the incorrect diagnosis of ventricular fibrillation (VF). Therapies are delivered in absence of previous ill feeling. In some cases, deep breathing may reproduce oversensing (preferentially P-wave oversensing).

Chest radiography
Chest radiography can be helpful for diagnosing lead fracture, lead dislodgement, lead malposition, or loose pin connection in the header, but a normal appearance cannot exclude a lead failure.

No specific radiographic signs can be observed in cases of T-wave oversensing or double counting of the R-wave. In contrast, oversensing of the P-wave occurs preferentially when the defibrillation coil of an integrated bipolar lead (the anode of the sensing circuit is the defibrillation electrode of the right ventricular lead) is straddling the tricuspid valve. Chest radiography typically shows the tip of the ventricular lead near the tricuspid valve.

The chest radiograph was normal in this patient.

Pacing parameters
An initial and essential step in troubleshooting is to retrieve the information from the device (programmed parameters, battery and capacitor status, system data, event logs, system component testing, including sensing and pacing thresholds).

T-wave oversensing often occurs in presence of a low-amplitude R-wave, because the gain adjusts the sensitivity automatically, based on the amplitude of the sensed R-wave. In this patient, the ventricular sensing capacities were altered (R-wave 2.6 mV at rest with a probable decrease during exercise). The pacing and defibrillation impedances and the pacing thresholds were normal.

Analysis of stored EGMs
Interval plot Interval plots are available in ICDs manufactured by Medtronic and Boston Scientific but not in St. Jude Medical ICDs. As shown in another example of a patient with a Medtronic device and double counting of the R-wave (**Fig. 1**), the plot gives essential information in patients with oversensing of a cardiac signal. The episode plot clearly shows the characteristic short-long cycle alternation observed in presence of oversensing of a cardiac signal other than the R-wave (P-wave, T-wave, R-wave double counting) with a typical railroad track pattern. The magnitude of alternation between the 2 cycles may be smaller

Treated VT/VF Episode #1047

Device: **Virtuoso DR D164AWG**   Date of Visit: **14-Mar-2011 11:50:40**

Patient: ID: Physician:

Type	ATP Seq	Shocks	Success	ID#	Date	Time hh:mm	Duration hh:mm:ss	Avg bpm A/V	Max bpm A/V	Activity at Onset
VF	0	35J	Yes	1047	26-Jul-2010	20:57	:20	115/240	---/---	Active

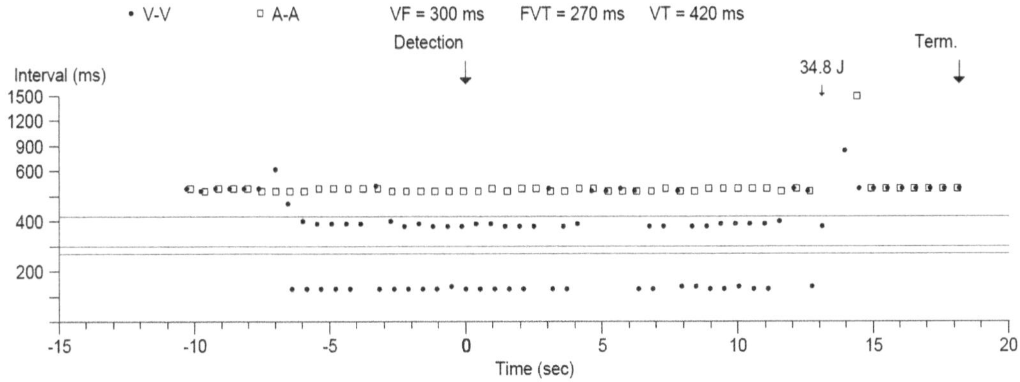

• V-V   □ A-A   VF = 300 ms   FVT = 270 ms   VT = 420 ms

Detection

Fig. 1. The episode plot (Medtronic device) clearly shows the characteristic short-long cycle alternating observed in presence of oversensing of a cardiac signal other than the R-wave (P-wave, T-wave, R-wave double counting) with a typical railroad track pattern.

in cases of T-wave versus P-wave or R-wave oversensing. This type of episode plot is different from that observed in presence of electromagnetic interference (several very fast identical signals during the same cardiac cycle) or lead failure (short nonphysiologic cycles of variable amplitude).

EGMs In the tracing shown in **Fig. 2**A, the EGM channel corresponds to the ventricular pace/sense channel. The amplification (here, 6.7 mm/mV) of the signals must be known to correctly evaluate the amplitude of the various signals. In this tracing, intermittent sensing of 2 signals of different morphology is observed within a single cardiac cycle with alternating short and longer cycles. Oversensing of the T-wave after a spontaneous ventricular event occurs preferentially in presence of a low-amplitude R-wave. Two T-waves are not oversensed, when the R-wave seems to be of higher amplitude. Sensitivity and gain are adjusted automatically, based on the amplitude of the R-wave that was just sensed: when that amplitude is low, the likelihood is high of subsequently and rapidly reaching the highest sensitivity. The episode that was detected fell initially in the VT monitor zone, avoiding the delivery of any inappropriate therapy. Subsequently, the heart rate increased with persistence of oversensing, and the episode was detected in the VF zone, explaining the delivery of a shock.

The same episode and tracing are shown at an amplification of 1 mm/mV, which facilitates the measurement of the various signals, showing the

very low amplitude of the ventricular EGM (see **Fig. 2**B).

Proposed solution In this patient, any decrease in the ventricular sensitivity to prevent T-wave oversensing would incur a serious risk of VF underdetection, because the amplitude of the ventricular EGM during sinus rhythm was already low. Furthermore, as shown by the tracing, sensing of the ventricular EGM was modified by exercise, with relatively wide amplitude variations from 1 ventricular complex to the other. Modifications in the threshold level and decay delay eliminated oversensing of the T-wave, including during a confirmatory exercise test. However, the low quality of ventricular EGM sensing remains troublesome in this patient, and a search for an alternative sensing site must be strongly considered.

The number of cycles that determines the return of sinus rhythm (reprogrammed at 3 in this patient) is a key programming point when confronted with this issue in St. Jude Medical devices, because, in presence of intermittent oversensing, it directly influences the likelihood of inappropriate therapy.

Algorithms available in the new range of defibrillators (Medtronic and St. Jude Medical) may solve this problem. The T-wave oversensing algorithm (Medtronic) integrates a fully automatic frequency analysis instead of a manual adjustment of the sensitivity to anticipate and prevent inappropriate shocks caused by T-wave oversensing. The discrimination of T-waves assumes that R-waves and T-waves are physically different; the slew

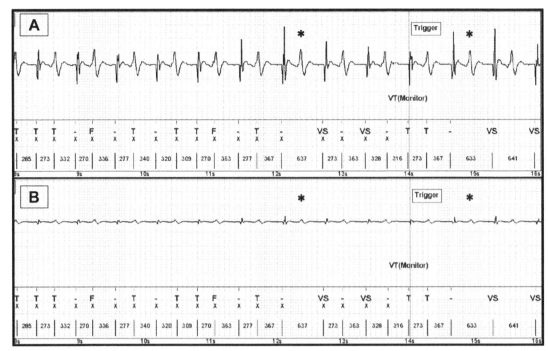

Fig. 2. (A) The EGM channel corresponds to the ventricular pace/sense channel (amplification: 6.7 mm/mV). We observed intermittent sensing of 2 signals of different morphology within a single cardiac cycle with alternating short and longer cycles: oversensing of the T-wave. Two T-waves are not oversensed (*asterisk*), where the R-wave seems to be of higher amplitude. The episode that was detected fell initially in the VT monitor zone. (B) The same episode at an amplification of 1 mm/mV.

rate of the R-wave is generally higher than that of the T-wave, a difference that can be amplified by a high-pass differential filter, which examines differences in amplitude, slew rate, and pattern to distinguish R from T. The SecureSense algorithm (St. Jude Medical) compares the bipolar channel (RV distal to RV ring) with the unipolar channel (RV coil to can/RV distal to can). When rapid signals are sensed on the bipolar but not on the unipolar channel, therapy is inhibited. This algorithm was initially designed to avoid inappropriate therapies related to lead fractures but may also enable the prevention of therapies because of T-wave, P-wave, or R-wave oversensing.

In case of P-wave oversensing, several solutions can be considered (lower ventricular sensitivity or forced atrial pacing with dynamic overdrive mode), but the ventricular lead often has to be repositioned to eliminate oversensing entirely.

In cases of R-wave double counting, a prolongation of the ventricular blanking is required.

LEAD DYSFUNCTION

Multiple shocks can be related to incessant ventricular arrhythmias, VT, or VF with ineffective shocks, inappropriate therapies (electromagnetic interference, lead fracture, oversensing of myopotentials or physiologic cardiac signals, supraventricular tachycardia). The shocks can also be proarrhythmic and create, accelerate, or disorganize an arrhythmia.

Patient 2: Lead Fracture and Multiple Shocks

A 74-year-old man, recipient of a Virtuoso DR dual-chamber defibrillator (Medtronic) for ischemic cardiomyopathy and syncope caused by VT was seen in the ambulatory department after receiving several shocks in the absence of previous symptoms.

Clinical history and physical examination

In case of lead fractures, inappropriate therapies are usually delivered in absence of previous ill feeling. Multiple shocks without previous symptoms may be caused by lead failure. Manipulation of the device or the lead in the pocket may elicit electrical lead artifact. In this patient, particular motions of the ipsilateral arm or shoulder could reproduce oversensing with very short RR intervals (<150 milliseconds).

Chest radiography

Chest radiographs show fracture lines in less than half of instances of lead fracture. In this patient, the chest radiograph was normal.

Pacing parameters

A pacing less than 200 Ohms or shock impedance less than 25 Ohms increase the likelihood of a breakdown in lead insulation as the source of extracardiac signals. In contrast, a pacing greater than 2000 Ohms or shock impedance greater than 100 Ohms increases the likelihood of a conductor fracture. A sudden variation in the impedance curves (>30%) is important to identify, even if it remains within the normal range. On the other hand, the normal impedance found in this case without measured important variations does not exclude this diagnosis. The sensing and pacing thresholds were also normal.

Analysis of stored EGMs

Interval plot The interval plot is consistent with a fracture of the ventricular lead conductor or a faulty lead connection (**Fig. 3**). It shows a very irregular ventricular rate, with alternation between short (close to the sensed ventricular blanking period) and normal cycles. Oversensing is prolonged, and 3 shocks of maximal strength are delivered.

EGMs In the tracing shown in **Fig. 4A**, the EGM channels correspond to the atrial and ventricular pace/sense channels. Extracardiac signals are recognizable by the absence of correlation with the intrinsic cardiac cycle. The tracing suggests a lead fracture (short cycles, intermittent oversensing within the cardiac cycle, disorganized ventricular EGMs of variable amplitude, with intermittent large complexes saturating the amplifiers).

Proposed solution This patient underwent the extraction of this defective lead, and a new ICD lead was implanted. Different algorithms can be programmed to decrease the occurrence of inappropriate therapies in case of lead fracture. The Lead Integrity Alert algorithm (Medtronic) is based on the detection of abnormal impedance, very short ventricular cycles, and presence of nonsustained VT. It delays the diagnosis of VF by automatically increasing the number of cycles required for the diagnosis (to 30/40). A noise detection algorithm is also available in the newest Medtronic defibrillators (see **Fig. 4B**: example of a patient with a new device and lead fracture). The function of this algorithm is similar to the Secure-Sense algorithm (St. Jude Medical) with comparison between bipolar and shock channels. The algorithm compares the sensed right ventricular bipolar EGM with the shock/morphology EGM, and if the right ventricular lead is functioning properly, these signals both show high amplitude. If the RV sense signal shows electrical signals on the rate sense lead and no activity on the shock/morphology EGM, then the device determines that lead noise is present and therapy is withheld. If the lead noise alert is programmed on, the device sounds a patient alert tone.

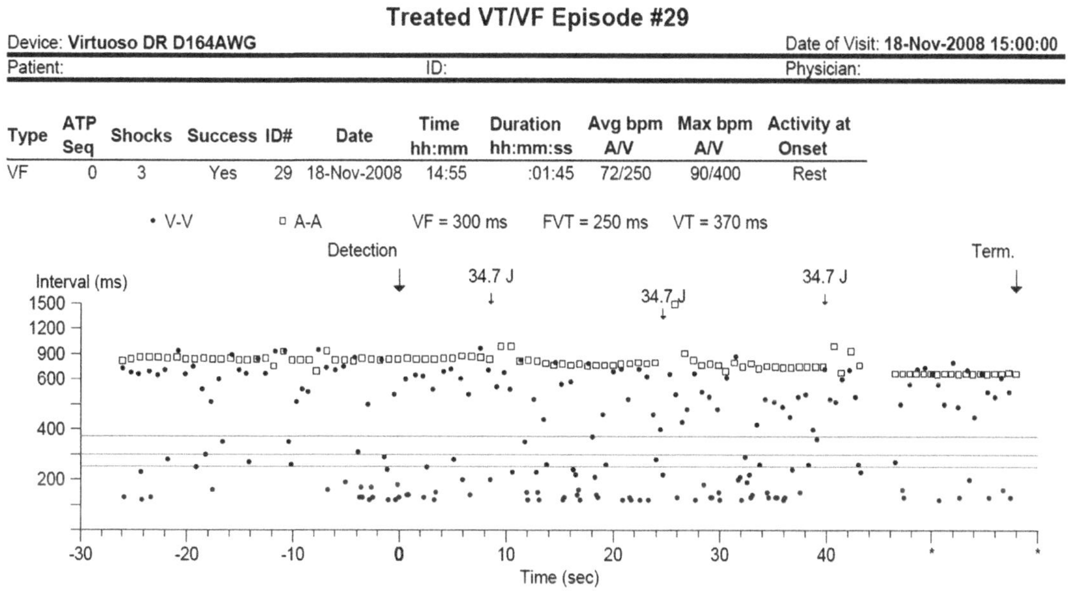

Fig. 3. The interval plot shows a very irregular ventricular rate, alternating between short (close to the sensed ventricular blanking period) and normal cycles: lead fracture. Oversensing was prolonged and 3 shocks of maximal strength (34.7 J) were delivered.

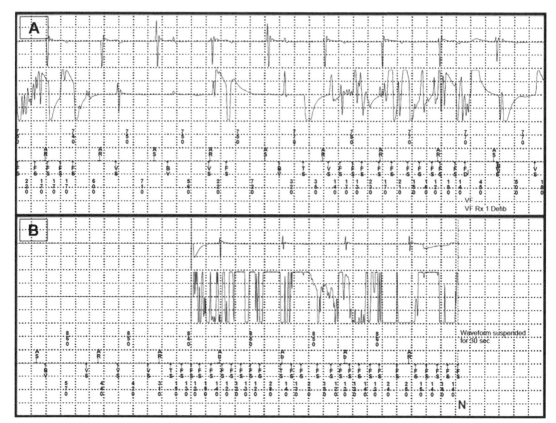

Fig. 4. (A) In this tracing, the EGM channels correspond to the atrial (*upper tracing*) and ventricular (*lower tracing*) pace/sense channels. The tracing suggests a lead fracture (short cycles, intermittent within the cardiac cycle, disorganized, of variable amplitude, some large complexes saturating the amplifiers). (B) Example of patient with a new device and a diagnosis of lead fracture (N, noise) by the device. No shock is delivered.

ELECTROMAGNETIC INTERFERENCE

Cardiac defibrillators are vulnerable to magnetic interferences, because they are designed to detect small, fast signals and require programming of high sensitivity and automatic threshold adaptation. The bandwidths are also broad to detect high frequencies during VF. Some devices contain noise reversion capacities, but the protection is often imperfect.

Patient 3: 50-Hz Oversensing and Shock

A 34-year-old male recipient of a single-chamber ICD (Atlas, St. Jude Medical), implanted after he suffered an episode of aborted sudden death, experienced an electrical shock while operating a power saw in the rain.

Clinical history and physical examination
The determinant point of this episode is the exposure to a source at the time of the event.

Chest radiography
In this patient, the chest radiograph was normal.

Pacing parameters
Electrical tests (sensing and pacing thresholds, impedances) were normal.

Analysis of stored EGMs
Interval plot The interval plot is not available for this manufacturer but would probably have shown presence of very short cycles.

EGMs The tracing in **Fig. 5**A shows the usual characteristics observed in patients presenting with electromagnetic interference and oversensing of external high-frequency electrical noise, a typical pattern of intermittent sensing of 50 Hz signal, sensing of very rapid regular signals spanning the entire cardiac cycle; these signals heavily saturate the baseline, although the QRS complexes remain visible. A few seconds later, there was further oversensing and diagnosis of a VF episode, start of the charge of the capacitors, and delivery of a 36-J shock.

The tracing was identical with the previous tracing, although the faster sweep speed (see **Fig. 5**B) showed the characteristic sinusoidal

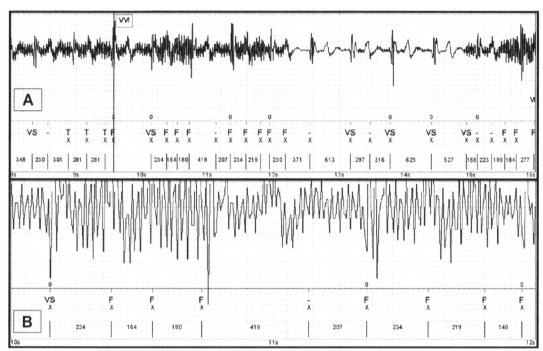

Fig. 5. (*A*) This tracing shows the typical pattern of intermittent sensing of a 50-Hz signal: sensing of very rapid regular signals spanning the entire cardiac cycle. (*B*) Tracing identical to the previous tracing, although the faster sweep speed shows the characteristic sinusoidal aspect of a 50-Hz alternating current, with a 20-minute interval between each signal.

aspect of a 50-Hz alternating current, with a 20-m interval between each signal.

On a dual-chamber ICD, the signals are usually visible on both the atrial and the ventricular channels, and are larger on the shocking (widely spaced electrodes) than on the sensing lead channel (closely spaced electrodes).

Proposed solution The main preventive measures consist of finding the emitting source and avoiding the use of poorly insulated instrumentation/appliances.

VENTRICULAR ARRHYTHMIA AND MULTIPLE SHOCKS
Patient 4: Electrical Shock for Fast VT Inducing VF and Prompting Multiple Shocks

A 55-year-old overweight man received a Marquis VR single-chamber ICD (Medtronic) in the context of an old anterior myocardial infarction, 40% left ventricular ejection fraction, and episodes of VT at 200 bpm during an electrical storm. He was on a regimen of amiodarone. He presented after suffering a 2-hour episode of chest pain, followed by prolonged syncope and, according to his wife, several body jolts consistent with the delivery of electrical shocks.

Clinical history and physical examination
Syncope preceding discharge strongly suggested therapies for fast ventricular arrhythmias or oversensing in a patient dependent on his ICD for bradycardia pacing (misdiagnosis of ventricular arrhythmia leading to pacing inhibition, syncope, and shock).

Chest radiography
In this patient, the chest radiograph was normal.

Pacing parameters
The electrical tests (sensing and pacing thresholds, impedances) were normal.

Analysis of stored EGMs
Interval plot The episode started with a regular, monomorphic fast VT at a rate near 210 bpm detected in the VF zone; the first shock disorganized the VT and induced VF (faster and irregular); VF persisted after the delivery of 3 additional shocks at maximal strength; VF was terminated by a fifth maximal shock (**Fig. 6**).

EGMs The initial arrhythmia was a regular, monomorphic VT at a rate near 210 bpm. The first shock delivered on the R-wave disorganized the VT and induced VF (**Fig. 7A**). VF was terminated by the fifth maximal shock (see **Fig. 7B**).

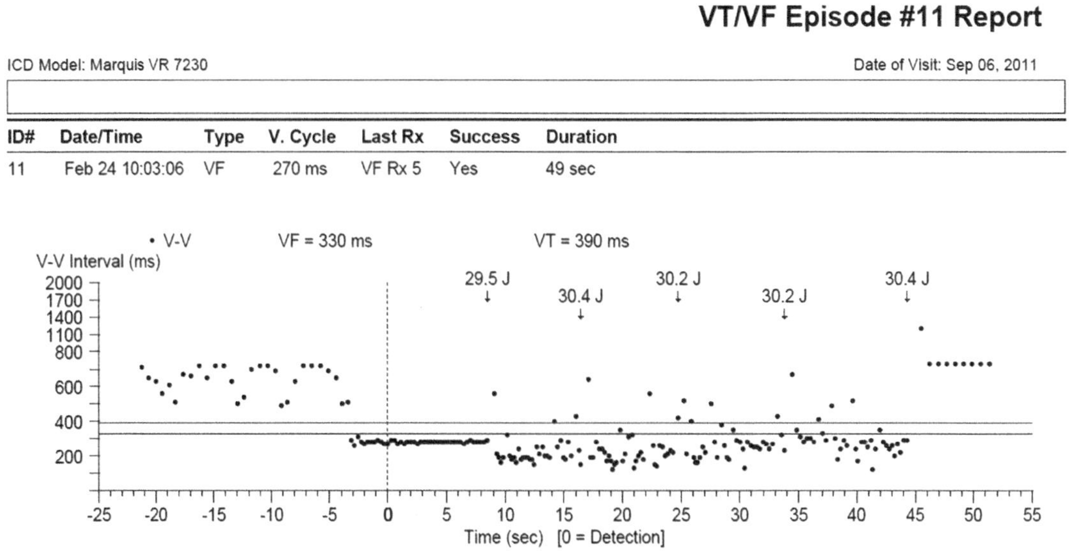

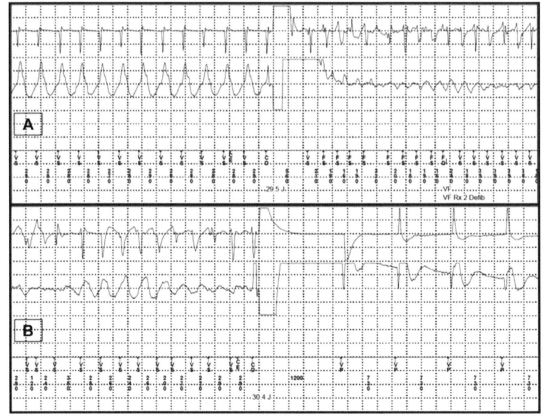

Fig. 6. The episode started with a regular, monomorphic fast VT at a rate near 210 bpm detected in the VF zone; the first shock (29.5 J) disorganized the VT and induced VF (faster and irregular); VF persisted after the delivery of 3 additional shocks at maximal strength (30.2 J–30.4 J); VF was terminated by a fifth maximal shock (30.4 J).

Fig. 7. (A) The initial arrhythmia was a regular, monomorphic VT at a rate near 210 bpm. The first shock (29.5 J) delivered on the R-wave disorganized the VT and induced VF. (B) VF was terminated by the fifth maximal shock (30.4 J).

Proposed solution This tracing shows 3 key elements:

1. The delivery of a shock is the primary function of an ICD. Shocks terminate tachyarrhythmias in most cases. However, on rare occasions, the shocks are proarrhythmic and, as in this case, transform an organized VT into life-threatening VF.
2. A major goal, when programming an ICD, is to decrease the likelihood of shock delivery without compromising the patient's safety. Many tachyarrhythmias detected in the VF zone are organized, monomorphic, and can be terminated by ATP. Its programming during capacitor charging does not delay the shock delivery, if needed. The detection of VF simultaneously triggers ATP and the charge of the capacitors. If ATP terminates the tachycardia, all other therapies are withheld, preserving the patient's quality of life. On the other hand, the charge of the capacitors drains energy, which can be problematic, if frequent. Programming before charge meets 2 important goals: the delivery of fewer shocks and less drain of the battery.
3. This arrhythmic event is worrisome because it was not terminated before the full-strength fifth shock. In Medtronic and St. Jude Medical ICDs, the number of shocks for a single arrhythmic episode of VF is limited to 6 (8 in Boston Scientific devices). The likelihood of a successful shock after 6 failed attempts at maximum strength is limited. On the other hand, the number of shocks delivered inappropriately needs to be limited. This tracing underscores the noncorrespondence of the defibrillation threshold to a fixed value. In this case, several maximum energy shocks were unsuccessful, whereas the fifth shock, of the same strength, resolved a troublesome situation. In this patient, the safety margin was limited by the presence of factors associated with high defibrillation thresholds. Although some of these factors, such as the substrate of ischemic cardiomyopathy and obesity can not easily be modified, others are more manageable. For instance, treatment with amiodarone could be eliminated, which would likely decrease the defibrillation threshold (there is some evidence to suggest that chronic amiodarone therapy may increase defibrillation thresholds in older defibrillators), although with a risk of increasing the incidence of ventricular arrhythmias. The shocks delivered were biphasic, anodal in polarity (anode in the ventricle, cathodal pulse generator for the first phase) for shocks 1, 3,

and 5, cathodal in polarity for shocks 2 and 4, dual coil, and fixed tilt. In Medtronic devices, there are not many possibilities in terms of optimization of the waveform (tilt fixed and not programmable, cathodal or anodal, single or double coil).

The normal shock impedance that was measured suggests that an optimization of these settings, for example the programming of a fixed pulse duration, had little chance of increasing the likelihood of successful defibrillation. In this patient, an additional coil was placed inside the coronary sinus. A shock delivered between a pair of electrodes in contact with, or in the immediate proximity of, the cardiac mass is likely to be more effective by spreading the induced electrical field over a larger volume.

SUMMARY

The increased complexity of ICD devices requires a systematic and stepwise approach to troubleshooting and a detailed knowledge and understanding of the specificities of the different manufacturers.

REFERENCES

1. Mirowski M, Mower MM, Reid PR, et al. Implantable automatic defibrillators: their potential in prevention of sudden coronary death. Ann N Y Acad Sci 1982;382:371–80.
2. Mirowski M. The automatic implantable cardioverter-defibrillator: an overview. J Am Coll Cardiol 1985;6: 461–6.
3. Goldberger Z, Lampert R. Implantable cardioverter-defibrillators: expanding indications and technologies. JAMA 2006;295:809–18.
4. Gregoratos G, Abrams J, Epstein AE, et al, American College of Cardiology/American Heart Association Task Force on Practice Guidelines/North American Society for Pacing and Electrophysiology Committee to Update the 1998 Pacemaker Guidelines. ACC/AHA/NASPE 2002 guideline update for implantation of cardiac pacemakers and antiarrhythmia devices: summary article: a report of the American College of Cardiology/American Heart Association Task Force on practice guidelines (ACC/AHA/NASPE Committee to update the 1998 pacemaker guidelines). Circulation 2002;106:2145–61.
5. Epstein AE, DiMarco JP, Ellenbogen KA, et al. ACC/AHA/HRS 2008 guidelines for device-based therapy of cardiac rhythm abnormalities: a report of the American College of Cardiology/American Heart Association Task Force on practice guidelines (Writing Committee to revise the ACC/AHA/NASPE 2002 guideline update for implantation of

cardiac pacemakers and antiarrhythmia devices) developed in collaboration with the American Association for Thoracic Surgery and Society of Thoracic Surgeons. J Am Coll Cardiol 2008; 51:1–62.

6. Epstein AE, DiMarco JP, Ellenbogen KA, et al, American College of Cardiology Foundation, American Heart Association Task Force on Practice Guidelines, Heart Rhythm Society. 2012 ACCF/AHA/HRS focused update incorporated into the ACCF/AHA/HRS 2008 guidelines for device-based therapy of cardiac rhythm abnormalities: a report of the American College of Cardiology Foundation/American Heart Association Task Force on practice guidelines and the Heart Rhythm Society. J Am Coll Cardiol 2013;61:6–75.

7. Koneru JN, Swerdlow CD, Wood MA, et al. Minimizing inappropriate or "unnecessary" implantable cardioverter-defibrillator shocks: appropriate programming. Circ Arrhythm Electrophysiol 2011;4:778–90.

8. Tan VH, Wilton SB, Kuriachan V, et al. Impact of programming strategies aimed at reducing nonessential implantable cardioverter defibrillator therapies on mortality: a systematic review and meta-analysis. Circ Arrhythm Electrophysiol 2014;7:164–70.

9. Mansour F, Khairy P. ICD monitoring zones: intricacies, pitfalls, and programming tips. J Cardiovasc Electrophysiol 2008;19:568–74.

10. Moss AJ, Schuger C, Beck CA, et al, MADIT-RIT Trial Investigators. Reduction in inappropriate therapy and mortality through ICD programming. N Engl J Med 2012;367:2275–83.

Troubleshooting the Malfunctioning CRT-D Device: A Systematic Approach

Ammar M. Killu, MBBS, Yong-Mei Cha, MD*

KEYWORDS

- CRT • Resynchronization • Pacemaker • ICD • Malfunction • Troubleshoot • Therapy
- Heart failure

KEY POINTS

- Inability to cannulate the coronary sinus occurs in fewer than 5% of patients.
- Extracardiac stimulation, including diaphragmatic stimulation, occurs in less than 6% of patients.
- The use of a device and leads with multiple programmable pacing configurations may mitigate the need for lead repositioning at a later date.
- Capture should be checked using alternate vectors, and cathodal capture should be confirmed.
- Any factor that reduces ventricular pacing will hamper resynchronization/CRT; the goal is resynchronization 100% of the time.
- Sensing problems in an implantable cardioverter defibrillator may result in either inappropriate therapy or failure to deliver appropriate therapy.
- Oversensing can originate from intracardiac signals (eg, P waves), or extracardiac signals (eg, pectoral muscle potentials).
- Electromagnetic inference and radiation therapy may have adverse effects on cardiovascular implantable electronic device function.

INTRODUCTION

In more than a decade, the invention of transvenous left ventricular (LV) pacing integrated to a conventional pacemaker (cardiac resynchronization pacemaker, CRT-P) or an implantable cardioverter defibrillator (CRT-D) has offered effective alternative therapy for patients with mild to severe heart failure (HF).[1–5] One of the fundamental pathophysiological processes in HF is conduction system disease, often manifesting as left bundle branch block (LBBB), resulting in delayed electrical excitation and myocardial contraction at the LV lateral wall and, in turn, a reduction of cardiac output. By pacing the LV free wall and right ventricular septum simultaneously, CRT is able to resynchronize both ventricular excitation and contraction. The acute hemodynamic benefit is apparent, including improvement in ventricular contractility and cardiac output, as well as reduction in mitral regurgitation and LV filling pressure. It has now been clearly proven that CRT can improve chronic LV systolic dysfunction with evidence of reverse LV remodeling, thereby reducing HF symptoms, HF readmission, and mortality.[1,2,4–7] Like other cardiovascular implantable electronic devices (CIED), CRT-D malfunction may occur during the chronic course of therapy. A systemic approach on trouble-shooting CRT-D device malfunction is discussed in this article.

The authors have nothing to disclose.
Division of Cardiovascular Diseases, Department of Internal Medicine, Mayo Clinic, 200 First Street Southwest, Rochester, MN 55905, USA
* Corresponding author.
E-mail address: ycha@mayo.edu

cardiacEP.theclinics.com

COMMON CAUSES OF CRT MALFUNCTION

The commonly encountered causes of CRT malfunction are listed in **Box 1**. A general approach is outlined in **Fig. 1**.

PACING MALFUNCTION
Noncapture

Case: A 69-year-old woman with NYHA class III HF secondary to dilated cardiomyopathy received a CRT-D implant. At 3-month follow-up, she reported little improvement and it was noted that the LV lead (placed in the lateral vein at the basal anterolateral wall) had dislodged, causing high pacing threshold 6.0 mv/1.0 ms with intermittent failure to capture. Fig. 2 shows sequential ECG recordings. Before CRT, the patient had sinus rhythm, LBBB, and QRS duration of 214 ms. After CRT, biventricular pacing resulted in a paced RBBB morphology and QS wave in lead I, suggesting the presence of LV pacing. Three months later, repeat ECG indicated a paced LBBB morphology and loss of QS, evidence consistent with failure

---

Box 1
Commonly encountered causes of CRT malfunction

Pacing malfunction
- Elevated LV pacing threshold or loss of LV capture
- Diaphragmatic stimulation
- Anodal stimulation

Sensing malfunction
- Double-counting
- Oversensing
- Undersensing

Generator malfunction
- Failure output
- Battery depletion

Loss of synchronization
- Long programed AV delay or AV search hysteresis
- Conduction of rapid atrial/supraventricular arrhythmias
- Premature ventricular complexes
- Low maximal tracking rate
- Prolonged postventricular atrial refractory period
- Rate smoothing algorithms

---

of LV capture and RV pacing only. The patient underwent LV lead revision. Coronary venogram showed a large lateral coronary vein with an acute curve at the take-off of this branch (U shape). An Easy Track 3 LV lead (Boston Scientific Inc, Natick, MA, USA) was placed in the lateral vein with satisfactory thresholds. Cine showed appropriate LV lead position in both RAO and LAO views (Fig. 3). Following this, she felt clinically improved with NYHA class I symptoms at 6-month follow-up.

LV lead dislodgment occurs in greater frequency than right-sided leads. A meta-analysis including 7 CRT trials revealed an LV lead dislodgment rate of 5.7% (range 2.8%–10.6%).[8] Causes of LV lead dislodgment include poor lead redundancy (overredundant or underredundant), unstable lead location, use of a spiral lead in a short vein segment, and unfavorable vein anatomy. Unfavorable vein anatomy entails wide-caliber veins, proximity to the coronary sinus, and an upward course/flat take-off to a posterolateral site. Spiral curved leads or angled lead tips enhance lead stability; although it requires an optimal vein length to accommodate the entire spiral part, this permits the lead to be wedged into side branches. On occasion, active fixation leads, such as the Starfix lead (Medtronic Inc, St. Paul, MN, USA), may be suitable for recurrent LV lead dislodgment. Although noncapture may be transient, biventricular capture should be assessed at regular intervals with 12-lead electrocardiography (ECG) analysis to confirm the presence of LV capture, as shown in **Fig. 2**. Loss of q/Q wave in lead I is 100% predictive of loss of LV capture. Hemodynamic deterioration following a period of initial improvement may also raise a concern of loss in LV pacing.

Inability to cannulate the coronary sinus occurs in fewer than 5%. Although LV lead can be successfully placed in the lateral vein in more than 80% of cases, some patients present small and/or torturous coronary veins that preclude LV lead placement. Furthermore, fluoroscopy is not able to determine the presence of scar, and what seems to be a perfect lead location fluoroscopically may in fact be an area of high threshold due to the presence of underlying myocardial damage or scar necessitating repositioning. If the coronary venous approach fails, consideration for surgical epicardial lead placement is an alternative option.

Other causes of LV lead noncapture are shown in **Box 2**. All patients should undergo ECG, device interrogation, and chest radiograph within 24 hours of device implantation to identify acute lead dislodgment as well as other potential complications. Air trapped in the device pocket or a loose-set screw results in acute loss of LV capture, usually occurring immediately after the procedure.

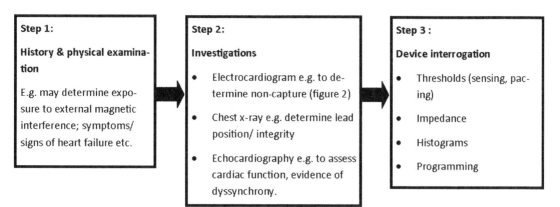

Step 1:	Step 2:	Step 3 :
History & physical examination	**Investigations**	**Device interrogation**
E.g. may determine exposure to external magnetic interference; symptoms/ signs of heart failure etc.	• Electrocardiogram e.g. to determine non-capture (figure 2) • Chest x-ray e.g. determine lead position/ integrity • Echocardiography e.g. to assess cardiac function, evidence of dyssynchrony.	• Thresholds (sensing, pacing) • Impedance • Histograms • Programming

Fig. 1. Algorithmic approach to the malfunctioning implantable cardiac device, including CRT-D.

Lead fracture often develops in the chronic course of device therapy, as shown in **Fig. 4**. Severe acidosis, hyperkalemia, and drug toxicity can cause acute loss of myocardial capture with pacing. Loss of LV capture is transient and will resolve when the metabolic disturbance is corrected. Although micro-dislodgment, as indicated by increased thresholds or noncapture without

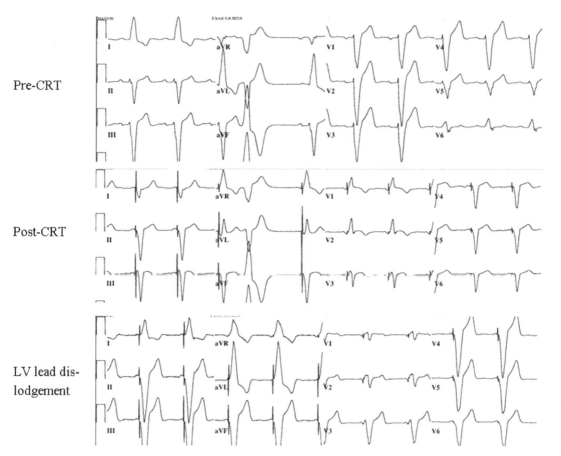

Pre-CRT

Post-CRT

LV lead dislodgement

Fig. 2. Noncapture. (*Top panel*) Before CRT, the patient had sinus rhythm, LBBB, and QRS duration of 214 ms. The LV lead was placed in the lateral vein at the basal LV lateral wall tributary. (*Middle panel*) After CRT, biventricular pacing resulted in a paced right bundle branch block morphology and QS wave in lead I, suggesting the presence of LV pacing. (*Bottom panel*) Three months later, repeat ECG indicates a paced LBBB morphology and loss of QS, evidence consistent with failure of LV capture.

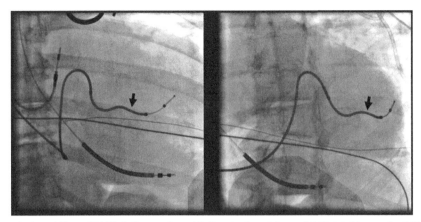

Fig. 3. Right anterior oblique (RAO) (*left panel*) and left anterior oblique (LAO) (*right panel*) of LV lead placed (Guidant bipolar left ventricular lead 4549, Natick, MA) in the lateral vein (*arrows*). Also seen are the right atrial lead and RV ICD lead.

evidence of gross lead position change, can occasionally be managed by device reprogramming (for example, to adjust the pacing output, pacing configuration, or both), macrodislodgment necessitates lead revision. During lead revision, alternative vein branches may be used. If, however, the same branch is desired, a different lead may be used.

Elevated Pacing Threshold

High pacing thresholds may be avoided by careful selection of the pacing site. If a suitable location is difficult to find, the use of a device and leads with

---

Box 2
Causes of noncapture according to time course

Early noncapture (less than 1 week)

- Lead dislodgment
- Air in pocket
- Loose setscrew

Subacute noncapture (1–6 weeks)

- Exit block

Late noncapture (after 6 weeks)

- Lead fracture/insulation failure (see **Fig. 4**)
- Battery depletion

Noncapture at any time

- Metabolic/drug effect
- Circuit failure
- Pseudomalfunction (apparent pacing system malfunction is suggested clinically, although is actually normal pacemaker programing function aimed to maximize intrinsic conduction)

---

multiple programmable pacing configurations may mitigate the need for lead repositioning at a later date. If this approach is ineffective, lead revision or epicardial lead placement should be considered. LV leads implanted via coronary sinus tributaries may have less stable tip contact than right ventricular endocardial leads, which results in greater threshold fluctuations.[9] Unfortunately, even with a modest elevation in the threshold, battery longevity is compromised. During implantation, high pacing threshold (the incidence of which may be as high as 20%[10]) in what otherwise appears to be a suitable vein for LV lead positioning relates to the presence underlying scar on the epicardial surface beneath the target vein. However, as most myocardial infarcts result in scar/fibrosis in sites other than the LV free wall, this does not pose a problem.[11] Another cause of high threshold is the presence of epicardial fat, the volume of which may be sufficient to prevent electrical capture without increasing the threshold. If exit block were to occur, for example, in the LV lead, the relative contribution to depolarization of the LV would diminish and would resemble right-ventricular–only pacing. Options include (1) increasing the pacing output (not ideal because battery life will be reduced), and (2) offsetting LV pacing (ie, pacing the LV before the RV), allowing for increased capture latency of the LV, before RV pacing.

Diaphragmatic Stimulation

Extracardiac stimulation, including diaphragmatic stimulation, occurs in less than 6% of patients.[12] Because it is poorly tolerated, roughly one-third will require lead revision after failure of reprogramming. Diaphragmatic stimulation usually occurs due to the LV pacing site being in close proximity

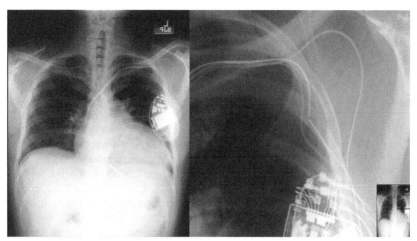

Fig. 4. PA chest radiograph (*left*) with close-up image (*right*) showing LV lead fracture that subsequently required lead replacement.

to the phrenic nerve, for example, in a posterolateral or posterior vein (**Fig. 5**). Most often, diaphragmatic stimulation can be identified by high-voltage output pacing intraprocedurally (typically 10 V). Placing the lead into a different venous branch tributary, or programing bipolar pacing in a different configuration, can be a good solution. **Fig. 6** shows a Quartet Quadpolar LV lead (St. Jude Medical, Little Canada, MN, USA) placed in the lateral coronary vein in a 73-year-old woman with idiopathic dilated cardiomyopathy. Diaphragmatic stimulation was apparent when pacing pole 2 or 3 at 2 V/0.5 ms or greater (*black arrows*), but absent when pacing pole 1 or 4 at 10 V/0.5 ms (*red arrows*). Multiple bipolar configurations (4 of 10 programmable configurations allow LV pacing

in this case) provide more options to avoid phrenic nerve stimulation. Although intraprocedural assessment of phrenic nerve stimulation via high-voltage output is a routine test, diaphragmatic stimulation may only manifest itself in the postprocedural period due to a change in patient position illustrating an alteration in the relative position of the lead to the phrenic nerve. Similarly, it could be an indicator of lead dislodgment/migration. Sometimes, intercostal stimulation may occur with (most often when lying on left side) or without changing the body position. Several management

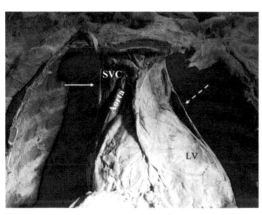

Fig. 5. Gross anatomic specimen showing the course of the right (*solid arrow*) and left (*broken arrow*) phenic nerves. The LV pacing lead through the coronary sinus is usually in close proximity to the left phrenic nerve and thus may cause diaphragmatic stimulation. SVC, superior vena cava.

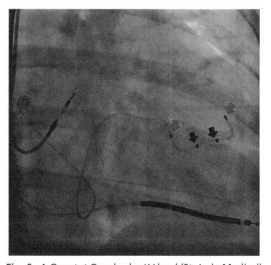

Fig. 6. A Quartet Quadpolar LV lead (St. Jude Medical) placed in the lateral coronary vein (RAO view). (*Black arrows*) LV lead pole 2 and pole 3, which are in the vicinity of the phrenic nerve with apparent diaphragmatic stimulation. (*Red arrows*) Lead pole 1 and pole 4, where diaphragmatic stimulation is not present. These leads can be programed for biventricular pacing.

strategies may overcome this problem noninvasively, as shown in **Table 1**. However, on occasion, lead repositioning is required when a safe difference in capture threshold between the LV and phrenic nerve is not possible.

Anodal Capture

CRT devices allow the option of programing LV lead pacing with the configuration of LV tip electrode (cathode) to right ventricular lead coil or ring (anode) as an alternative to improve pacing thresholds. Anodal stimulation is defined as a capture at the pacing anode instead of the cathode. If anodal stimulation occurs when a CRT device is programed to the LV tip to RV coil or ring, the RV is unintentionally captured instead of the LV.

Fig. 7 illustrates the LV lead position and ECG tracings of a 68-year-old man with ischemic cardiomyopathy in whom a Medtronic 7991 ID pulse generator (Medtronic Inc) was placed. He had a Medtronic 6947 Sprint Quattro Secure RV defibrillator lead positioned in the RV apex. The LV lead (Boston Scientific Easy Track 2; Boston Scientific) was positioned in the basal lateral location. The minimum threshold of the LV lead after testing various pacing configurations was 2.4 V at 0.50 ms with LV tip to RV coil pacing. Pacing from this location would be expected to have a negative QRS complex in lead I and positive R wave in V1. In this patient, the anode (RV coil) was captured during LV pacing, resulting in positive QRS in lead I. The narrow QRS could have been due to capture of the RV septum, or from capture at both the cathode (LV tip) and the anode (RV coil), as seen in fused anodal stimulation and shown in **Fig. 8**.

Anodal capture is more frequent in true bipolar pacing (ring-tip electrode) in which a high current density due to the small surface area is found, compared with an integrated bipolar system where a defibrillation coil is used as the RV anode (large surface area, low current density) (see **Fig. 8**). Commonly underrecognized,[13] loss of resynchronization may occur if the RV anodal capture is incorrectly recognized as LV cathodal capture, and the pacing output is programed at a value that is subthreshold for the LV. Capture should be checked using alternate vectors, and cathodal capture should be confirmed. Without LV pacing, anodal stimulation at the RV only will not achieve optimal CRT outcome. As such, it could be a potential cause of nonresponse to CRT.

Percentage Biventricular Pacing

To maximize the benefit from CRT, the frequency of biventricular pacing needs to be optimized. Studies have shown that the minimum goal is to deliver CRT, that is, synchronize the ventricles, greater than 92% of the time.[14,15] Some studies expand on this by showing that pacing greater than 98% of the time is associated with an even better outcome.[16] Essentially, any factor that reduces ventricular pacing will hamper resynchronization and therefore limit the degree of benefit obtained from CRT. Programing choices following CRT implantation include the choice of pacing mode, upper and lower rate limits, and atrioventricular (AV) delay.

Pacing mode should be set at VVIR (ventricular pacing and sensing, inhibition in response to sensing, and rate modulation) in patients with chronic atrial fibrillation, and DDDR (dual chamber pacing and sensing, dual [inhibition and triggering] response to sensing, and rate modulation) in those with paroxysmal atrial fibrillation. The upper rate limit should be programed relative to the patient's age and activity level. Otherwise, if the atrial rate exceeds the programed upper tracking rate, a pacemaker Wenckebach response (if P-P interval remains longer than the total atrial refractory period [TARP]) or fixed ratio block (if P-P interval is shorter than the TARP) may be encountered.[17]

Although many factors can affect synchrony, intrinsic AV conduction that may occur if the programed AV delay is too long, or if the patient conducts a rapid atrial or supraventricular arrhythmia, accounts for the majority. Atrial fibrillation is the most common atrial arrhythmia, the frequency of which increases in patients with progressively severe HF. It can reduce the frequency of biventricular pacing and, therefore, CRT response. Available studies suggest that rate control with AV node

Table 1	
Phrenic nerve stimulation	
Cause	**Troubleshooting**
Excess pacing output	Decrease pacing output (may capture LV but not phrenic nerve)[a] Alter the pacing vector
Device maintenance function	Disable lead integrity testing
Lead migration/ dislodgment	If above measures fail, lead repositioning

[a] In patients with LV thresholds <2 V in whom phrenic nerve stimulation is an issue, a safety margin of 1 V is adequate to ensure LV capture. However, in those with higher thresholds, a greater safety margin is required due to larger fluctuation in threshold over time.[25]

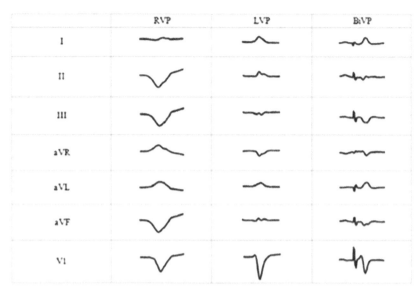

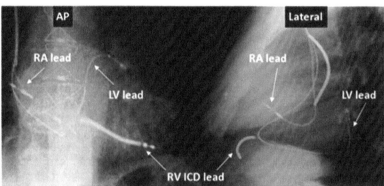

Fig. 7. Anodal stimulation in a 68-year-old man with ischemic cardiomyopathy (left ventricular ejection fraction 23%), QRS duration 138 ms, and New York Heart Association class III functional status on maximal medical therapy status post CRT-D implantation. The LV lead (Boston Scientific Easy Track 2) was positioned in the basal lateral location. The minimum LV lead threshold after testing various pacing configurations was 2.4 V at 0.50 ms and was in the LV tip to RV (right ventricle) coil pacing configuration. The final LV pacing output was programed LV tip to RV coil at 5.0 V, 0.50 ms. See text for further details. AP, anteroposterior; BiVP, biventricular pacing; LVP, left ventricular pacing; RA, right atrium; RVP, right ventricular pacing. (Adapted from Dendy KF, Powell BD, Cha YM, et al. Anodal stimulation: an underrecognized cause of nonresponders to cardiac resynchronization therapy. Indian Pacing Electrophysiol J 2011;11:64–72.)

ablation, which would ensure 100% pacing requirement, is superior to medical management,[18,19] whereby a greater survival benefit and HF improvement is attained than compared with medical therapy. The role of pulmonary vein isolation in such patients has yet to be fully determined, however.[20] Although mode switching may be effective in preventing rapid ventricular rates during paroxysmal atrial fibrillation in those with AV block, newer algorithms have been developed to allow continual biventricular pacing during atrial arrhythmias when the QRS is sensed. However, the sensed LV is delayed (therefore, so too is resynchronization) and may reduce the true biventricular pacing efficiency. Frequent ventricular premature contractions (PVC)

are a second common cause of dampening adequate CRT. The frequency of PVCs can be greater than 10,000 per day, or greater than 10% of total heart beats. PVC suppression by antiarrhythmic drugs or ablation is recommended to maximize biventricular pacing.[21]

SENSING PROBLEMS

As with implantable cardioverter defibrillators (ICDs), sensing problems in CRT-D may result in either inappropriate therapy or failure to deliver appropriate therapy. Supraventricular tachycardia-ventricular tachycardia (SVT-VT) discrimination in part relies on comparison of atrial and

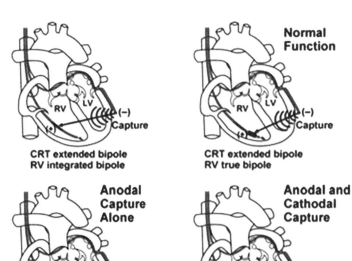

CRT extended bipole
RV integrated bipole

Normal
Function

CRT extended bipole
RV true bipole

Anodal
Capture
Alone

CRT extended bipole
RV true bipole

Anodal and
Cathodal
Capture

CRT extended bipole
RV true bipole

Fig. 8. The upper 2 figures demonstrate normal cathodal capture in the setting of integrated and dedicated bipolar RV leads. The lower left figure is an illustration of attempted pacing from the LV electrode resulting instead in anodal stimulation of the RV ring electrode. The lower right figure illustrates fusion, resulting from capture of both the cathode (LV electrode) and the anode (RV ring electrode). (*From* Swerdlow CD, Friedman PA. Advanced ICD troubleshooting: Part II. Pace 2006;29(1): 86; with permission.)

ventricular rates. However, if atrial electrogram sensing is inaccurate (for example, as seen with lead dislodgment, R-wave oversensing, or atrial event undersensing [as may occur in postventricular atrial blanking]), then the true underlying rhythm may be misclassified. Current devices primarily use the right ventricular lead bipole to detect the heart rate (R-R interval).

Double-Counting

Patients with CRT are particularly prone to double-count as they already have interventricular (and intraventricular) delay (hence why they are candidates for CRT). This conduction delay may cause the same impulse to be counted twice by RV lead sensing, for example, from the RV to the LV. Furthermore, these patients are more likely to have PVCs and supraventricular tachyarrhythmia, which may inhibit pacing for brief periods.[21] R-wave double-counting in SVT may lead to inappropriate detection of ventricular tachycardia/ventricular fibrillation (VT/VF) and therapy. Pacing 100% of the time (see above), if possible, can mitigate such issues. Synchronization of LV and RV, coupled with optimal refractory periods, should help prevent double-counting.

Oversensing

Oversensing can originate from intracardiac signals (eg, P waves), or extracardiac signals (eg, pectoral muscle potentials). This oversensing

may result in several problems including inappropriate delivery of VT/VF therapy, inhibition of pacing, or inappropriate mode switch in which there is loss of AV synchronous pacing, therefore impairing AV synchrony. Loss of P-synchronous pacing may also occur with lead dislodgment and may be particularly troublesome in an extended bipolar setting; for example, the LV lead dislodges proximally into the coronary sinus and leads to left atrial P-wave over-sensing. If atrial oversensing occurs, options include increasing the postventricular atrial blanking period, or reducing sensitivity. If this does not resolve the issue, lead repositioning should be considered. If ventricular oversensing occurs, options include reducing ventricular sensitivity and adjusting refractory periods. If this fails to resolve the issue, lead repositioning should be considered.

Undersensing

If atrial undersensing occurs, loss of ventricular tracking will result. In the setting of an intact AV conduction system, intrinsic ventricular activation may ensue, thereby inhibiting ventricular pacing. It is important to ensure that atrial sensitivity is optimized; lead repositioning may be required, as appropriate. Ventricular undersensing can result in an inappropriate pacing interval following an intrinsic QRS. If pacing decreases on the T wave, at the vulnerable time of ventricular repolarization, ventricular fibrillation may occur, as shown in **Fig. 9.**

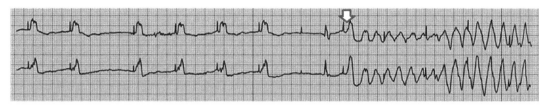

Fig. 9. Ventricular undersensing is seen. A pacing spike is delivered earlier than the programed R-R interval. It decreases on the T wave (*red arrow*), resulting in ventricular fibrillation. Note this tracing also shows ventricular pacing noncapture (the pacing spike preceding the intrinsic QRS). RV, right ventricle.

GENERATOR

In order for the device to function properly, a full and secure connection between the leads and generator is mandated, usually with the use of setscrews. Failure to do so may result in an "open-circuit" (if there is no contact), leading to absence of electrical continuity and, therefore, function. Intermittent contact may inhibit pulse generator output through the detection of potentials mistaken as intrinsic electrical activity. Loose setscrews can result in noise detection and subsequent inappropriate ICD therapy.

Although there may be differences in battery longevity by manufacturer,[22] premature display of end-of-life/elective replacement indicators (ERI) characteristics warrants further investigation. Generator malfunction, excess pacing output, frequent mode switching or shock therapy, and lead problems can all lead to premature battery depletion. Although end of life denotes pacemaker malfunction or loss of function, ERI highlights the need for consideration of generator replacement within a short period of time (usually 3 months), which may vary depending on the amount of antibradycardia pacing and antitachycardia therapies required. Certainly, the requirement for near 100% biventricular pacing places considerable drain on battery life. Although some changes once ERI is reached are universal across manufacturers (eg, pacing rate in response to magnet placement, rate response features, storage features), others (eg, pacing mode) are manufacturer-specific and are beyond the scope of this article; the reader is directed to consult with the respective manufacturer for further details.

ELECTROMAGNETIC INTERFERENCE AND RADIATION EFFECT

Electromagnetic inference (EMI) and radiation therapy may have adverse effects on CIED function. Several sources of EMI may be encountered in clinical practice, especially within the hospital setting. EMI can cause inappropriate ICD detection and therapy delivery. Magnetic resonance imaging, extracorporeal shock wave lithotripsy, radiofrequency ablation (including electrocautery), and radiation therapy all have the potential to modify device function. The susceptibility of CIEDs to radiation therapy may occur either from direction irradiation or due to scatter radiation. Certainly, this can cause electrical components to fail.[23] Radiation therapy, via ionizing radiation, may result in sensing interference, and therefore, inappropriate antitachycardia therapy.[24] If a sufficient ionizing dose is delivered, the CIED may fail altogether. Indeed, the device should be interrogated following each radiation therapy session; however, one should be aware of the possibility of late device malfunction following radiation exposure.

SUMMARY

The development of novel CRT-D algorithms has improved the ways in which common problems encountered in HF patients can be addressed and effectively managed. However, this comes at the expense of increasingly complex device function and troubleshooting. As such, physicians require not only a thorough understanding of CRT-D devices but also a systematic approach in addressing any malfunction.

REFERENCES

1. Bristow MR, Saxon LA, Boehmer J, et al. Cardiac-resynchronization therapy with or without an implantable defibrillator in advanced chronic heart failure. N Engl J Med 2004;350:2140–50.
2. Cleland JG, Daubert JC, Erdmann E, et al. The effect of cardiac resynchronization on morbidity and mortality in heart failure. N Engl J Med 2005;352: 1539–49.
3. Epstein AE, DiMarco JP, Ellenbogen KA, et al. 2012 ACCF/AHA/HRS focused update incorporated into the ACCF/AHA/HRS 2008 guidelines for device-based therapy of cardiac rhythm abnormalities: a report of the American College of Cardiology Foundation/American Heart Association Task Force on

Practice Guidelines and the Heart Rhythm Society. Circulation 2013;127:e283–352.

4. Linde C, Abraham WT, Gold MR, et al. Randomized trial of cardiac resynchronization in mildly symptomatic heart failure patients and in asymptomatic patients with left ventricular dysfunction and previous heart failure symptoms. J Am Coll Cardiol 2008;52: 1834–43.

5. Moss AJ, Hall WJ, Cannom DS, et al. Cardiac-resynchronization therapy for the prevention of heart-failure events. N Engl J Med 2009;361: 1329–38.

6. Abraham WT, Fisher WG, Smith AL, et al. Cardiac resynchronization in chronic heart failure. N Engl J Med 2002;346:1845–53.

7. Tang AS, Wells GA, Talajic M, et al. Cardiac-resynchronization therapy for mild-to-moderate heart failure. N Engl J Med 2010;363:2385–95.

8. van Rees JB, de Bie MK, Thijssen J, et al. Implantation-related complications of implantable cardioverter-defibrillators and cardiac resynchronization therapy devices: a systematic review of randomized clinical trials. J Am Coll Cardiol 2011;58:995–1000.

9. Alonso C, Leclercq C, d'Allonnes FR, et al. Six year experience of transvenous left ventricular lead implantation for permanent biventricular pacing in patients with advanced heart failure: technical aspects. Heart 2001;86:405–10.

10. Gurevitz O, Nof E, Carasso S, et al. Programmable multiple pacing configurations help to overcome high left ventricular pacing thresholds and avoid phrenic nerve stimulation. Pacing Clin Electrophysiol 2005;28:1255–9.

11. Xu YZ, Cha YM, Feng D, et al. Impact of myocardial scarring on outcomes of cardiac resynchronization therapy: extent or location? J Nucl Med 2012;53: 47–54.

12. Killu AM, Wu JH, Friedman PA, et al. Outcomes of cardiac resynchronization therapy in the elderly. Pacing Clin Electrophysiol 2013;36:664–72.

13. Dendy KF, Powell BD, Cha YM, et al. Anodal stimulation: an underrecognized cause of nonresponders to cardiac resynchronization therapy. Indian Pacing Electrophysiol J 2011;11:64–72.

14. Gasparini M, Auricchio A, Regoli F, et al. Four-year efficacy of cardiac resynchronization therapy on exercise tolerance and disease progression: the importance of performing atrioventricular junction ablation in patients with atrial fibrillation. J Am Coll Cardiol 2006;48:734–43.

15. Koplan BA, Kaplan AJ, Weiner S, et al. Heart failure decompensation and all-cause mortality in relation to percent biventricular pacing in patients with heart failure: is a goal of 100% biventricular pacing necessary? J Am Coll Cardiol 2009;53:355–60.

16. Hayes DL, Boehmer JP, Day JD, et al. Cardiac resynchronization therapy and the relationship of percent biventricular pacing to symptoms and survival. Heart Rhythm 2011;8:1469–75.

17. Leclercq C. Problems and troubleshooting in regular follow-up of patients with cardiac resynchronization therapy. Europace 2009;11(Suppl 5):v66–71.

18. Dong K, Shen WK, Powell BD, et al. Atrioventricular nodal ablation predicts survival benefit in patients with atrial fibrillation receiving cardiac resynchronization therapy. Heart Rhythm 2010;7:1240–5.

19. Gasparini M, Auricchio A, Metra M, et al. Long-term survival in patients undergoing cardiac resynchronization therapy: the importance of performing atrioventricular junction ablation in patients with permanent atrial fibrillation. Eur Heart J 2008;29:1644–52.

20. Khan MN, Jais P, Cummings J, et al. Pulmonary-vein isolation for atrial fibrillation in patients with heart failure. N Engl J Med 2008;359:1778–85.

21. Lakkireddy D, Di Biase L, Ryschon K, et al. Radiofrequency ablation of premature ventricular ectopy improves the efficacy of cardiac resynchronization therapy in nonresponders. J Am Coll Cardiol 2012; 60:1531–9.

22. Alam MB, Munir MB, Rattan R, et al. Battery longevity in cardiac resynchronization therapy implantable cardioverter defibrillators. Europace 2014;16(2):246–51.

23. Kapa S, Fong L, Blackwell CR, et al. Effects of scatter radiation on ICD and CRT function. Pacing Clin Electrophysiol 2008;31:727–32.

24. Hurkmans CW, Scheepers E, Springorum BG, et al. Influence of radiotherapy on the latest generation of implantable cardioverter-defibrillators. Int J Radiat Oncol Biol Phys 2005;63:282–9.

25. Burri H, Gerritse B, Davenport L, et al. Fluctuation of left ventricular thresholds and required safety margin for left ventricular pacing with cardiac resynchronization therapy. Europace 2009;11:931–6.

Specialized Functions of Cardiac Implantable Devices and How They Can Mimic Malfunction

Taylor Lebeis, MD, Michael S. Lloyd, MD, FHRS*

KEYWORDS

- Pacemaker • Implantable cardioverter defibrillator • Algorithms • Malfunction

KEY POINTS

- Understanding common algorithms and features of cardiac implantable electronic devices is necessary to recognize their appearance on telemetry.
- Although many specialized functions are helpful, many have not been shown to benefit patients in randomized trials.
- Automated and programmable features have dramatically increased in number and complexity.

90% of pacemaker malfunction is a lack of understanding on the physician's behalf. The Third Law of Electrophysiology according to Jonathan J. Langberg, MD.

INTRODUCTION

With each new generation of cardiac implantable electronic devices (CIED) comes an increasing number of special features designed for safety, diagnostic, and therapeutic purposes. A specialized function of a CIED can be defined as an automated or programmable function beyond fundamental pacemaker behavior as would otherwise be explained by the North American Pacing and Electrophysiology/British Pacing and Electrophysiology Group coding system and rate response.[1] These numerous features can pose challenges when assessing normal device function. Many modern CIED features automatically reprogram device settings, which can be mistaken for abnormal CIED function. Familiarity with these algorithms is critical for the care of any patient with a CIED.[2] However, the abundance of these functions, as seen in **Box 1**, makes it difficult to understand each nuance of every feature. Instead of an exhaustive review of each algorithm, this article categorizes some popular functions that commonly cause confusion in the clinical setting because of automatic transient or permanent changes to normal programmed parameters (**Table 1**).

ALGORITHMS THAT DECREASE RIGHT VENTRICULAR PACING

Because of data suggesting that right ventricular (RV) pacing increases mortality,[3] attempts by manufacturers to allow for intrinsic atrioventricular (AV) nodal conduction have resulted in several automated features. Some of these features allow for transient AV block, which has caused safety concerns because of long-short cardiac

M.S. Lloyd discloses minor consulting fees from St. Jude Medical, minor consulting and research support from Medtronic, and minor consulting fees from Boston Scientific. T. Lebeis has nothing to disclose.
Division of Clinical Cardiac Electrophysiology, Emory University Hospital, 1364 Clifton Road, Northeast, Atlanta, GA 30322, USA
* Corresponding author. 1364 Clifton Road, Northeast, Suite F424, Atlanta, GA 30322.
E-mail address: mlloyd2@emory.edu

cardiacEP.theclinics.com

Box 1
A selected, noncomprehensive sample of currently available special CIED features from 3 major device manufacturers

+PVARP on PVC	Conducted Atrial Fibrillation Response	Rate Response (RR)
10 beats >PMT	Impedance Monitoring	Rate Responsive AV delay
A Blanking after V Pace	Dynamic AV Delay	Rate Responsive PVARP
A-Tachycardia Response	Dynamic PVARP	Rate smoothing
Auto Capture	Hysteresis rate	Rest rate
AdaptivCRT	Hysteresis with Search	Runaway Protection
Adaptive-Rate Sensors	I-Opt	RV Lead Integrity Alert
Advanced Hysteresis	LV Capture Management	RV Lead Noise Discrimination
ATR Fallback Mode	Managed Ventricular Pacing	RV/LV Capture Confirmation
ATR Mode Switch	Mode Switch	SafeR
Atrial Dynamic Overdrive	MRI SureScan	Safety Switch
AF Suppression	Negative AV Hysteresis with Search	Search AV+
Atrial Flutter Response	Noncompetitive Atrial Pacing	Sensing Assurance
Atrial Pace on PMT	PMT Intervention	Rate Hysteresis
Atrial Pace on PVC	Post Mode Switch Overdrive Pacing	Sinus Preference
Atrial Preference Pacing	PVARP after PVC/PAC	Sleep Function
Atrial Protection Interval	PVC Response	Sudden Bradycardia Response
Atrial Rate Stabilization	QuickOpt	V Blanking after A Pace
Atrial Tachy Response	Rate Adaptive AV	Ventricular Capture Management
Atrial Tracking Recovery	Rate Branch SVT Discriminator	Ventricular Intrinsic Pacing
Mode Switch	Automatic Mode Switching	Ventricular Rate Regulation
Auto Ventricular Blanking	AutoIntrinsic Conduction Search	Ventricular Safety Pacing
AV Search Hysteresis		Ventricular Sense Response

Some terms listed above are registered trademarks of Boston Scientific Corporation, Medtronic Corporation, and St. Jude Medical.

Abbreviations: AV, atrioventricular; LV, left ventricular; PMT, pacemaker-mediated tachycardia; PVARP, postventricular atrial refractory period; PVC, premature ventricular contraction; RV, right ventricular; SVT, supraventricular tachycardia.

---

sequences.[4] However, in those with intact AV nodal conduction, these features are frequently enabled. They are a common cause of confusion on telemetry wards, because they may manifest as repeated cycles of varying AV delays or apparent inappropriate inhibition of ventricular output and transient AV block.

Novel Pacing Modes to Reduce RV Pacing

Managed Ventricular Pacing (MVP) mode (Medtronic, Minneapolis, MN) is 1 popular algorithm to reduce RV pacing by maximizing the amount of time spent in an AAI/R pacing mode and switching to DDD/R during periods of AV block. This mode is commonly referred to as AAI(R)/DDD(R) and has been shown to decrease RV pacing.[5] This mode monitors for ventricular sensed events after each atrial event. If no ventricular sensed beat occurs, the pacemaker delivers a ventricular paced beat after the next atrial event with a very short AV delay (80 milliseconds). This short AV delay paced sequence is followed by another check for intrinsic conduction. If 2 of 4 consecutive cardiac cycles do not have a sensed ventricular pacing event, DDD(R) mode continues for 1 minute, with a short AV delay, with subsequent conduction checks at

progressively lengthening intervals thereafter (**Fig. 1**).

The Reverse Mode Switch and Rhythmiq algorithms (Boston Scientific, Natick MA) operate in the AAI(R) mode with backup VVI pacing at 15 beats per minute (BPM) lower than desired base pacing rate. The algorithm switches from AAI(R) to DDD(R) if loss of AV conduction is detected. Loss of AV conduction is defined by 3 slow ventricular beats (any backup ventricular pacing beat or any ventricular sensed beat slower than the base rate + 150 milliseconds) occurring in a window of 11 ventricular beats. If 25 or more ventricular sensed events are sensed via AV hysteresis, the mode returns from DDD(R) to AAI(R). There has been concern that this algorithm is frequently fooled by the presence of premature ventricular contractions (PVCs), which trigger slow ventricular beat counts and cause unnecessary DDD(R) pacing.[6] Like the MVP mode, this specialized mode has had reports of ventricular proarrhythmia.[7]

AV Conduction Hysteresis and Variants

Each manufacturer has 1 or more branded versions of AV conduction hysteresis to promote intrinsic conduction whenever possible (**Table 2**).

Table 1
Categories of specialized CIED functions and some of their telemetry manifestations

Functions	Feature Types	Clinical Manifestations
Features designed to minimize RV apical pacing	AAIR/DDDR mode (Managed Ventricular Pacing) Reverse Mode Switch (RMS, Rhythmiq) AV hysteresis Rate hysteresis	Transient AV block allowed. Sudden changes to pacing mode with short AV delays Transient decreases in the programmed base rate to allow for intrinsic conduction Ventricular pacing at slower than expected rates
Features intended to maximize biventricular pacing	Attempted resynchronization of intrinsic ventricular events Negative AV hysteresis Atrial tracking recovery	Pacing stimulus within the QRS of an intrinsic ventricular event, usually a PVC (apparent ventricular undersensing) Shorter than programmed AV delay Shortening of AV delay after nonsustained VT or SVT Sudden BiV pacing after a salvo of intrinsic ventricular rhythm
Automated AV and VV optimization functions	Rate adaptive AV delay EGM-based AV, VV optimization LV fused vs BiV pacing	Shortening of AV interval with increased heart rates Varying AV intervals and VV intervals Alternating LV only and BiV pacing patterns with varying AV and VV intervals
Automated sensing and capture assurance	Sensing and impedance assurance Capture assurance	Alternating atrial and ventricular sensitivities. Unexplained scheduled pacing output, occasionally at moderately high stimulus strengths Unexpected pacing and loss of capture, usually in the nighttime hours
Automated features for atrial fibrillation	See **Table 3**	See **Table 3**
Features that decrease or increase pacing rate not explained by rate response	Rest or sleep rates Rate drop response	Lower-than-expected base pacing rate at night Sudden increase in pacing rate after a decrease in heart rate
Algorithms to avoid noise or cross talk	Safety pacing Noise reversion modes ICD lead noise algorithms	AV pacing stimuli at short AV intervals, usually in response to a PVC that occurred simultaneous to an atrial paced event Change in pacing mode or pacing rate. Apparent loss of sensing Automatic prolongation of detection intervals for VF. Delay or inhibition of ICD therapy
Features for the prevention of endless loop tachycardias	PVARP extension Atrial pacing on PMT	Lack of otherwise expected atrial tracking after PVCs Atrial pacing at shorter than expected coupling intervals
Automated device alarms		Scheduled audible or vibratory cue detected by patient

Abbreviations: AV, atrioventricular; BiV, biventricular; ICD, implantable cardioverter defibrillator; LV, left ventricular; PMT, pacemaker-mediated tachycardia; PVARP, postventricular atrial refractory period; RV, right ventricular; SVT, supraventricular tachycardia; VF, ventricular fibrillation; VT, ventricular tachycardia.

In general, this function gradually extends the AV delay to a programmable maximum limit to determine if ventricular sensed events follow atrial events, indicating that intrinsic conduction is intact. If there is ventricular sensing, the AV interval remains prolonged to promote intrinsic conduction. AV search hysteresis has been shown to reduce the amount of RV pacing.[8] This feature manifests in the monitored patient as prolongation of the paced AV delay (**Fig. 2**).

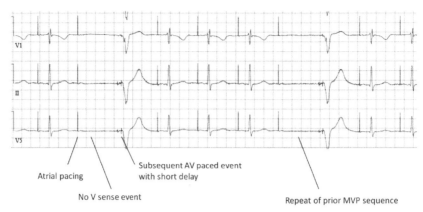

Atrial pacing

No V sense event

Subsequent AV paced event
with short delay

Repeat of prior MVP sequence

Fig. 1. An electrocardiographic example of the MVP algorithm. An atrial event is followed by the absence of a ventricular sensed event. The subsequent atrial event is followed by a ventricular paced event with a characteristically short AV delay of 80 ms. Had either of the 2 subsequent atrial paced events been nonconducted, the device would have reverted to DDD mode for 1 minute. After 1 minute, the pacemaker inhibits ventricular pacing for 1 cycle to monitor for intact AV conduction. The pacemaker proceeds with conduction checks at doubling time intervals thereafter (2 minutes, 4 minutes, and so on). If AV conduction is verified, the pacemaker proceeds in AAIR pacing mode.

Rate Hysteresis

Single-chamber or rate hysteresis is also designed to minimize RV pacing in the setting of single-chamber pacing, as in the case of permanent atrial fibrillation (AF). This feature transiently increases the lower rate interval (resulting in a slower base rate) if there is a sensed ventricular event. For example, if the base rate were programmed at 60 BPM (1000 milliseconds), a device with rate hysteresis would automatically prolong this interval to a programmed hysteresis value (eg, 50 BPM [1200 milliseconds]), if sensed ventricular events occurred. This feature encourages intrinsic rhythm, but can mimic pacemaker oversensing because it manifests as a lower-than-expected pacing rate.

A similar algorithm is available for the atrial pacing channel, in which the programmed base pacing rate of the atrium is decreased to allow for atrial intrinsic conduction in response to sensed

Table 2
Common AV hysteresis modes

Mode	Manufacturer	Function
AV Search+	Boston Scientific	Allows AV delay to lengthen for at most 8 consecutive paced or sensed cardiac cycle
Search AV+	Medtronic	Searches for patient's intrinsic AV conduction by a scanning window of 16 cycles. Adjusts AV delay according to programmable maximum based on amount of ventricular sensed or ventricular paced beats in previous scanning window
Autointrinsic Conduction Search (AICS)	St. Jude Medical	Increases the AV delay to sense for intrinsic conduction within a programmable extension value every 5 min. If detected, it adjusts settings to allow intrinsic conduction
Intrinsic Rhythm Support	Biotronik	Extends the set AV delay to monitor for intrinsic AV conduction more than 1–10 consecutive cycles. If present, it allows native conduction. It also automatically extends AV delay after 180 cycles of ventricular pacing for 1–10 cycles to monitor for intermittent AV conduction
Ventricular Intrinsic Preference	St. Jude Medical	Operates in a similar fashion to AICS but operates at higher heart rates and has upper limit of AV extension to 350 ms

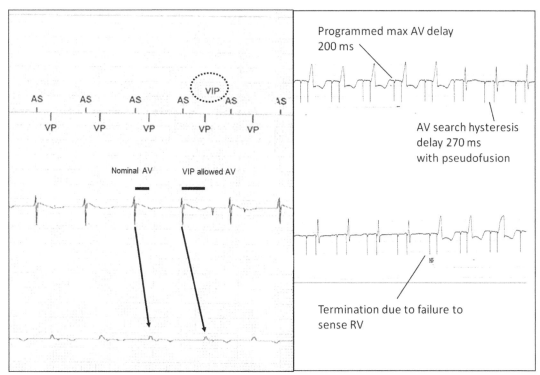

Fig. 2. Two examples of AV hysteresis. (*Left*) A St. Jude model Accent DR 2110 pacemaker was enabled with the ventricular intrinsic preference (VIP, circled). After several cycles of a programmed AV delay, the feature activates and extends the AV delay to a programmable length (*black arrows*). (*Right*) A Boston Scientific dual-chamber pacemaker with a base AV delay of 200 ms is shown. The AV delay increases to almost 270 ms, 30% longer than the programmed AV delay for 8 cycles. In this case, the algorithm failed to sense the intrinsic narrow QRS as it fell just beyond the extended AV delay, resulting in pseudofusion. Because of the lack of sensing during the 8 cycles, the AV delay then shortens to the programmed delay of 200 ms and reattempts the algorithm in 32 cycles. AS, atrial sensed; VP, ventricle sensed.

atrial events. This feature was designed in response to some data suggesting that sinus rhythm is preferable to sensor-based atrial pacing during exercise.[9]

ALGORITHMS DESIGNED TO MAXIMIZE BIVENTRICULAR PACING

Published trials of cardiac resynchronization therapy (CRT) have shown that those with less biventricular pacing have increased mortality and worsened symptoms than those who are nearly 100% biventricular paced.[10] This dose-response effect of CRT has led to algorithms devised to maximize biventricular pacing at all costs, even attempting to resynchronize premature ventricular beats and conducted AF.

Automated Pacing Responses to Ventricular Sensed Events

Most CRTs have a feature that is enabled by default that paces into or chases a sensed ventricular event in hopes of resynchronizing rapid AF or

PVCs. The sensing occurs in the RV channel and triggers a pacing spike several milliseconds after a native ventricular beat. The chasing pacer stimulus can be biventricular, left ventricular (LV) only, or programmable depending on manufacturer. Occasionally, the stimuli appear late after QRS onset and may mimic a form of ventricular undersensing or atrial oversensing of a ventricular event (**Fig. 3**).

Variations of rate smoothing functions have been developed in hopes of increasing biventricular pacing to maximize CRT even during rapid or irregularly conducted AF. A function that is frequently enabled for those with AF and CRT devices is a form of rate smoothing algorithm in response to irregularly conducted AF (Conducted AF Response, Medtronic, Minneapolis, MN). This feature, in response to 3 sensed beats while in a nontracking mode (such as those programmed during AF), increases the base pacing rate up to 3 BPM and decreases the rate progressively if pacing occurs without breakthrough of the intrinsic rhythm. This feature manifests as varying

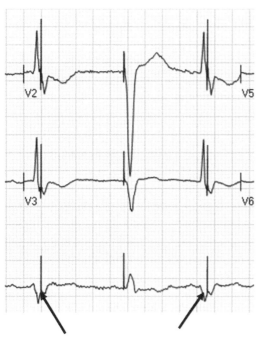

Biventricular stimuli delivered relatively late to "resynchronize" intrinsic ventricular event

Fig. 3. An example of automated resynchronization of ventricular sensed events. These features frequently appear as late stimulus artifacts within ventricular ectopy (*arrows*) and represent the attempt of the devices to resynchronize the ventricular event. They sometimes occur late within the PVC and can be mistaken for undersensing.

ventricular pacing rates at higher than expected values in the setting of underlying AF and can be thought of as the reverse of single-chamber rate hysteresis.

Automated shortening of the postventricular atrial refractory period (PVARP) can occur in response to a series of ventricular sensed events in CRT devices. If greater than 8 cycles of ventricular sensed events within the acceptable tracking rates followed by refractory atrial events are seen, Atrial Tracking Recovery (Medtronic, Minneapolis, MN) shortens the PVARP to allow for resumption of biventricular pacing.

Negative or Reverse AV Hysteresis

As its name implies, 1 algorithm intentionally shortens paced AV intervals to promote ventricular pacing (St. Jude Medical, Sylmar, CA). In response to a sensed ventricular event, the algorithm automatically shortens the A-sense V-paced interval and the A-paced, V-paced interval by a programmable preset value. When enabled, this feature manifests as shorter than expected AV intervals.

AUTOMATED AV AND VV OPTIMIZATION ALGORITHMS

Data examining the benefits of echocardiographically guided manual AV and VV optimization (in the case of biventricular systems) have been disappointing. A large meta-analysis of AV and VV optimization in a population of patients with heart failure with CRT devices failed to show benefit.[11] Nonetheless, manufacturers continue to generate devices capable of adjusting timing based on measurements that correlate with hemodynamic events.

Rate Adaptive AV Delays

To mimic the shortened AV times seen with exercise, most CIEDs with at least dual-chamber pacing capabilities have rate adaptability of programmed AV delays. This feature shortens the paced and sensed AV delays beyond the programmed baseline values according to rate. This feature is meant to mimic the physiologic decrease in AV nodal conduction time during physiologic stress. Although this feature has shown to benefit those with RV-only pacing in older literature, it is still present in both dual-chamber pacing and CRT devices.[12] The degree of AV shortening is programmable with most devices (**Fig. 4**).

Automated AV Optimization and VV Optimization

AV optimization for dual-chamber systems has declined in popularity in light of data that avoidance of RV pacing altogether has shown mortality benefits. However, in the population with CRT, automated AV and VV optimization functions are available. One push-button AV and VV optimization algorithm (QuickOpt, St. Jude Medical, Sylmar CA), uses analysis of the intracardiac electrocardiogram timing to infer data about right to left intra-atrial conduction times as well as RV to LV activation times and adjusts intervals accordingly. It can be repeated and has been shown to be equivalent to echo-guided methods at improving echo measures of LV function. Another algorithm is a modification of an earlier pacing feature that uses data of the intrinsic AV interval and the QRS duration to predict optimum AV delays. In a trial comparing a fixed AV delay of 120 milliseconds, echocardiographic guided AV and VV optimization, and an automated algorithm of AV optimization (SmartDelay, Boston Scientific, Natick, MA), showed no difference in heart failure end points among those with empirical, echocardiography-guided and algorithm-guided AV interval optimization.[13]

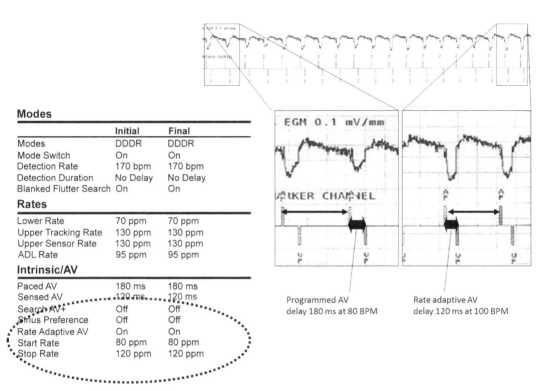

Modes

	Initial	Final
Modes	DDDR	DDDR
Mode Switch	On	On
Detection Rate	170 bpm	170 bpm
Detection Duration	No Delay	No Delay
Blanked Flutter Search	On	On

Rates

Lower Rate	70 ppm	70 ppm
Upper Tracking Rate	130 ppm	130 ppm
Upper Sensor Rate	130 ppm	130 ppm
ADL Rate	95 ppm	95 ppm

Intrinsic/AV

Paced AV	180 ms	180 ms
Sensed AV	120 ms	120 ms
Search AV+	Off	Off
Sinus Preference	Off	Off
Rate Adaptive AV	On	On
Start Rate	80 ppm	80 ppm
Stop Rate	120 ppm	120 ppm

EGN 0.1 mV/mm

MARKER CHANNEL

Programmed AV delay 180 ms at 80 BPM

Rate adaptive AV delay 120 ms at 100 BPM

Fig. 4. An example of rate adaptive AV delay on 1 continuous strip. In this case, a dual-chamber pacemaker programmed DDDR had rate adaptive AV delay programmed at rates of 80 to 120 BPM (*circle*). In the top strip, the sensor-based atrial rate gradually increases from about 80 BPM to 105 BPM and the programmed AV paced delay shortens from about 180 ms to 120 ms (*arrows* and *insets*). Rate adaptive AV delay algorithms have programmable degrees of shortening and may manifest as very short (down to 30 ms) AV intervals during intrinsic or sensor-driven high atrial rates.

Automated LV Fused Pacing and Biventricular Pacing

A newer feature available in attempts to optimize CRT pacer timing cycles is the AdaptivCRT algorithm (Medtronic, Minneapolis, MN). This feature has been developed in response to published data that suggest that it may be advantageous to fuse an LV paced beat with intrinsic rhythm rather than force biventricular (RV + LV) pacing when AV conduction is normal.[14–16] The algorithm on a minute-by-minute basis assesses the intrinsic AV interval, the atrial electrogram width, and ventricular electrogram width and adjusts any 3 of the following parameters: AV delay, VV timing, or LV only pacing. Knowledge of this common feature in modern CRT devices is crucial, because the telemetry appearance of this algorithm regularly shows shifts in pacing configuration, AV, and VV timing (**Fig. 5**).

AUTOMATED THRESHOLD AND SENSING ASSURANCE

Regular assurance of proper sensing and capture can now be automated in most CIEDs. These

features are a frequent source of confusion on telemetry wards, typically in the nighttime hours with unexplained salvos of ventricular pacing and bizarre pacing patterns. These features are particularly useful in pacemaker-dependent patients and in CIEDs using leads with a higher rate of dislodgement, such as LV leads for CRT devices.

Automatic Capture Confirmation Algorithms

Since the original algorithms using enhancements in sense amplifiers to detect evoked potentials after large pacing stimuli in the mid-1990s,[17] most manufacturers have evolved their own version of automatically, periodically, and independently measuring and adjusting atrial, RV, and LV output. In some algorithms, this feature can manifest as unexpected or unexplained pacing output.

One example of how these features could be misinterpreted is the LV Capture Management algorithm (LVCM, Medtronic, Minneapolis, MN). The algorithm measures the threshold for LV pacing every day at 1:00 AM. Details of the algorithm and an example are shown in **Fig. 6**. These

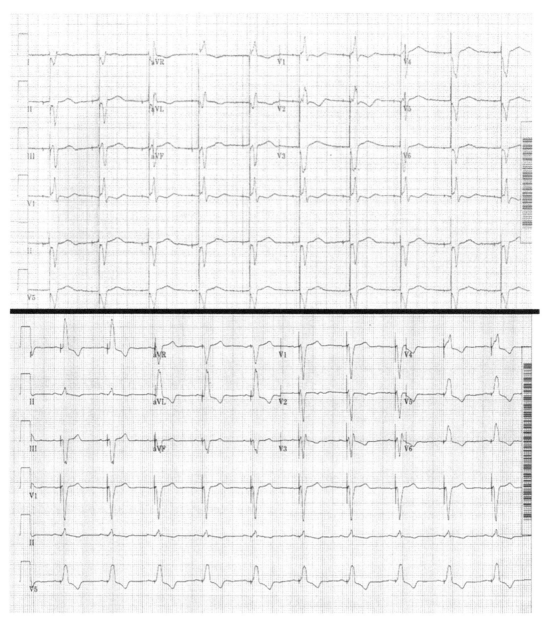

Fig. 5. An example of the electrocardiographic manifestations of the AdaptivCRT algorithm. This algorithm can change AV delays and pacing configurations on a minute-by-minute basis from biventricular pacing (*upper panel*) to LV only pacing fused with intrinsic rhythm (*lower panel*). This algorithm is relatively new and has led to confusion with intermittent loss of LV capture.

features manifest as bizarre or erratic pacing behaviors, typically in the nighttime hours.

Sensing and Impedance Algorithms

Devices regularly and automatically ensure appropriate sensing and lead impedance.[18] These functions occur continuously or at scheduled times on the pacemaker clock at a typical frequency of every 3 to 4 hours. One way these features can manifest clinically is during lead impedance monitoring in an otherwise sensed chamber. To check impedance, an electrical stimulus of moderate to high intensity (eg, 5 V at 1 millisecond, Medtronic) is delivered through the lead for several cycles. Rarely, this may cause symptoms in the patient who is sensitive to higher output pacing in chambers not regularly being paced. These scheduled

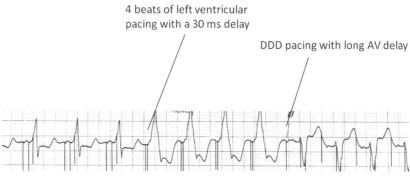

4 beats of left ventricular
pacing with a 30 ms delay

DDD pacing with long AV delay

Fig. 6. An example of LV autocapture algorithm. There are 4 stages that comprise this method: stability check, LV-RV conduction test, AV conduction test, and LV pacing threshold search. During the stability check, 12 cycles of the pacer are assessed to ensure stability. During the LV-RV and AV conduction tests, the interval from when the LV is stimulated to when the RV captures is measured for 4 consecutive cycles. This measurement allows for the capture and loss of capture windows to be defined. The current output setting is used for the test pulse. If there is no capture, then a backup pace is used with the permanent settings. The AV conduction is tested as well while the device uses overdrive pacing. The LV pacing threshold search then uses a series of test paces with different voltages to determine the LV threshold. The testing starts 1 V lower than the last determined threshold. The final setting is based on a series of 2 or 3 test paces.

checks may also lead to confusion on telemetry monitoring.

Sensing assurance algorithms can automatically adjust the sensitivity for atrial and ventricular leads to a target safety margin. For 1 manufacturer, if a series of consecutive beats is less than 4 times the programmed sensitivity of the device, the sensitivity is automatically set to a lower value (higher sensitivity). Alternatively, if a series of sensed beats are greater than 5.6 times the programmed value, the sensitivity automatically adjusts to a higher value (lower sensitivity).

FUNCTIONS FOR AF AND SPECIAL ATRIAL PACING ALGORITHMS

AF and other atrial arrhythmias are commonly encountered in those with CIEDs. Beyond specific antitachycardia pacing algorithms not discussed here, other specialized functions have been designed in attempts to both prevent AF and reduce symptoms associated with irregular ventricular contraction (**Table 3**).

Mode Switching

One of the older and most useful automated features of CIEDs is the ability to detect rapid atrial events and automatically change pacing mode. This feature prevents rapid tracking of the atrium by the ventricular pacing channel. When the atrial channel senses a series of rapid atrial events at a programmable rate (or rate average in 1 manufacturer's case), this feature automatically switches pacing mode from a tracking mode, such as DDD, to an inhibited mode (eg, DDI). To avoid

potential abrupt changes in rate from switching to a nontracking mode, many mode switch algorithms gradually decrease the pacing rate from the rapid, tracked rate down to the programmed base rate. One caution of this feature is that the default settings of the nonatrial tracking mode may be at a different rate than the tracking mode and may not have rate response enabled. Many mode switching functions are now available, with the option of programming a period of higher pacing rate after the mode switch episode terminates (eg, Post Mode Switch Overdrive Pacing, Medtronic).

Antiarrhythmic Atrial Pacing Algorithms

In addition to specific antitachycardia pacing functions, several pacing algorithms are in use for prevention and reduction of atrial arrhythmia.[19] These algorithms are based on evidence that AF episodes can be initiated by premature atrial contractions, by pauses, and by bradycardia-provoked immediate recurrences.[20–23] Clinically, these features are important to consider in a patient with an unexplained increased pacing rate at rest.

Certain AF algorithms change pacing behavior in response to atrial ectopy. One such feature increases the heart rate for several beats on detection of a premature atrial contraction (PAC).[24] Others prevent pauses after a PAC. Prevention of immediate recurrence of AF by high-rate atrial pacing after an episode of AF is also commonly used to prevent AF.[25] These algorithms are frequently the culprits of atrial pacing at relatively high rates (nominally 80 BPM, programmable up to 120 BPM) that are otherwise unexplained.

Table 3
Specialized CIED functions for atrial arrhythmias[a]

Function Name	Brief Description	Effects
Atrial Rate Smoothing	Paces atrium a certain percentage of a preceding interval followed by gradual return to the base or sensor-indicated pacing rate	May prevent atrial arrhythmias by avoiding atrial long-short sequences May reduce palpitations from irregularity
Ventricular Rate Smoothing	Ventricular pacing at a specified percentage of the preceding VV interval	Intended to reduce palpitations and manifest as higher than expected ventricular pacing
Mode Switch	Switches from an atrial tracking mode to a nonatrial tracking mode in response to detection of atrial events faster than a programmable high rate or averaged high rate	Prevents rapid ventricular pacing because of tracking of atrial arrhythmias
Post Mode Switch High Rate Pacing	After a mode switch event, the base rate is increased higher than expected values and gradually returns to base or sensor-indicated pacing rate	Increased pacing rates after resolution of atrial arrhythmias may reduce recurrence of arrhythmia and may reduce symptoms related to abrupt changes in rate
Preferential atrial pacing	Forced atrial pacing at rates higher than the intrinsic rate	Intended to suppress atrial fibrillation, but has been shown to be ineffective and increases battery drain[43]
Atrial pacing algorithms in response to PVC and PACs	Forced atrial paced events in response to an atrial refractory event after a PVC Forced pacing after atrial premature beats	Intended to reduce atrial pacing-induced proarrhythmia and results in unexpected atrial paced beats after PVCs and PACs

[a] Excluding specific antitachycardia pacing therapies.

Most trials have not shown any difference in the AF burden when features like these are enabled, including a large randomized trial by Healey and colleagues.[26–31]

Some of the most confusing algorithms alter pacing timing cycles in response to PVCs. This feature is intended to avoid pacing-induced arrhythmia from a short coupled retrograde atrial beat and a subsequent atrial paced beat. One such algorithm (noncompetitive atrial pacing) has a specified time window, at which rate-indicated pacing is inhibited after an atrial sensed event during the PVARP of the preceding ventricular event. Another algorithm, the A Pace after PVC (St. Jude Medical), is designed to avoid pacemaker-mediated tachycardia (PMT) and to avoid delivering atrial stimuli at short coupling intervals to undetected intrinsic atrial activity that occurs in the PVARP (**Fig. 7**). Although this feature is intended to be antiarrhythmic, we have described an unintended propensity for it be proarrhythmic by inducing PMT.[32]

Rate Smoothing Algorithms

Rate smoothing algorithms are designed to regularize irregular rates or abrupt changes in heart rate such as those seen in AF. When enabled, they increase the base pacing rate in response to a series of ventricular sensed events.[33,34] Alternatively, when there are consecutive ventricular paced events, the pacemaker gradually decreases the pacing rate. Ventricular rate stabilization algorithms have not been shown to significantly affect the severity of reported symptoms.[35] Aggressive programming of rate smoothing algorithms in implantable cardioverter defibrillators (ICDs) may result in undersensing of slower monomorphic ventricular tachycardias.

NOISE DETECTION AND NOISE DISCRIMINATION ALGORITHMS

Cross talk, the inadvertent sensing of the ventricular channel of an atrial pacing stimulus, is rarely an issue in CIEDs. However, features designed to avoid this potentially disastrous phenomenon still exist and can manifest as apparent ventricular undersensing. More importantly, algorithms designed to discriminate noise from true cardiac events are now a common feature in most CIEDs. This feature is most relevant to ICDs in which noise could cause inappropriate shocks.

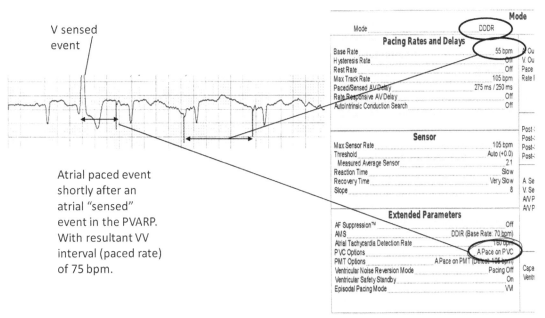

Fig. 7. Example of a pace on PVC. Undersensing of the PVC by the ventricular lead does not account for the time between the last sinus beat and the atrial paced event, which exceeds the paced rate. The PVC is appropriately sensed and, because of an A pace on PVC option, paces the atrium after detection of an atrial event in the PVARP. This feature extends the PVARP after a PVC to 475 ms, which is intended to prevent pacemaker-mediated tachy-cardia. It nonetheless allows sensing of the atrial channel during this time. If any atrial event is sensed within that period, the PVARP is terminated and the atrium is paced 330 ms after the atrial sensed event.

Cross Talk Avoidance Algorithms

Ventricular safety pacing is the intentional delivery of a ventricular pacing stimulus after a ventricular sensed event that occurs shortly after an atrial paced event. This feature has existed for several generations of pacing devices and is designed to avoid the inappropriate inhibition of ventricular output caused by ventricular sensing of the atrial stimulus (ie, cross talk). The most common clinical context in which this feature occurs is a fortuitously timed PVC that is sensed immediately after delivery of an A pacing stimulus. The hallmark of 1 common safety pacing algorithm is a very short AV delay, to distinguish it from a truly blanked event (**Fig. 8**).[36]

Noise/Magnet Detection and Reversion Modes

Noise detection algorithms are nonprogrammable features that have been present in pacing systems for many years.[37] This feature is meant to

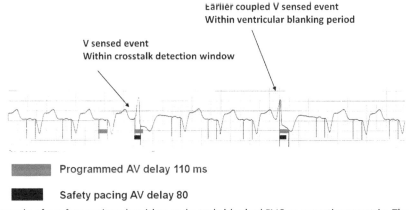

Fig. 8. An example of a safety pacing algorithm and a truly blanked PVC on a continuous strip. The most frequent manifestation of safety pacing is a PVC simultaneous with an atrial paced event. The safety paced event (*left arrow*) has a classic very short AV interval.

distinguish true cardiac depolarization events from noise. Examples of noise can originate from physiologic events, such as skeletal muscle myopotentials, or from nonphysiologic events, like conductor fractures or electromagnetic interference. Many manufacturers' noise reversion feature is triggered by multiple detections of events within a narrow time window after a previous sensed event, such as the atrial refractory period or ventricular refractory period. If this situation occurs, the feature reverts to pacing at a base rate or sensor-indicated rate mode to avoid inappropriate inhibition of pacing.

ICD Noise Detection Resulting in Automated Reprogramming

Details of ICD detection and arrhythmia discrimination represent a topic too expansive for this review and have been reviewed elsewhere,[38] but there are certain features that result in automatic reprogramming of device parameters and thus warrant mention. Noise discrimination algorithms (RV Lead Noise Discrimination, Secure Sense, St. Jude Medical) compare signals detected on the local bipole with far-field signals. Another separates sensed events into frequency bands and, if noise is detected, automatically increases the maximum sensitivity (Dynamic Noise Algorithm, Boston Scientific, Natick, MA). In some algorithms, ICD shocks or therapy can be withheld. A newer ICD noise detection feature may automatically prolong detection intervals (Lead Integrity Alert, Medtronic, Minneapolis, MN) (**Fig. 9**). This algorithm was the first to automatically change the programming of an ICD feature based on a triggered detection of a potential abnormal finding by the algorithm.

OBSERVATIONS (11)
· Alert: RV defib lead impedance warning on 03-Aug-2013.
· Alert: SVC lead impedance warning on 03-Aug-2013.
· Alert: RV Lead Integrity warning on 03-Aug-2013 (2 or more criteria met). Review VT-NS episodes, Sensing Integrity Counter (Short V-V Intervals) and RV Lead Impedance. VF Initial Beats to Detect may have extended to 30/40 (if applicable).
· 48 days with more than 6 hr AT/AF.
· Avg. Ventricular Rate >= 100 bpm for 6 hr during AT/AF.
· V. Pacing less than 90%.

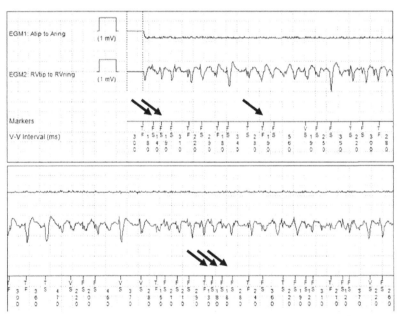

Fig. 9. Example of an unintended consequence of Lead Integrity Alert feature. This feature monitors for abnormal RV lead impedance, detection of short VV intervals numbering >30 within 3 consecutive days, and ≥2 nonsustained ventricular arrhythmia episodes with rates of <220 ms (heart rate >272 BPM). If ≥2 of any of these criteria are met, detection criteria are automatically prolonged for ventricular tachycardia (VT) and ventricular fibrillation (VF) therapies and patient alerts are given. Although this feature may avoid inappropriate shocks caused by noise, it may also delay appropriate therapy for true VT or VF and may manifest as unexpected prolongation of VF and VT detection. Here, the true VF intervals are <220 ms (*arrows*) and the RV lead impedance was 380 Ω, which was less than the alert cutoff. This feature triggered the device to extend intervals to 30 of 40 (*boxed text in interrogation printout*). Because of low intrinsic R waves, there was undersensing of VF.

Retrograde atrial event is sensed and tracked by DDD pacemaker

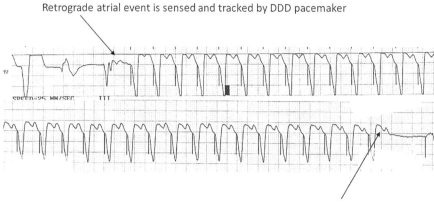

PVARP is automatically extended after PMT criteria
are met and endless loop tachycardia terminates.

Fig. 10. Example of automated pacemaker-mediated tachycardia termination algorithm. When a series of ventricular paced beats track an atrial sensed event at a programmable threshold rate, the algorithm automatically extends the PVARP to prevent tracking of the following atrial event and terminate endless loop tachycardias. Most manufacturers' algorithms trigger the PVARP extension within 8 beats to 16 beats of the tachycardia, but some algorithms require stability of the VA intervals (Boston Scientific), which can prolong PMT episodes before intervention.

SLEEP RATES AND RATE DROP RESPONSE

One common reason for pacing rates below that of the programmed lower rate limit is the so-called sleep or rest rate.[39] This feature allows a decrease in pacemaker rate to a programmable value lower than the lower rate limit during nighttime hours or prolonged rest. This function may work in conjunction with a physiologic sensor to detect periods of rest. Although this type of feature may aid in restorative sleep, patients with extremely compromised cardiac outputs and pacemaker dependence may complain of worsening symptoms at this lower rate.[40] In this clinical context, the feature can cause symptoms, which may be confused with orthopnea, because the function is on usually during the night while the patient is recumbent.

A function that results in transient increased pacing rate is rate drop response, which detects a sudden decline in the sensed atrial rate and triggers pacing at a programmable higher rate and programmable duration. This feature is intended to address the cardioinhibitory response of vasovagal episodes and can manifest as sudden increases in pacing rate not explained by patient activity.[41] This feature is incompatible with certain other features, such as mode switching from DDD, and specialized pacing modes, like AAIR/DDDR.

ALGORITHMS USED FOR THE PREVENTION OF ENDLESS LOOP TACHYCARDIAS

Most dual-chamber pacing systems automatically extend the PVARP after a PVC (**Fig. 10**). This

feature reduces the chance of the atrial lead sensing a retrograde atrial event and triggering PMT. Although this algorithm has proved fruitful in reducing PMT, other PMT avoidance algorithms may also allow for pacing at unexpected rates (A Pace on PMT, St. Jude Medical).[42]

AUDIBLE AND VIBRATORY DEVICE ALARMS

The automatic detection of an anomalous or unacceptable parameter of a lead, battery, or significant arrhythmia can now alert the patient, either by an audible or vibratory cue, to seek medical attention for most defibrillators and some pacemakers. These alarms are given usually at a programmable time and can monitor the following: lead diagnostics, battery voltage, excessive charge times, anomalous or dangerous programmed pacing parameters, electrical device reset, ventricular fibrillation therapy turned off, and arrhythmia episodes. In the clinical setting, it is useful to remind or demonstrate these alerts to patients as audible alarms can be confused for external noises and vice versa, and vibratory alarms can be confused for ICD shocks.

SUMMARY

The number of specialized features available in modern CIEDs places a significant strain on the ability of a clinician to manage patients with these devices effectively. Many special CIED features are enabled as default settings. Many of these functions, such as mode switching and capture verification, have a clear role for use in most CIEDs. However, the few randomized trials examining many of these features have had lackluster results, and the tax of these functions on device battery life is uncertain. Although it would be virtually impossible to be familiar with all CIED algorithms, the several features discussed here are frequently encountered and have key clues that aid in their recognition and result in better patient care. A basic understanding of specialized CIED functions allows the clinician to select appropriate features and avoid unnecessary or potentially harmful bells and whistles.

ACKNOWLEDGMENTS

The authors are grateful to the technical support teams of device companies for their assistance with this article. Many of the examples provided are adapted from another review on the topic published by the authors.[2] There are many features from many device companies that may not be directly disclosed within this review. This article was not edited or reviewed by any device manufacturer employee or representative, and the authors take full responsibility with respect to the accuracy or completeness regarding trademarked or proprietary features.

REFERENCES

1. Bernstein AD, Camm AJ, Fletcher RD, et al. The NASPE/BPEG generic pacemaker code for antibradyarrhythmia and adaptive-rate pacing and antitachyarrhythmia devices. Pacing Clin Electrophysiol 1987;10:794–9.
2. Lloyd MS, El Chami MF, Langberg JJ. Pacing features that mimic malfunction: a review of current programmable and automated device functions that cause confusion in the clinical setting. J Cardiovasc Electrophysiol 2009;20:453–60.
3. Wilkoff BL, Cook JR, Epstein AE, et al. Dual-chamber pacing or ventricular backup pacing in patients with an implantable defibrillator: the dual chamber and VVI implantable defibrillator (DAVID) trial. JAMA 2002;288:3115–23.
4. Sweeney MO, Ruetz LL, Belk P, et al. Bradycardia pacing-induced short-long-short sequences at the onset of ventricular tachyarrhythmias: a possible mechanism of proarrhythmia? J Am Coll Cardiol 2007;50:614–22.
5. Sweeney MO, Ellenbogen KA, Casavant D, et al. Multicenter, prospective, randomized safety and efficacy study of a new atrial-based managed ventricular pacing mode (MVP) in dual chamber ICDs. J Cardiovasc Electrophysiol 2005;16:811–7.
6. Akerstrom F, Arias MA, Pachon M, et al. The reverse mode switch algorithm: how well does it work? Heart Rhythm 2013;10:1146–52.
7. MAUDE–manufacturer and user facility device experience. Available at: www.accessdata.fda.gov. Record 2521280. 2012.
8. Olshansky B, Day J, McGuire M, et al. Reduction of right ventricular pacing in patients with dual-chamber ICDs. Pacing Clin Electrophysiol 2006;29: 237–43.
9. Byrd CL, Schwartz SJ, Gonzales M, et al. DDD pacemakers maximize hemodynamic benefits and minimize complications for most patients. Pacing Clin Electrophysiol 1988;11:1911–6.
10. Hayes DL, Boehmer JP, Day JD, et al. Cardiac resynchronization therapy and the relationship of percent biventricular pacing to symptoms and survival. Heart Rhythm 2011;8:1469–75.
11. Auger D, Hoke U, Bax JJ, et al. Effect of atrioventricular and ventriculoventricular delay optimization on clinical and echocardiographic outcomes of patients treated with cardiac resynchronization therapy: a meta-analysis. Am Heart J 2013;166: 20–9.
12. Sheppard RC, Ren JF, Ross J, et al. Doppler echocardiographic assessment of the hemodynamic benefits of rate adaptive AV delay during exercise in paced patients with complete heart block. Pacing Clin Electrophysiol 1993;16:2157–67.
13. Ellenbogen KA, Gold MR, Meyer TE, et al. Primary results from the SmartDelay determined AV optimization: a comparison to other AV delay methods used in cardiac resynchronization therapy (SMART-AV) trial: a randomized trial comparing empirical, echocardiography-guided, and algorithmic atrioventricular delay programming in cardiac resynchronization therapy. Circulation 2010;122:2660–8.
14. van Gelder BM, Bracke FA, Meijer A, et al. The hemodynamic effect of intrinsic conduction during left ventricular pacing as compared to biventricular pacing. J Am Coll Cardiol 2005;46:2305–10.
15. Kurzidim K, Reinke H, Sperzel J, et al. Invasive optimization of cardiac resynchronization therapy: role of sequential biventricular and left ventricular pacing. Pacing Clin Electrophysiol 2005;28:754–61.
16. Lee KL, Burnes JE, Mullen TJ, et al. Avoidance of right ventricular pacing in cardiac resynchronization therapy improves right ventricular hemodynamics in heart failure patients. J Cardiovasc Electrophysiol 2007;18:497–504.
17. Clarke M, Liu B, Schuller H, et al. Automatic adjustment of pacemaker stimulation output correlated with continuously monitored capture thresholds: a multicenter study. European Microny Study Group. Pacing Clin Electrophysiol 1998;21:1567–75.
18. Wood MA. Automated pacemaker function. Cardiol Clin 2000;18:177–91, ix.

19. Mitchell AR, Sulke N. How do atrial pacing algorithms prevent atrial arrhythmias? Europace 2004; 6:351–62.

20. Guyomar Y, Thomas O, Marquie C, et al. Mechanisms of onset of atrial fibrillation: a multicenter, prospective, pacemaker-based study. Pacing Clin Electrophysiol 2003;26:1336–41.

21. Ogawa H, Ishikawa T, Matsushita K, et al. Effects of right atrial pacing preference in prevention of paroxysmal atrial fibrillation: Atrial Pacing Preference study (APP study). Circ J 2008;72:700–4.

22. Levine PA, Wachsner R, El-Bialy A. Pacing for the suppression of paroxysmal atrial fibrillation in an 87-year-old patient. Indian Pacing Electrophysiol J 2003;3:88–90.

23. Carlson MD, Ip J, Messenger J, et al. A new pacemaker algorithm for the treatment of atrial fibrillation: results of the atrial dynamic overdrive pacing trial (ADOPT). J Am Coll Cardiol 2003;42:627–33.

24. Hettrick DA. Implantable Device Therapy. In: Schwartzman D, Zenati MA, editors. Innovative Management of Atrial Fibrillation. Malden, Massachusetts: Blackwell Publishing; 2007. p. 113–30. http://dx.doi.org/10.1002/9780470994818.ch8.

25. Purerfellner H, Ruiter JH, Widdershoven JW, et al. Reduction of atrial tachyarrhythmia episodes during the overdrive pacing period using the post-mode switch overdrive pacing (PMOP) algorithm. Heart Rhythm 2006;3:1164–71.

26. Healey JS, Connolly SJ, Gold MR, et al. Subclinical atrial fibrillation and the risk of stroke. N Engl J Med 2012;366:120–9.

27. Popovic ZB, Mowrey KA, Zhang Y, et al. Slow rate during AF improves ventricular performance by reducing sensitivity to cycle length irregularity. Am J Physiol Heart Circ Physiol 2002;283:H2706–13.

28. Israel CW, Gronefeld G, Ehrlich JR, et al. Prevention of immediate reinitiation of atrial tachyarrhythmias by high-rate overdrive pacing: results from a prospective randomized trial. J Cardiovasc Electrophysiol 2003;14:954–9.

29. Wiberg S, Lonnerholm S, Jensen SM, et al. Effect of right atrial overdrive pacing in the prevention of symptomatic paroxysmal atrial fibrillation: a multicenter randomized study, the PAF-PACE study. Pacing Clin Electrophysiol 2003;26:1841–8.

30. Blanc JJ, De Roy L, Mansourati J, et al. Atrial pacing for prevention of atrial fibrillation: assessment of simultaneously implemented algorithms. Europace 2004;6:371–9.

31. Sulke N, Silberbauer J, Boodhoo L, et al. The use of atrial overdrive and ventricular rate stabilization pacing algorithms for the prevention and treatment of paroxysmal atrial fibrillation: the Pacemaker Atrial Fibrillation Suppression (PAFS) study. Europace 2007;9:790–7.

32. Velasquez-Castano JC, Lloyd MS. Palpitations after a pacemaker generator exchange: a new algorithm-induced cause of endless loop tachycardia. Heart Rhythm 2009;6:1380–2.

33. Wood MA. Trials of pacing to control ventricular rate during atrial fibrillation. J Interv Card Electrophysiol 2004;10(Suppl 1):63–70.

34. Lian J, Mussig D, Lang V. Ventricular rate smoothing for atrial fibrillation: a quantitative comparison study. Europace 2007;9:506–13.

35. Tse HF, Newman D, Ellenbogen KA, et al. Effects of ventricular rate regularization pacing on quality of life and symptoms in patients with atrial fibrillation (Atrial fibrillation symptoms mediated by pacing to mean rates [AF SYMPTOMS study]). Am J Cardiol 2004;94:938–41.

36. Ajiki K, Sagara K, Namiki T, et al. A case of a pseudomalfunction of a DDD pacemaker. Pacing Clin Electrophysiol 1991;14:1456–60.

37. Glikson M, Trusty JM, Grice SK, et al. Importance of pacemaker noise reversion as a potential mechanism of pacemaker-ICD interactions. Pacing Clin Electrophysiol 1998;21:1111–21.

38. Koneru JN, Swerdlow CD, Wood MA, et al. Minimizing inappropriate or "unnecessary" implantable cardioverter-defibrillator shocks: appropriate programming. Circ Arrhythm Electrophysiol 2011;4: 778–90.

39. Duru F, Bloch KE, Weilenmann D, et al. Clinical evaluation of a pacemaker algorithm that adjusts the pacing rate during sleep using activity variance. Pacing Clin Electrophysiol 2000;23:1509–15.

40. Greco OT, Bittencourt LR, Vargas RN, et al. Sleep parameters in patients using pacemakers with sleep rate function on. Pacing Clin Electrophysiol 2006;29: 135–41.

41. Gammage MD. Rate-drop response programming. Pacing Clin Electrophysiol 1997;20:841–3.

42. Barold SS, Levine P. Pacemaker repetitive nonreentrant ventriculoatrial synchronous rhythm. A review. J Interv Card Electrophysiol 2001;5:59–66.

43. Hohnloser SH, Healey JS, Gold MR, et al. Atrial overdrive pacing to prevent atrial fibrillation: Insights from assert. Heart Rhythm 2012;9:1667–73.

Remote Monitoring
Technology and Evolving Use

Jane Chen, MD, FHRS

KEYWORDS

- Implantable devices • Remote monitors • Atrial arrhythmias • Congestive heart failure
- Lead integrity

KEY POINTS

- Remote monitors are transmitters that can download stored diagnostic data from patients' cardiovascular implantable electronic devices to physicians' offices.
- Clinical trials have shown that monitoring implantable devices remotely can lead to earlier detection of clinically relevant events that may result in medical intervention.
- Clinically relevant events that may require action include new-onset atrial arrhythmias, early signs of congestive heart failure, shocks from defibrillators (either appropriate or inappropriate), and compromise in device hardware system.
- Whether early intervention of clinically relevant events using remote monitors can actually lead to a reduction in health care utilization remains inconclusive.

INTRODUCTION

Since the implantation of the first pacemaker in 1958, cardiovascular implantable electronic devices (CIEDs) have expanded in use and in complexity. The implantation of these devices requires technical expertise for appropriate positioning of leads, avoidance of infection, and tailored programming of the pulse generator. Equally important is the appropriate monitoring of these devices to ensure early detection of device malfunction. Current generations of implantable devices have incorporated extensive monitoring tools that may be used clinically to evaluate patients. In the last decade, remote monitors have been developed by all device manufacturers to download stored information from these devices. These monitors transmit information from patients' homes to physicians' offices, allowing notification of patients' clinical status without additional office visits. This article discusses the utility of these remote monitors in various disease states, their

potential impact on health care resources, and possible future benefits.

TRADITIONAL DEVICE FOLLOW-UP

Pacemakers traditionally were checked from patient's homes via transtelephonic monitoring, which transmitted a snapshot of the heart rhythm and battery status of the pacemaker. In addition, patients were routinely seen in outpatient office visits every 6 to 12 months. Defibrillators did not have transtelephonic monitoring capabilities, and patients were seen in clinic every 3 to 6 months. With the expansion of indications for device implantation over the last 2 decades, these routine device-related office visits have significantly increased outpatient volume. Current devices are also equipped with extensive monitoring capabilities, such as thoracic impedance monitoring for volume overload, onset and duration of atrial arrhythmias, lead integrity alerts, and percentage of pacing. With outpatient follow-up alone, any

Disclosure: The author receives speaker honoraria from Medtronic and St. Jude Medical, and participates in clinic trials with Medtronic, St. Jude, Biotronik, and Boston Scientific.
Cardiovascular Division, Department of Medicine, Washington University School of Medicine, 660 South Euclid Avenue, Campus Box 8086, St Louis, MO 63110, USA
E-mail address: janechen@dom.wustl.edu

cardiacEP.theclinics.com

clinical changes stored in the devices are not usually detected until the following office visit. The current recommendations for routine follow-up of implantable devices are listed in **Table 1**.[1]

REMOTE MONITORING BY MANUFACTURER

At present all device manufacturers have created remote monitors for implantable devices, and each has its own unique features (**Table 2**). Remote monitors are available for all devices, including pacemakers, defibrillators, cardiac resynchronization devices, and implantable loop recorders. Contemporary remote monitors use encrypted radiofrequency signals that allow for transmission and receipt of stored data. Most transmitters require the use of analog phone lines, and data can be uploaded manually or wirelessly to a secure central station where the data are processed. The information is stored on a secure Web site, which is accessible by the patient's following physician and support team. Routine transmissions are usually scheduled by the physician's office. The physician's office can also be notified of any alerts, which are programmable parameters indicating any hardware abnormalities or arrhythmias that may require urgent attention (**Box 1**).

The Biotronik (Berlin, Germany) Home Monitoring is currently the only truly portable system, as it uses the Global System for Mobile communication (GSM) cellular network system for all transmissions. Therefore, an analog telephone line is not required. Automatic transmissions are uploaded every 24 hours, and any alerts are sent to the physician's office. Routine transmissions may be scheduled by the physician's office, or the accumulated daily collected data may be accessed by the physician at any time for review.

The Boston Scientific (Natick, MA) Latitude system has a unique feature that allows for wireless transmission of blood pressure and weights. In addition, patients can answer a set of questions regarding symptoms, including edema, fatigue, and shortness of breath (**Table 3**). The blood pressure, weight, and questionnaire answers may be transmitted separately to the patient's general cardiologist, without the additional arrhythmia data.

Medtronic (Minneapolis, MN) CareLink allows a detailed report via the Cardiac Compass visualization system, which shows up to 14 months of accumulated parameters. In addition it shows an OptiVol sensor graph, which illustrates changes in intrathoracic impedance as a potential marker for fluid accumulation and congestive heart failure.

REMOTE MONITORING TRIALS FOR PACEMAKERS

Current generations of pacemakers are more than just pacing systems, as they have sophisticated monitoring software that can be used for disease management. Remote monitors may assist physicians in more rapidly obtaining these comprehensive data, without the need for more office visits. The Pacemaker REmote Follow-up Evaluation and Review (PREFER) trial[2] was a multicenter, randomized, prospective trial to determine the utility of remote monitoring for the diagnosis of clinically actionable events (CAEs) compared with transtelephonic monitoring (TTM) plus office visits in 897 patients with Medtronic pacemakers. CAEs are defined as events for which a clinical decision may be made and may alter a patient's clinical management (see **Box 1**). Mean time to detection of any CAE was significantly shorter in the remote group than in the TTM group (5.7 vs 7.7 months). TTM identified only 2% of events, whereas remote

Table 1
Current recommendations for follow-up of implantable devices in person or with remote monitoring

Pacemakers/ICDs/CRT	
Within 72 h of CIED implantation	In person
2–12 wk postimplantation	In person
Every 3–12 mo pacemaker/ CRT-P	In person or remote
Every 3–6 mo ICD/CRT-D	In person or remote
Annually until battery depletion	In person
Every 1–3 mo at signs of battery depletion	In person or remote
Implantable loop recorder	
Every 1–6 mo depending on patient symptoms and indication	In person or remote
Implantable hemodynamic monitor	
Every 1–6 mo depending on indication	In person or remote
More frequent assessment as clinically indicated	In person or remote

Abbreviations: CIED, cardiovascular implantable electronic device; CRT, cardiac resynchronization therapy; CRT-D, cardiac resynchronization therapy defibrillator; CRT-P, cardiac resynchronization therapy pacemaker; ICD, implantable cardioverter-defibrillator.

From Epstein AE, DiMarco JP, Ellenbogen KA, et al. 2012 ACCF/AHA/HRS Focused update incorporated into the ACCF/AHA/HRS 2008 guidelines for device-based therapy of cardiac rhythm abnormalities. J Am Coll Cardiol 2013;61:e35.; with permission.

Table 2
Specific features of remote monitors per manufacturer

Manufacturer	FDA Approval Date	Cell Phone Transmission	Real-Time Electrogram	Blood Pressure/ Weight	Intrathoracic Impedance Measurements	Manual and Auto Transmissions
Biotronik (Home Monitoring)	2001	√[a]	√			√
Boston Scientific (Latitude)	2006		√	√		√
Medtronic (CareLink)	2005		√		√	√
St. Jude (Merlin.net)	2007		√		√	√
Sorin (SmartView)	2013		√			√

Abbreviation: FDA, Food and Drug Administration.
[a] Although most manufacturers have cell phone adapters for remote transmission, only Biotronik routinely utilizes cell phone transmissions without additional coats to patients.

monitoring identified 66% of events. The study was not intended to detect any overall survival benefit, reduced incidence of stroke, or hospitalizations for congestive heart failure. The investigators concluded that remote monitoring of pacemakers resulted in more rapid detection of clinical events, and that TTM is really only useful for determination of battery status.

The COMPArative follow-up Schedule with Home Monitoring (COMPAS) trial[3] randomized 538 patients with Biotronik pacemakers to remote monitoring versus routine. Patients in the remote group were monitored daily without any scheduled outpatient visits. Patients in the remote monitoring arm had fewer major adverse events, hospitalizations for arrhythmias and stroke, and unscheduled office visits. The office visits in the remote group, however,

were more medically appropriate because they resulted in more reprogramming and medication changes. The COMPAS trial confirmed that remote monitoring without routine office visits is a safe method of monitoring patients with pacemakers, and results in fewer but more effective office visits.

REMOTE MONITORING TRIALS FOR DEFIBRILLATORS

Care of patients with implantable defibrillators presents even more of a challenge than pacemakers. Appropriate shocks for ventricular arrhythmias, inappropriate shocks caused by atrial arrhythmias or noise, and compromise of lead integrity should ideally be detected and treated as soon as possible. Early signs of congestive heart failure as suggested by changes in intrathoracic impedance, suboptimal percentage of biventricular pacing in cardiac resynchronization devices, or a high percentage of unnecessary right ventricular pacing are also parameters that should prompt attention. Earlier detection of clinically relevant events should decrease hospitalizations and improve mortality. However, data as to whether remote monitoring with defibrillators actually improves these objective outcomes remain contradictory.

The Lumos-T Safely Reduces Routine Office Device Follow-up (TRUST) trial[4] was the first large-scale study to assess the safety of home monitoring for defibrillators. Patients with Biotronik Lumos single-chamber or dual-chamber defibrillators were randomized to remote monitoring versus routine office visits. Not surprisingly, remote monitoring transmission schedules were maintained by patients more consistently than office visits. Remote monitoring reduced hospital encounters for device interrogations by 45% without an increase in adverse events. More than 90% of

---

Box 1
Programmable parameters that may trigger alerts on remote monitors

- New onset atrial arrhythmias
- Duration of atrial arrhythmias
- Atrial fibrillation with rapid ventricular response
- Right ventricular pacing over a programmable percentage
- Biventricular pacing under a programmable percentage
- Increasing pacing thresholds
- Significant changes in lead impedances
- Nonsustained ventricular tachycardia
- ICD shocks
- Generator replacement indicator or end of life

Table 3
Example of weekly symptoms questionnaire, and wirelessly transmitted blood pressure and weight, in a Boston Scientific Latitude remote monitoring system

	24 Sep 2013 10:35 AM	02 Oct 2013 1:14 PM	08 Oct 2013 8:45 AM	16 Oct 2013 10:39 AM	22 Oct 2013 9:37 PM
Feeling unusually fatigued?	No	No	No	No	No
Faint or dizzy over past few days?	No	No	No	No	No
Swelling over past few days?	Remained same	Remained same	Remained same	Remained same	Remained same
Ability to walk or climb past few days?	Remained same	Remained same	Remained same	Remained same	Remained same
Pillows used last night?	None or 1	None or 1	None or 1	None or 1	None or 1
Woke up breathless last night?	None	None	None	None	None

Date	Weight (lb)	Systolic (mm Hg)	Diastolic (mm Hg)
22 Oct 2013	265.2	113	74
21 Oct 2013			
20 Oct 2013			
19 Oct 2013			
18 Oct 2013			
17 Oct 2013			
16 Oct 2013		103	76
15 Oct 2013			
14 Oct 2013			
13 Oct 2013			
12 Oct 2013			
11 Oct 2013			
10 Oct 2013			
09 Oct 2013			
08 Oct 2013		110	78
07 Oct 2013			

scheduled transmissions did not require any action. Problems, however, were discovered 30 days earlier with remote monitors.

Patients with a Medtronic implantable cardiac defibrillator (ICD) or cardiac resynchronization therapy defibrillator (CRT-D) were evaluated in the Clinical Evaluation of Remote Notification to Reduce Time to Clinical Decision (CONNECT) Trial.[5] Remotely monitored patients had decreased length of stay in hospital, with an estimated cost saving of $1793. No mortality benefit was noted in patients followed remotely compared with those who visited the office.

The largest study to date of remote monitoring of ICD and cardiac resynchronization therapy (CRT) patients involved 185,778 patients followed in the ALTITUDE study.[6] All patients had Boston Scientific devices and were randomized to either remote monitoring 3 to 4 times per month plus office visits twice a year, or to routine office visits alone. The study found a 50% reduction in mortality at 1 and 5 years. The lowest mortality was noted in patients who transmitted weight and blood pressure, suggesting that improved survival in this study may be attributable to increased patient self-care rather than remote monitoring itself.

REMOTE MONITORING FOR DISEASE MANAGEMENT

A major goal of remote monitoring is the earlier detection of clinically relevant events, which may lead to earlier initiation or adjustment of medications. This proactive approach may reduce hospitalizations, health care utilization, and mortality. Specific scenarios that may benefit from remote monitors are congestive heart failure, atrial arrhythmias, ICD shocks, and lead integrity issues.

Congestive Heart Failure

It has been estimated that in Medicare patients discharged from the hospital after admission with exacerbation of heart failure, 21% were readmitted within 30 days.[7] Early and frequent communication by telephone between patients and congestive heart failure coordinators can significantly reduce hospital readmission and all-cause mortality.[8]

Continuous monitoring capabilities within implantable devices can offer even more data that may be helpful in the treatment of patients with heart failure. For example, decreased patient-activity level and reduced heart rate variability may predict heart-failure decompensation. Intrathoracic impedance, measured between the tip of the right ventricular lead and the pulse generator, may be a surrogate for pulmonary vascular fluid status. For example, in the Medtronic OptiVol system, measurements of thoracic impedance are compared against a baseline. The difference is plotted against a programmable threshold, and alerts may be triggered if the threshold is crossed (**Fig. 1**). It should be noted that transthoracic measurements may not reliably indicate worsening congestion, and may be influenced by pneumonia, pleural effusion, pocket edema, or inflammation. An alert for threshold crossing should prompt an evaluation of the patient rather than reflex adjustment of medications.

In a large study of patients 532 patients who had audible alerts for OptiVol threshold crossing turned "ON" versus "OFF," hospitalization for congestive heart failure was significantly lower in the ON group.[9] However, in the Diagnostic Outcome Trial for Heart Failure (DOT-HF),[10] audible alerts increased outpatient visits (250 vs 84, $P<.0001$) and increased hospitalizations for heart failure (hazard ratio 1.79, $P = .022$), without any changes in mortality. An ongoing study, The Optimization of Heart Failure Management using Optivol Fluid Status Monitoring and Carelink (OptiLink HF study),[11] is planning to enroll at least 1000 patients to answer the question of whether use of OptiVol reduces mortality and hospitalizations for congestive heart failure.

The use of multiple variables may improve the predictive value of impedance measurements for exacerbation of heart failure. In the Program to Access and Review Trending Information and Evaluate Correlation to Symptoms in Patients with Heart Failure (PARTNERS HF) trial,[12] 694 patients with CRT-Ds were evaluated. Patients with a fluid index of more than 100 or any 2 of the following were identified: long duration of atrial fibrillation (AF), AF with rapid ventricular response, fluid index higher than 60, low patient activity, high nighttime heart rate, low heart-rate variability, low CRT pacing, or ICD shocks. Patients with combined factors had a 5.5-fold increased risk of hospitalization for heart failure within the subsequent 30 days.

Atrial Fibrillation

An unexpected finding in the Atrial Fibrillation Follow-up Investigation of Rhythm Management (AFFIRM) trial[13] was that the risk of stroke was similar in both the rhythm control group and the rate control group. The risk of stroke does not appear to be related to the concomitant presence of AF. In fact, 64% of patients in the rhythm control group were in sinus rhythm at the time of stroke. Undetected AF likely contributes to the risk of stroke.

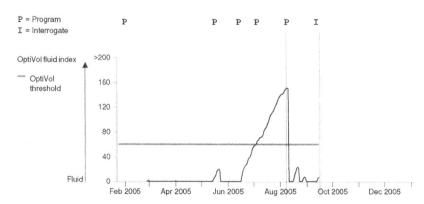

Fig. 1. OptiVol fluid index is a measurement of the difference between the daily and reference impedances. In this example, notification was sent when the OptiVol fluid index crossed the preset threshold of 60, prompting an unscheduled office visit to assess the patient's clinical status.

Many clinical trials using implantable devices as continuous monitors suggest that the duration of AF relates to stroke rate. The minimum duration of AF that increases the risk for stroke is unclear. The TRENDs study[14] was a prospective observational study of patients with pacemakers and ICDs, with or without AF, but with at least 1 risk factor for stroke. The study found that the annual thromboembolic risk was significantly higher for patients with a high burden of AF, defined as more than 5.5 hours in the prior 30 days, compared with patients with a low burden (<5.5 hours in prior 30 days) or zero burden. The ASSERT investigators[15] noted that in 2580 patients with pacemakers or ICDs but without a prior history of AF, AF duration of more than 6 minutes was associated with an increased risk of ischemic stroke and thromboembolism. A recently published pooled analysis from 3 major clinical trials of more than 10,000 patients with implantable devices and without permanent AF showed that over a 24-month follow up period, 43% of patients had a least 1 day of AF lasting more than 5 minutes. Moreover, AF duration of longer than 1 hour was associated with increased thromboembolic events. In addition, for every additional hour increase in the daily maximum AF burden, the relative risk for stroke increased by 3%.[16] These studies support the ongoing search for specific AF burden that may be associated with a significant increase in the risk for stroke.

Remote monitors can be programmed to alert physicians' offices for AF episodes of new onset and any programmable duration, allowing for earlier detection of asymptomatic episodes (**Fig. 2**). In the AWARE trial of more than 11,000 patients with the Biotronik Home Monitoring system,[17] approximately 65% of automatically transmitted alerts were for AF, and more than 10% of those episodes were for AF over 2.5 hours. In a study of ICD patients, detection of AF was significantly higher when patients were followed with remote monitoring (45%) in comparison with quarterly office visits (26%).[18] Thus, remote monitors can alert physicians to new-onset AF as soon as possible, and may lead to earlier initiation of appropriate anticoagulation.

Whether the earlier detection of asymptomatic AF episodes and earlier initiation of appropriate anticoagulation may result in reduction in strokes and mortality remains unknown. The ongoing IMPACT trial[19] recently completed enrollment of 2718 patients with cardiac resynchronization defibrillators. In this trial, initiation and withdrawal of anticoagulation will be based on AF duration and burden as documented by remote monitoring. The outcomes of strokes, thromboembolism, and bleeding will be compared with a control group in which anticoagulation is offered via routine detection and office visits. The results of the IMPACT trial will offer insights as to whether anticoagulation based on earlier detection of AF by remote monitors will in fact change the clinical outcome.

ICD Shocks

A special consideration for patients with implantable defibrillators is to monitor shocks. In addition to being a source of anxiety and discomfort to patients, shocks, both appropriate and inappropriate, may affect mortality. Patients with shocks from recurrent ventricular arrhythmias should be evaluated for precipitating causes such as ischemia and exacerbation of heart failure. Inappropriate shocks should prompt a thorough review to rule out lead integrity issues and to adjust ICD programming. In the ALTITUDE study of almost 70,000 ICD and CRT-D patients followed by the Boston Scientific Latitude remote system,[6] the incidence of appropriate shocks at 5-year follow-up was 23%. The incidence of inappropriate shock at 5 years was 17%. It is interesting that shocks, both appropriate and inappropriate, predicted mortality although shocks for oversensing did not, suggesting that shocks may cause mortality as a result of underlying conditions. Not surprisingly, time to discovery of ICD shocks has not been shown to significantly differ between remote monitoring and routine office visits, because most patients are aware of ICD shocks and will actively seek medical care.

Hardware Integrity

Sophisticated systems such as implantable devices require routine surveillance to ensure proper functioning of components. In addition to notification of pulse generators that have reached elective replacement indicators, remote monitors may alert physicians to early lead failure. Fracture of conductors or insulation breach in pacing leads may result in failure to capture. Oversensing and inhibition of pacing may be catastrophic in pacer-dependent patients. Conductor fracture of defibrillation leads may lead to inappropriate shocks from noise. Alerts for a sudden increase in lead impedance can result in earlier management of lead fracture and avoidance of multiple inappropriate shocks (**Fig. 3**). Remote monitors have been shown to identify lead issues 54 days earlier than traditional follow-up, and inappropriate shocks attributable to lead fracture were reduced from 53% with traditional follow-up to 27% in remote monitoring.[20,21]

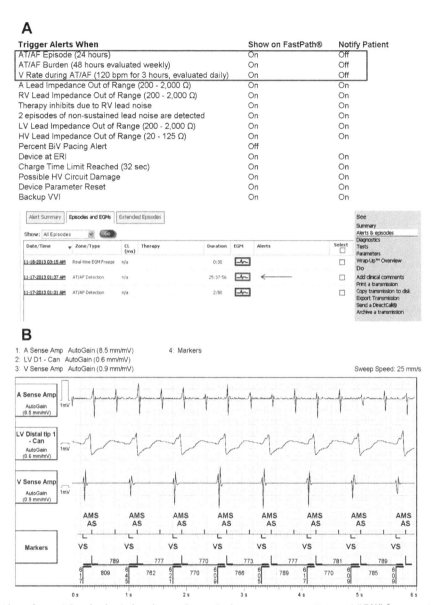

A

Trigger Alerts When	Show on FastPath®	Notify Patient
AT/AF Episode (24 hours)	On	Off
AT/AF Burden (48 hours evaluated weekly)	On	Off
V Rate during AT/AF (120 bpm for 3 hours, evaluated daily)	On	Off
A Lead Impedance Out of Range (200 - 2,000 Ω)	On	On
RV Lead Impedance Out of Range (200 - 2,000 Ω)	On	On
Therapy inhibits due to RV lead noise	On	On
2 episodes of non-sustained lead noise are detected	On	On
LV Lead Impedance Out of Range (200 - 2,000 Ω)	On	On
HV Lead Impedance Out of Range (20 - 125 Ω)	On	On
Percent BiV Pacing Alert	Off	
Device at ERI	On	On
Charge Time Limit Reached (32 sec)	On	On
Possible HV Circuit Damage	On	On
Device Parameter Reset	On	On
Backup VVI	On	On

B

1: A Sense Amp AutoGain (8.5 mm/mV)   4: Markers
2: LV D1 - Can AutoGain (0.6 mm/mV)
3: V Sense Amp AutoGain (0.9 mm/mV)   Sweep Speed: 25 mm/s

Fig. 2. (A) Alerts for atrial arrhythmia burden and ventricular rates are programmed "ON" for a patient without history of AF. One episode of AT/AF is shown to last more than 25 minutes. (B) Stored electrogram of the AT/AF episode above (*arrow in A*) demonstrates atrial tachycardia with 2:1 ventricular conduction. The ventricular rate exceeded the lower rate limit and reduced the percentage of biventricular pacing. Source of screen shot was from an actual patient interrogation. AMS, automatic mode switching; AS, atrial sense; AT/AF, atrial tachycardia/fibrillation; BiV, biventricular; ERI, elective replacement indicator; HV, high-voltage; LV, left ventricular; RV, right ventricular; V, ventricular; VS, ventricular sense; VVI, VVI mode.

IMPACT ON WORKFLOW

A main impetus for the use of remote monitors is to reduce office visits, which can be burdensome given the increasing number of implantable devices over the last decade. However, for remote data to be appropriately processed an adequate number of trained personnel is required. Whether the shift from in-person office visits to Internet-based monitoring actually reduces resource utilization is a matter of controversy. In a study of 500 remote transmissions from the Cleveland Clinic,[22] mean time spent on each remote transmission was significantly shorter, at 11.5 ± 7.7 minutes, compared with in-office interrogations, which took a mean of 27.7 ± 9.9 minutes. However, remote transmissions containing clinically important findings still took a mean of 21.0 ± 7.4 minutes each. Of

RV Pacing Impedance

At Implant	736 ohms	Highest	736 ohms
Last	>2500 ohms	Lowest	392 ohms

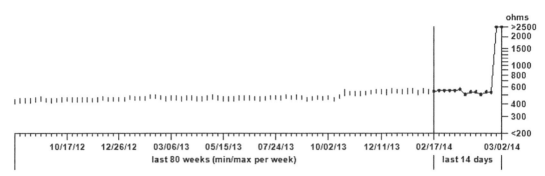

Fig. 3. Automatic lead impedance alert on a defibrillation lead. A sudden increase in lead impedance of greater than 2000 Ω suggests conductor fracture. No shocks were delivered. The patient underwent lead extraction and reimplantation of a new lead without complications.

significance, almost 50% of scheduled transmissions were missed because of patient noncompliance. Follow-up of these missed transmissions took almost 1 hour per day of telephone time by staff. In addition to patient noncompliance, failure of transmissions may also result from connection issues with monitors. In the CONNECT trial,[5] up to 45% of automatic alerts failed to transmit because the monitors were not set up properly or were unplugged from the landline. The increasing availability of wireless transmissions and the increasing reliability of transmissions by cellular phones should improve successful transmissions.

Successful transmission of data would not result in medical interventions without timely review. At present, there are no guidelines as to the acceptable time delay from time of data acquisition to physician response. In the CONNECT trial,[5] the time between transmission to physician review was less than 1.5 days in 70% of the cases, and the mean time to clinical decision was 4 to 6 days in the remote arm compared with 22 days in the office arm. In the COMPAS trial of pacemakers,[3] the time between warning message and medical intervention was reduced from 139 days in the control group to 17 days in the remote group. Whether this reduction in time to action translates to a significant impact on clinical outcome, however, is unknown. In one study of remote monitoring versus office visits, remote data were required to be reviewed by the physicians within 2 days. Despite this rapid response, there were no differences in overall mortality, hospitalizations, or quality of life of patients.[18]

MEDICOLEGAL ISSUES

As of now there is no specific recommendation on frequency of follow-up using only remote

monitors. Patients do not sign any informed consents for having their information stored on Web sites. Confidentiality by device companies, potential for hackers and database vulnerability, and licensing issues with physicians monitoring patients in states where they are not licensed to practice are issues that are yet to be resolved.[23] The liability of physicians and their representatives in processing the data is not defined. Potential legal implications if the physician misses an urgent alert and a patient undergoes a catastrophic event require serious consideration.

SUMMARY

CIEDs are sophisticated appliances with diagnostic capabilities that can assist in disease management. Convenience of use to the patient is improved with wireless transmissions, and can be further increased with the use of cellular phone transmissions. Remote monitors can alert physicians to abnormalities in the diagnostic data sooner, without an increase in office visits. However, the quantity of data that requires processing by trained personnel, and the time necessary for physicians to review these data, may be shifting the workload from face-to-face time with patients to computer work rather than decreasing the overall burden. Because the overwhelming majority of routine transmissions does not require any action, the possibility and safety of abolishing routine transmissions altogether, and only using remote monitors for alerts of CAEs, may warrant further scrutiny. Objective end points of earlier detection of these CAEs, such as reductions in stroke rates, hospitalizations for heart failure, and overall mortality, continue to be an area of active investigation.

REFERENCES

1. Epstein AE, DiMarco JP, Ellenbogen KA, et al. 2012 ACCF/AHA/HRS Focused update incorporated into the ACCF/AHA/HRS 2008 guidelines for device-based therapy of cardiac rhythm abnormalities. J Am Coll Cardiol 2013;61:e6–75.
2. Crossley GH, Chen J, Choucair W, et al, for the PREFER study investigators. Clinical benefits of remote versus transtelephonic monitoring of implanted pacemakers. J Am Coll Cardiol 2009;54:2012–9.
3. Mabo P, Victor F, Bazin P, et al, for the COMPAS trial investigators. A randomized trial of long-term remote monitoring of pacemaker recipients (the COMPAS trial). Eur Heart J 2012;33:1105–11.
4. Varma N, Epstein AE, Irimpen A, et al, for the TRUST investigators. Efficacy and safety of automatic remote monitoring for implantable cardioverter-defibrillator follow-up: the Lumos-T safely reduces routine office device follow-up (TRUST) trial. Circulation 2010;122:325–32.
5. Crossley GH, Boyle A, Vitense H, et al, for the CONNECT investigators. The CONNECT (Clinical evaluation of remote notification to reduce time to clinical decision) trial. J Am Coll Cardiol 2011;57:1181–9.
6. Saxon LA, Hayes DL, Gilliam R, et al. Long-term outcome after ICD and CRT implantation and influence of remote device follow-up: the ALTITUDE survival study. Circulation 2010;122:2359–67.
7. Hernandez AF, Greiner MA, Fonorrow GC, et al. Relationship between early physician follow-up and 30-day readmission among Medicare beneficiaries hospitalized for heart failure. JAMA 2010;303:1716–22.
8. Inglis SC, Clark RA, McAlister FA, et al. Structured telephone support or telemonitoring programmes for patients with chronic heart failure. Cochrane Database Syst Rev 2010;(8):CD007228.
9. Catanzariti D, Lunati M, Landolina M, et al, Italian Clinical Service Optivol-CRT Group. Monitoring intrathoracic impedance with an implantable defibrillator reduces hospitalizations in patients with heart failure. Pacing Clin Electrophysiol 2009;32:363–70.
10. van Veldhuisen DJ, Braunschweig F, Conraads V, et al. DOT-HF investigators. Intrathoracic impedance monitoring, audible patient alerts, and outcome in patients with heart failure. Circulation 2011;124:1719–26.
11. Brachmann J, Böhm M, Rybak K, et al. Fluid status monitoring with a wireless network to reduce cardiovascular-related hospitalizations and mortality in heart failure: rationale and design of the OptiLink HF study (Optimization of heart failure management using OptiVol fluid status monitoring and CareLink). Eur J Heart Fail 2011;13:796–804.
12. Whellan DJ, Ousdigian KT, Al-Khatib SM, et al. Combined heart failure device diagnostics identify patients at higher risk of subsequent heart failure hospitalizations: results from PARTNERS HF (Program to access and review trending information and evaluate correlation to symptoms in patients with heart failure) study. J Am Coll Cardiol 2010;55:1803–10.
13. Wyse DG, Waldo AL, DiMarco JP, et al, for the Atrial Fibrillation Follow-up Investigation of Rhythm Management (AFFIRM) Investigators. A Comparison of rate control and rhythm control in patients with atrial fibrillation. N Engl J Med 2002;347:1825–33.
14. Glotzer TV, Daoud EG, Wyse G, et al. The relationship between daily atrial tachyarrhythmia burden from implantable device diagnostics and stroke risk: the TRENDS study. Circ Arrhythm Electrophysiol 2009;2:474–80.
15. Healey JS, Connolly SJ, Gold MR, et al, for the ASSERT investigators. Subclinical atrial fibrillation and the risk of stroke. N Engl J Med 2012;366:120–9.
16. Boriani G, Glotzer TV, Santini M, et al. Device-detected atrial fibrillation and risk for stroke: an analysis of >10,000 patients from the SOS AF project (Stroke prevention strategies based on atrial fibrillation information from implanted devices). Eur Heart J 2014;35(8):508–16.
17. Lazarus A. Remote, wireless, ambulatory monitoring of implantable pacemakers, cardioverter defibrillators, and cardiac resynchronization therapy systems: analysis of worldwide database. Pacing Clin Electrophysiol 2007;30:S2–12.
18. Al-Khatib SM, Piccini JP, Knight D, et al. Remote monitoring of implantable cardioverter defibrillator versus quarterly device interrogations in clinic: results from randomized pilot clinical trial. J Cardiovasc Electrophysiol 2010;21:545–50.
19. Ip J, Waldo AL, Lip GY, et al, for the IMPACT investigators. Multicenter randomized study of anticoagulation guided by remote rhythm monitoring in patients with implantable cardioverter-defibrillator and CRT-D devices: rationale, design, and clinical characteristics of the initially enrolled cohort: the IMPACT study. Am Heart J 2009;158:363–70.
20. Neuzil P, Taborsky M, Walbrueck K. Early automatic remote detection of combined lead insulation defect and ICD damage. Europace 2008;10:556–7.
21. Marine JE. Remote monitoring for prevention of inappropriate implantable cardioverter defibrillator shocks: is there no place like home? Europace 2009;11:409–11.
22. Cronin EM, Ching EA, Varma N, et al. Remote monitoring of cardiovascular devices: a time and activity analysis. Heart Rhythm 2012;9:1947–51.
23. Vinck I, De Laet C, Stroobandt S, et al. Legal and organizational aspects of remote cardiac monitoring: the example of implantable cardioverter defibrillators. Europace 2012;14:1230–5.

The Implantable Loop Recorder
An Evolving Diagnostic Tool

Mikael Hanninen, MD, George J. Klein, MD, Jaimie Manlucu, MD*

KEYWORDS

• Implantable loop recorder • ILR • Clinical • Review • Syncope

KEY POINTS

- Implantable loop recorder (ILR) technology has undergone important improvements since first being used clinically in the late 1990s.
- In addition to a longer battery life and greater event storage capacity, improved arrhythmia-detection algorithms and remote monitoring capabilities have increased the number of potential applications of this prolonged rhythm monitoring strategy.
- Future iterations currently under development will result in further reduction in size, ease of implantation, and the addition of other sensors to expand usefulness.
- Although presently recommended by international guidelines primarily in the work-up of syncope, routine ILR implantation may gain greater acceptance in the future for other indications, including the work-up of cryptogenic stroke, atrial fibrillation monitoring following catheter ablation procedures, or to guide anticoagulant therapy and risk stratification for sudden cardiac death.

INTRODUCTION

Implantable loop recorders (ILRs) were initially developed in the 1990s, as microprocessor technology was being introduced into other cardiac implantable electronic devices. Automated event detection was made possible by heart rate–based algorithms that triggered recordings below or above a prespecified heart rate. Patient-triggered event detection (via a wireless device outside the body) was also featured, which allowed symptom-rhythm correlation. Since their first development, extensive clinical investigation and important improvements have made ILRs an integral part of modern cardiology practice. The ILR has traditionally been used in the work-up of recurrent, unexplained syncope, but recent studies have explored novel uses for the prolonged monitoring afforded by ILRs.

HOW IT WORKS

ILRs in current use for syncope (Medtronic Reveal DX, Medtronic Reveal XT, and St Jude Medical Confirm) are small, rectangular, titanium-encased devices with an estimated battery life of up to 3 years (**Fig. 1**). The devices are free from external conductors or leads and are therefore magnetic resonance imaging compatible (after an appropriate healing period following implantation). Subcutaneous placement parallel to the sternum usually allows adequate sensing of cardiac electrical activity, but surface estimation of the optimal sensing vector can also be performed. The sensing bipoles on the ILR are located on opposing ends of the device in order to maximize sensed electrical activity from the heart. As with other cardiac implantable electronic devices, sensed signals are amplified to allow

Conflicts of Interest: Dr G.J. Klein is a speaker for Medtronic and St Jude Medical, as well as a consultant for Medtronic.
Division of Cardiology, University of Western Ontario, London, Ontario N6A5A5, Canada
* Corresponding author. Arrhythmia Service, London Health Science Centre – University Hospital, 339 Windermere Road, Room B6-129B, London, Ontario N6G 5L5, Canada.
E-mail address: manlucuj@gmail.com

Card Electrophysiol Clin 6 (2014) 253–260
http://dx.doi.org/10.1016/j.ccep.2014.02.010

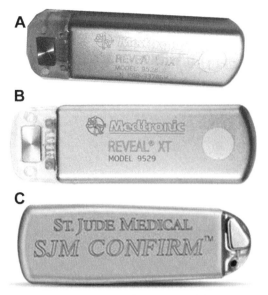

Fig. 1. ILRs in current use for syncope. (A) Medtronic Reveal DT, used for syncope. (B) Medtronic Reveal XT, used for syncope and/or atrial arrhythmia monitoring. (C) St Jude Medical Confirm, used for syncope and/or atrial arrhythmia monitoring. (Courtesy of [A, B] Medtronic, Minneapolis, MN. Copyright © Medtronic Inc. 2014; and [C] Confirm and St. Jude Medical are trademarks of St. Jude Medical or its related companies. Reprinted with permission of St. Jude Medical, © 2014. All rights reserved.)

signal processing and filtered to isolate the intrinsic deflection components of the electrogram.[1] The logic circuit is microprocessor driven and allows the identification and storage of rhythm recordings of interest. Early devices were limited in their storage capacity for rhythm events of interest, but this is not a major issue in modern devices.

Communication with the implanted device takes place via radiofrequency communication (telemetry). Options for ILR follow-up now include remote, transtelephonic monitoring in addition to standard, in-person device interrogation via a device programmer (Fig. 2). Patients who are followed remotely are provided with a home monitor, which transmits (automatically, in real time or at scheduled intervals) encrypted data via a standard telephone line. The transmitted data are stored on dedicated servers (Medtronic CareLink or St Jude Medical Latitude network) and can be accessed online by caregivers using a desktop computer or smartphone.[2] The potential benefits of remote ILR monitoring include patient convenience, the ability to provide constant surveillance, and early detection of asymptomatic arrhythmias.[3] However, criteria for automatic event detection and transmission must be carefully chosen in order to avoid the potential burden of analyzing excessive data.[4]

ILRs are also packaged with an external activator device that patients or bystanders can use to trigger a device recording in the event of a symptom (such as presyncope, palpitations, or syncope). Pressing the button on the activator while holding the device over the ILR triggers the ILR to save a SYMPTOM episode, with retrospective and prospective rhythm monitoring. This feature is particularly useful in that it allows patients to capture episodes despite a significant delay in signal transmission, which may occur with episodes of unheralded syncope.

The implantation procedure is generally well tolerated under local anesthesia and conscious sedation, with minimal risks aside from minor bleeding and, rarely, local infection. An injectable ILR (Medtronic Injectable Reveal) has been in development for several years and is expected to be released for clinical use in 2014.

CLINICAL APPLICATION
Syncope

Syncope remains the most extensively studied clinical indication for ILR implantation. In the largest published study of ILR use to date (the PICTURE registry), ILR data contributed to a definitive diagnosis in 78% of patients after a mean follow-up

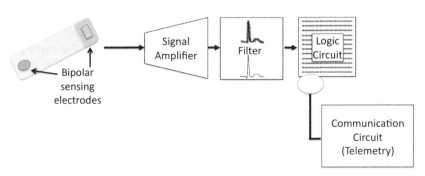

Fig. 2. Simplified ILR components.

of 10 months.[5] Longer monitoring periods seem to increase the diagnostic yield, with one group of investigators reporting that 26% of diagnoses were made more than 18 months after ILR implantation.[6] If an abnormal rhythm is detected during syncope, bradycardia is roughly 3 times more common than tachycardia (supraventricular or ventricular), although sinus rhythm is noted almost one-third of the time.[7]

Recent international guidelines on syncope have placed a greater emphasis on a rhythm-based diagnosis than in the past,[8,9] in part because of the publication of studies that have shown an increased rate of definitive diagnosis[10,11] and reduced cost per diagnosis.[12] Although commonly performed, Holter monitoring is inappropriate for symptom-rhythm correlation unless syncope occurs on an frequent basis (more than once per week). In contrast, an external loop recorder can be effective for syncope diagnosis in instances of weekly or monthly recurrence, although patient compliance (with wearing the recorder and with activating the device during symptoms) can be problematic.[13] For syncope occurring less frequently than once per month, the ILR is the most reasonable option to record a rhythm during symptoms. ILRs are recommended, with a class I recommendation, (1) in an early phase of evaluation in patients with recurrent syncope, (2) in high-risk patients following a negative in-hospital comprehensive evaluation, and (3) in patients with frequent or traumatic reflex (vasovagal) syncope to evaluate the contribution of bradycardia to symptoms.[8] Despite these recommendations, ILRs remain significantly underused.[14]

ILR recordings are thought to be diagnostic when syncope is correlated to a bradyarrhythmia or tachyarrhythmia and also when periods of high-grade (Mobitz II or type III) atrioventricular (AV) block, prolonged supraventricular tachycardia/ventricular tachycardia (SVT/VT), or prolonged ventricular pauses are observed in the absence of such correlation.[8] Representative recordings obtained from patients with ILRs implanted for syncope are shown in **Fig. 3**. Typical reflex (vasovagal) syncope is commonly associated with impressive sinus pauses (see **Fig. 3**A) and is classically preceded by progressive sinus bradycardia and PR interval prolongation. This pattern is important to recognize, because pacing is unlikely to eliminate recurrent syncope in these patients (although syncope frequency may be reduced by dual-chamber pacing in select patients[15]). In contrast, syncope from sinus node dysfunction (see **Fig. 3**B) or paroxysmal heart block with prolonged ventricular standstill should respond to demand pacing. Tachycardia (supraventricular or ventricular) may also be responsible

for syncope in some patients (see **Fig. 3**C), although this is rare.

Undersensing of cardiac electrical signals (see **Fig. 3**D, F) and oversensing of nonphysiologic signals (such as myopotentials and electromagnetic interference) remains a common limitation with implantable loop recordings. The large number of inappropriate automated device recordings generated has the potential of concealing clinically relevant events, because of limitations in storage capacity and prioritization of more recent events. It is important to ensure that the ILR device is implanted with the manufacturer's markings facing forward, because a device that is implanted backwards often has poor sensing parameters. Device repositioning with vector optimization may be required to alleviate this problem in some cases.

Risk Stratification After Myocardial Infarction

Despite modern reperfusion techniques for acute coronary syndromes, arrhythmias cause at least 30% to 50% of sudden deaths following myocardial infarction.[16,17] Prolonged monitoring of the heart rhythm with ILRs has significantly improved clinicians' understanding of life-threatening arrhythmias following myocardial infarction. The CARISMA trial followed 297 patients with ILRs for 1.9 years after myocardial infarction. All patients had a reduced ejection fraction ($\leq$40%), measured 3 to 21 days following their infarction. A large proportion (46%) of patients had arrhythmia detections, including new-onset atrial fibrillation (AF) with rapid ventricular response (>125 beats per minute) in 28%, prolonged sinus pauses ($\geq$5 seconds) or marked bradyarrhythmias (high-grade AV block or sinus bradycardia $\leq$30 beats per minute for $\geq$8 seconds) in 23%, nonsustained ventricular tachycardia ($\geq$16 beats) in 13%, and sustained ventricular tachycardia/ventricular fibrillation in 6%. Detected arrhythmias were associated with a high risk of cardiac death. Intermittent heart block, in particular, was associated with a hazard ratio of 6.75. Most of these events (86%) were asymptomatic.[18] In a subgroup analysis of patients who died during follow-up, bradyarrhythmias and ventricular tachyarrhythmias accounted for half of the rhythms detected at the time of death, with bradyarrhythmias and electromechanical dissociation being more commonly detected in nonsudden cardiac death (pump failure) and noncardiac death.[19]

At the present time, the role of ILR monitoring following myocardial infarction remains investigational. The usefulness of routine ILR monitoring in these patients remains uncertain and a significant

A

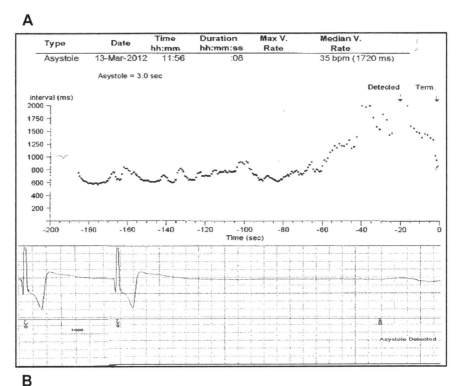

B

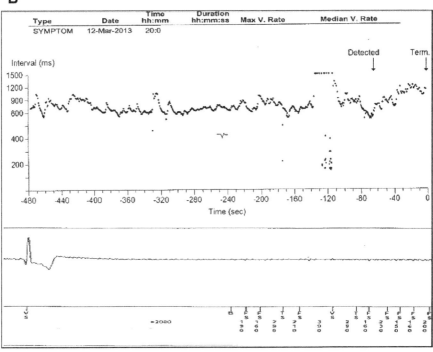

Fig. 3. Representative ILR recordings obtained from patients with syncope. (*A*) Reflex (vasovagal) syncope, characterized by gradual sinus bradycardia and a first degree AV block, which is followed by an impressive sinus pause. (*B*) Sinus node dysfunction with a sudden sinus arrest and oversensing of myopotentials from associated seizure activity. The external activator was triggered by a bystander and the event is recorded as a SYMPTOM episode. (*C*) Eight-second episode of wide-complex tachycardia, most likely nonsustained ventricular tachycardia. (*D*) Prominent sensed premature ventricular complex (PVCs) with undersensing of normal QRS complexes. The baseline sinus rate is appropriately 60 beats per minute (1000 milliseconds). Oversensing of nonphysiologic signals with extremely short cycle length (noise) is also observed on the dot plot. (*E*) Atrial fibrillation detection on a Reveal XT ILR. (*F*) Ventricular bigeminy with undersensing.

C

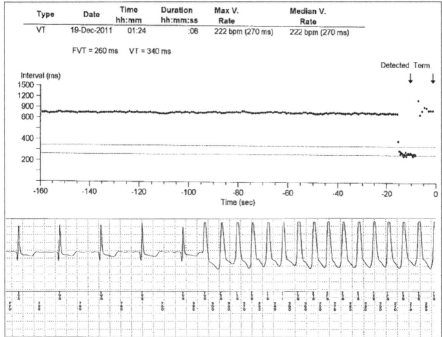

Type	Date	Time hh:mm	Duration hh:mm:ss	Max V. Rate	Median V. Rate
VT	19-Dec-2011	01:24	:08	222 bpm (270 ms)	222 bpm (270 ms)

FVT = 260 ms   VT = 340 ms

D

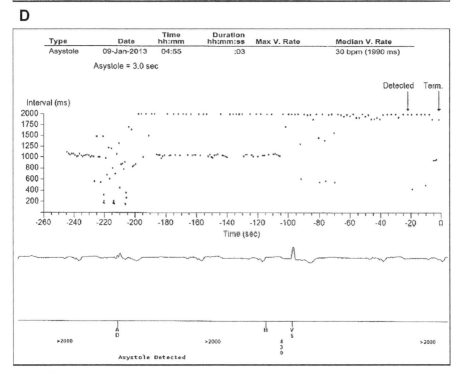

Type	Date	Time hh:mm	Duration hh:mm:ss	Max V. Rate	Median V. Rate
Asystole	09-Jan-2013	04:55	:03		30 bpm (1990 ms)

Asystole = 3.0 sec

Fig. 3. (continued)

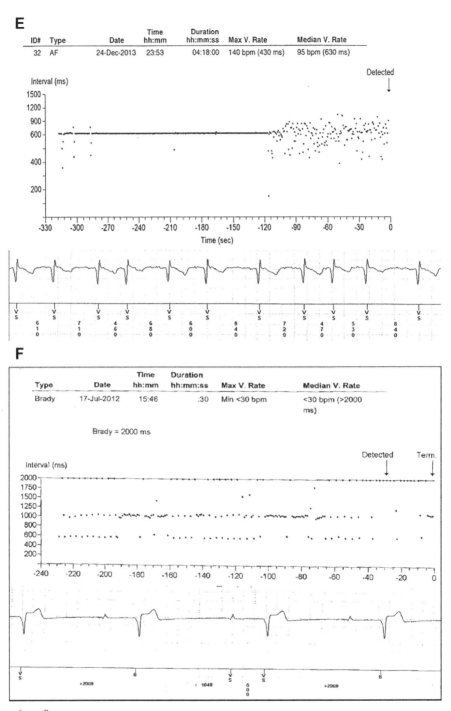

Fig. 3. (*continued*)

percentage of patients with reduced left ventricular function ultimately become candidates for primary prevention implantable-cardioverter defibrillator (ICD) implantation.[20] Further research is needed to determine whether ILR implantation can identify patients at high risk of malignant arrhythmias who are not current candidates for primary prevention ICD implantation (for instance, among patients with a left ventricular ejection fraction 36%–50%).

Atrial Arrhythmia Monitoring

A recent application of ILR technology is in the monitoring of AF (see **Fig. 3**E). Early ILR technology (Medtronic Reveal DX) used rate and irregularity algorithms to detect AF. These algorithms were more sensitive with rapid ventricular rates[17] than they were at detecting AF with controlled ventricular rates. Newer ILRs (Medtronic Reveal XT and St Jude Medical Confirm) are equipped with AF-detection algorithms that allow more accurate automatic detection of AF and a more accurate estimation of AF burden. Even among patients with highly symptomatic AF, asymptomatic AF episodes (detected by rhythm monitoring) are known to occur[21] and the underdetection of AF has important clinical implications.

Undetected paroxysmal AF is an important cause of cryptogenic stroke[22] and the detection rate of AF after stroke has been shown to increase with longer duration of cardiac monitoring.[23,24] Although the optimal method of monitoring remains uncertain, AF-detection rates as high as 25.5% have been shown with ILRs[25] and the role of prolonged cardiac monitoring in these patients will probably increase in the future.[26] An ongoing randomized prospective trial (CRYSTAL AF) is designed to further investigate the usefulness of ILR implantation (vs standard monitoring) in 450 patients with cryptogenic stroke.[27]

Prolonged ILR monitoring following atrial flutter ablation has recently shown that new AF detection can occur as late as 4 months after ablation. In a trial by Mittal and colleagues,[28] the rate of new AF diagnosis at 1 year was 55%, which is probably higher than the figure that has typically been quoted to patients undergoing atrial flutter ablation. The rate of AF detection has also been shown to be higher with ILR monitoring compared with standard rhythm monitoring following AF ablation.[29] It is logical that a strategy of routine prolonged monitoring after AF or atrial flutter ablation is useful in identifying patients who may safely discontinue their oral anticoagulation, a strategy under investigation in the current REACT COM trial.[30]

The use of ILR monitoring specifically to detect atrial arrhythmias remains under investigation and its use for this purpose is not yet advocated in national or international guidelines. Investigators have observed false-positive AF detections resulting from the automated AF-detection algorithms,[28,29] mainly related to oversensing of P waves and myopotentials, R wave undersensing, and frequent premature atrial contractions.[31] Software upgrades have been shown to improve the performance of AF-detection algorithms[31] and will become increasingly important if ILR monitoring for AF achieves widespread acceptance.

SUMMARY

ILR technology has undergone important improvements since it was first used clinically in the late 1990s. In addition to a longer battery life and greater event storage capacity, improved arrhythmia-detection algorithms and remote monitoring capabilities have increased the number of potential applications of this prolonged rhythm monitoring strategy. Future iterations currently under development will result in further reduction in size, ease of implantation, and the addition of other sensors to expand usefulness. Although presently recommended by international guidelines primarily in the work-up of syncope,[5] routine ILR implantation may gain greater acceptance in the future for other indications, including the work-up of cryptogenic stroke, AF monitoring following catheter ablation procedures, or to guide anticoagulant therapy and risk stratification for sudden cardiac death.

REFERENCES

1. Kenny T. The nuts and bolts of cardiac pacing. 2nd edition. Singapore: Wiley-Blackwell; 2008.
2. Dubner S, Auricchio A, Steinberg J, et al. ISHNE/ EHRA expert consensus on remote monitoring of cardiovascular implantable electronic devices (CIEDs). Europace 2012;14:278–93.
3. Varma N, Ricci R. Telemedicine and cardiac implants: what is the benefit? Eur Heart J 2013; 34(25):1885–95.
4. Arrocha A, Klein G, Benditt D, et al. Remote electrocardiographic monitoring with a wireless implantable loop recorder: minimizing the data review burden. Pacing Clin Electrophysiol 2010;13:1347–52.
5. Edvardsson N, Frykman V, van Mechelen R, et al. Use of an implantable loop recorder to increase the diagnostic yield in unexplained syncope: results from the PICTURE registry. Europace 2011;13(2):262.
6. Furukawa T, Maggi R, Bertolone C, et al. Additional diagnostic value of very prolonged observation by implantable loop recorder in patients with unexplained syncope. J Cardiovasc Electrophysiol 2012;23(1):67.
7. Krahn AD, Klein GJ, Fitzpatrick A, et al. Predicting the outcome of patients with unexplained syncope undergoing prolonged monitoring. Pacing Clin Electrophysiol 2002;25(1):37.
8. Moya A, Sutton R, Ammirati F, et al. Guidelines for the diagnosis and management of syncope. Eur Heart J 2009;30(21):2631–71.
9. Sheldon RS, Morillo CA, Krahn AD, et al. Standardized approaches to the investigation of syncope: Canadian Cardiovascular Society position paper. Can J Cardiol 2011;27(2):246–53.

10. Krahn AD, Klein GJ, Yee R, et al. Randomized assessment of syncope trial: conventional diagnostic testing versus a prolonged monitoring strategy. Circulation 2001;104(1):46–51.

11. Mitro P, Kirsch P, Valočik G, et al. A prospective study of the standardized diagnostic evaluation of syncope. Europace 2011;13(4):566–71.

12. Krahn AD, Klein GJ, Yee R, et al. Cost implications of testing strategy in patients with syncope: randomized assessment of syncope trial. J Am Coll Cardiol 2003;42(3):495–501.

13. Sivakumaran S, Krahn AD, Klein GJ, et al. A prospective randomized comparison of loop recorders versus Holter monitors in patients with syncope or presyncope. Am J Med 2003;115(1):1–5.

14. Vitale E, Ungar A, Maggi R, et al. Discrepancy between clinical practice and standardized indications for an implantable loop recorder in patients with unexplained syncope. Europace 2010;12(10):1475–9.

15. Brignole M, Menozzi C, Moya A, et al. Pacemaker therapy in patients with neurally mediated syncope and documented asystole: Third International Study on Syncope of Uncertain Etiology (ISSUE-3): a randomized trial. Circulation 2012;125(21):2566–71.

16. Adabag AS, Therneau TM, Gersh BJ, et al. Sudden death after myocardial infarction. JAMA 2008;300:2022–9.

17. Bloch Thomsen PE, Jons C, Raatikainen MJ, et al. Long-term recording of cardiac arrhythmias with an implantable cardiac monitor in patients with reduced ejection fraction after acute myocardial infarction: the Cardiac Arrhythmias and Risk Stratification After Acute Myocardial Infarction (CARISMA) study. Circulation 2010;122(13):1258–64.

18. Gang UJ, Jøns C, Jørgensen RM, et al. Heart rhythm at the time of death documented by an implantable loop recorder. Europace 2010;12(2):254–60.

19. Yap YG, Duong T, Bland M, et al. Temporal trends on the risk of arrhythmic vs. non-arrhythmic deaths in high-risk patients after myocardial infarction: a combined analysis from multicentre trials. Eur Heart J 2005;26:1385–93.

20. Russo AM, Stainback RF, Bailey SR, et al. ACCF/HRS/AHA/ASE/HFSA/SCAI/SCCT/SCMR 2013 appropriate use criteria for implantable cardioverter-defibrillators and cardiac resynchronization therapy: a report of the American College of Cardiology Foundation Appropriate Use Criteria Task Force, Heart Rhythm Society, American Heart Association, American Society of Echocardiography, Heart Failure Society of America, Society for Cardiovascular Angiography and Interventions, Society of Cardiovascular Computed Tomography, and Society for Cardiovascular Magnetic Resonance. Heart Rhythm 2013;10(4):e11–58.

21. Hindricks G, Piorkowski C, Tanner H, et al. Perception of atrial fibrillation before and after radiofrequency catheter ablation: relevance of asymptomatic arrhythmia recurrence. Circulation 2005;112(3):307–13.

22. Elijovich L, Josephson SA, Fung GL, et al. Intermittent atrial fibrillation may account for a large proportion of otherwise cryptogenic stroke: a study of 30-day cardiac event monitors. J Stroke Cerebrovasc Dis 2009;18:185–9.

23. Sposato LA, Klein FR, Jáuregui A, et al. Newly diagnosed atrial fibrillation after acute ischemic stroke and transient ischemic attack: importance of immediate and prolonged continuous cardiac monitoring. J Stroke Cerebrovasc Dis 2012;21(3):210–6.

24. Stahrenberg R, Weber-Kruger M, Seegers J, et al. Enhanced detection of paroxysmal atrial fibrillation by early and prolonged continuous Holter monitoring in patients with cerebral ischemia presenting in sinus rhythm. Stroke 2010;41:2884–8.

25. Cotter PE, Martin PJ, Ring L, et al. Incidence of atrial fibrillation detected by implantable loop recorders in unexplained stroke. Neurology 2013;80(17):1546–50.

26. Ritter MA, Kochhäuser S, Duning T, et al. Occult atrial fibrillation in cryptogenic stroke: detection by 7-day electrocardiogram versus implantable cardiac monitors. Stroke 2013;44(5):1449–52.

27. Sinha AM, Diener HC, Morillo CA, et al. Cryptogenic Stroke and underlying Atrial Fibrillation (CRYSTAL AF): design and rationale. Am Heart J 2010;160(1):36–41.

28. Mittal S, Pokushalov E, Romanov A, et al. Long-term ECG monitoring using an implantable loop recorder for the detection of atrial fibrillation after cavotricuspid isthmus ablation in patients with atrial flutter. Heart Rhythm 2013;10(11):1598–604.

29. Kapa S, Epstein AE, Callans DJ, et al. Assessing arrhythmia burden after catheter ablation of atrial fibrillation using an implantable loop recorder: the ABACUS study. J Cardiovasc Electrophysiol 2013;24(8):875–81.

30. Passman R. "ClinicalTrials.gov" Rhythm evaluation for AntiCoagulaTion with continuous monitoring (REACT COM). Northwestern University; 2013. Available at: http://clinicaltrials.gov/show/NCT01706146. Accessed October 10, 2013.

31. Eitel C, Hindricks G, Fruhauf M, et al. Performance of implantable automatic atrial fibrillation detection device: device impact of software adjustments and relevance of manual episode analysis. Europace 2011;13:480–5.

New Technology for Implantable Cardioverter Defibrillators

David Wilson, MD[a], Bengt Herweg, MD, FHRS[b],*

KEYWORDS

- Implantable cardioverter defibrillator • Cardiac resynchronization therapy • Remote monitoring
- Shock reduction • DF-4 connector • Subcutaneous implantable cardioverter defibrillator

KEY POINTS

- The DF-4 lead connector offers the advantage of a smaller, less complex header, requiring only a single set screw to connect all high and low voltage terminals. It reduces the possibility of lead/connector failure at the cost of decreased flexibility to selectively replace or substitute individual components of the implantable cardioverter defibrillator (ICD) lead.
- New floating atrial bipole single-lead ICD systems offer the benefits of dual-chamber sensing, including atrial tachyarrhythmia detection and improved supra ventricular tachycardia (SVT) discrimination, avoiding the disadvantages of an additional atrial lead. They are not suitable for atrial pacing.
- Novel shock reduction strategies include sophisticated T-wave discrimination algorithms, advanced lead integrity monitoring, and enhanced lead noise discrimination; they are further enhanced by remote ICD monitoring.
- Remote monitoring of ICD devices has been associated with a reduction in office visits and hospitalizations, improved battery life, and reduction in inappropriate ICD shocks.
- The subcutaneous ICD is a new effective alternative for patients who lack vascular access or when it seems beneficial to avoid transvenous lead placement.
- Up to 75% of cardiac implantable electronic device patients will need a magnetic resonance imaging scan (MRI) at some point in their life. MRI conditional ICD and cardiac resynchronization therapy (CRT) devices are under clinical investigation.

INTRODUCTION

During recent years, there has been dramatic progress in implantable cardioverter defibrillator (ICD) technology that has led to further reduction in generator size, improved ease of implantation, improved battery longevity, and reduction of inappropriate and unnecessary ICD therapies. These technological improvements have transformed the ICD into a reliable mainstream device now central to the therapy of heart failure patients. New technologies such as the subcutaneous ICD and the magnetic resonance imaging (MRI)-compatible ICD device offer treatment options to patient subgroups previously not considered for ICD therapy. The aim of this article is to summarize the

Disclosures: Dr B. Herweg reports receiving fellowship support from Medtronic, and minor consulting fees from St. Jude Medical and Biosense-Webster.
[a] Division of Cardiology, James A. Haley VA Medical Center, University of South Florida Morsani College of Medicine, 13000 Bruce B. Downs Boulevard, Tampa, FL 33612, USA; [b] Electrophysiology and Arrhythmia Services, Department of Cardiovascular Disease, Tampa General Hospital, University of South Florida Morsani College of Medicine, South Tampa Campus (5th Floor), Two Tampa General Circle, Tampa, FL 33606, USA
* Corresponding author.
E-mail address: bherweg@health.usf.edu

Card Electrophysiol Clin 6 (2014) 261–267
http://dx.doi.org/10.1016/j.ccep.2014.02.011

most recent advances in ICD technology that have led to this marked progress.

LEAD TECHNOLOGY

The transvenous lead remains a critical component of an ICD system. It serves as the critical interface allowing for communication of electrical signals between the myocardium and generator, for both, bradytherapy and tachytherapy. The connector is the interface between the lead and the pulse generator. Early on, it was recognized that a standard connector was required that could work across all manufacturers' ICD generators, similar to the IS-1 standard for bipolar pacing leads. This led to the development of the DF-1 standard, introduced in 1993.[1] The DF-1 connectors were utilized for the high voltage ports only, meaning that a dual-coil ICD lead would require 2 DF-1 and 1 IS-1 connector for the pace/sense portion of the lead. The lead separated with a trifurcation at the yoke (bifurcation for single coil leads). This design had several disadvantages, including increased pocket volume due to a large header accommodating multiple connectors, with the possibility of lead/connector failure at multiple sites due to shear stress and abrasion.[2] It also increased implant complexity with increased risk for setscrew problems and erroneous lead connections.

In response to these challenges, the DF-4 standard was developed. Initial discussions on this standard began with an industry-wide task force in 1998.[1] The first DF-4 connector was marketed by St. Jude Medical, St. Paul, MN with the Durata lead in June, 2009.[2] The DF-4 connector is a 4-pole in-line connector (**Fig. 1**), allowing for both high and low voltage terminals in 1 connector plug. The design is analogous to the similarly developed IS-4 standard, which holds 4 low voltage terminals for use with quadripolar pacing leads (see **Fig. 1**; **Fig. 2**).

The advantages of the DF-4 include significant reduction in both size and complexity of the header. Reduction in size is obvious, with a single connector requiring only a single set screw, reducing the risk of setscrew problems and eliminating the risk of port mismatch. The reduced pocket volume offers the potential for quicker, less traumatic implantation and improved patient comfort.

The DF-4 standard connector does pose some disadvantages. At the time of implantation, adapters are required to work with conventional alligator clips used for intraoperative testing. Also, there is less flexibility in dealing with undesirable clinical situations including high defibrillation thresholds. With a DF-1 standard connector, separate shocking coils can be connected allowing placement in various locations including the azygous vein, coronary sinus, or connection of a subcutaneous lead array (SQ array). This is not possible with a DF-4 lead and compatible device (at least not with currently available connectors). Secondly, there are situations in which isolated malfunction of the pace/sense portion of a high voltage lead can be identified. With a DF-1/IS-1 standard connector, addition of a bipolar pacing/sensing lead can be considered. This is not possible with a DF-4 lead. Therefore, in these situations, one may be more compelled to consider lead extraction and replacement over addition of a rate sensing lead, to avoid the risk of RV coil–coil contact leading to potential shunting of high voltage energy and lead noise in integrated bipolar designed systems.

Overall, the DF-4 standard offers several advantages going forward with a new ICD implantation. As with any new product, knowledge of its limitations and potential pitfalls is vital to ensure the best patient outcomes.

Another new lead technology available is the Biotronik Linoxsmart S DX ICD lead (Biotronik,

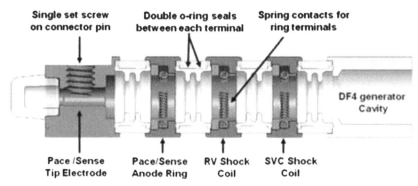

Fig. 1. DF-4 generator connector cavity shown. Note the spring contacts within each ring terminal with o-ring seals in between. RV, right ventricle; SVC, superior vena cava. (*From* Mond HG, Helland JR, Fischer A. The evolution of the cardiac implantable device connectory. Pacing Clin Electrophysiol 2013;36(11):1443; with permission.)

Lead Labeling

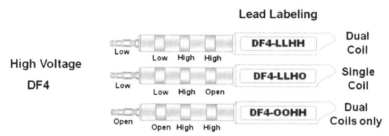

Fig. 2. DF-4 lead configuration with labeling. The lead labeling is required to be plainly visible on the grip zone of the lead adjacent to the connector plug. Low, low voltage connector; High, high voltage connector; Open, no connector. (*From* Mond HG, Helland JR, Fischer A. The evolution of the cardiac implantable device connectory. Pacing Clin Electrophysiol 2013;36(11):1442; with permission.)

Berlin, Germany). This single-coil ICD lead has an IS-1 and DF-1 standard connector and has a floating atrial bipole located either 15 cm or 17 cm proximal from the tip for atrial sensing (**Fig. 3**). This active fixation lead is only available at a length of 65 cm. It offers the benefits of dual-chamber sensing, including atrial tachyarrhythmia detection and improved SVT discrimination,[3] avoiding the disadvantages of an additional atrial lead.[4] The lead is used on the platform of the Biotronik DX family of devices, which are capable of processing varying atrial signals of different morphology and amplitude associated with the floating atrial bipole and perform a 4-fold amplification of the atrial signal.[5] Mean P-wave amplitudes during initial testing were 2.1 +/− 1.5 mV as measured by the PSA and 5.0 to 6.1 mV once amplified by the pulse generator.[2]

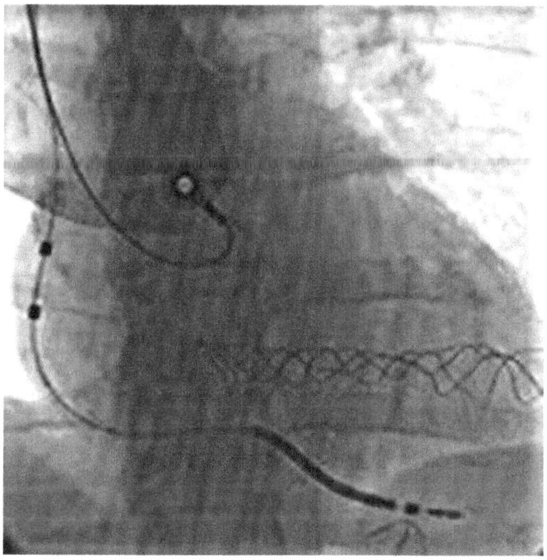

That study showed 93.8% appropriate atrial sensing 6 months after implantation.[5] It is important to emphasize that this lead is not intended for atrial pacing, should the patient require that at some point.

GENERATOR DESIGN

Improved battery design and increasing energy density have allowed for reduction in pulse generator volume over the last decades across all manufacturers. The latest generation of Medtronic ICD and CRT-D devices has been developed with a curved pulse generator can design with a contoured connector block and device body in order to reduce skin pressure. Internal testing by Medtronic yielded a 30% reduction in skin pressure when compared with noncurved designs. To date, there have been no outcome data associated with this design change.

SHOCK REDUCTION

Appropriately, shock reduction strategies have garnered a lot of attention in recent years. Associate relationships between ICD shocks, both appropriate and inappropriate, and a potential for increased mortality have been demonstrated in numerous retrospective studies.[6–9] However, there are currently no conclusive data from randomized controlled studies that ICD shocks lead to deterioration of cardiac function and increased mortality. As anticipated, shock reduction strategies have been shown to improve quality of life.[10]

A novel feature on the latest generation of Medtronic ICDs is a T-wave discrimination algorithm. This is relevant, as 6% of inappropriate shocks in the Sudden Cardiac Death in Heart Failure Trial (SCD-HeFT) study were adjudicated to be due to T-wave oversensing.[11,12] A novel T-wave discrimination algorithm analyzes the sensing electrogram

Fig. 3. CXR (PA view) of a patient implanted with the Biotronik Linoxsmart S DX ICD lead, demonstrating the floating atrial bipole in the midright atrium. (*Courtesy of* Biotronik S.E. & Co., Berlin, Germany.)

for alternating patterns of amplitude and frequency content by comparing the standard sensing signal to a first-order difference signal that attenuates the low-frequency content that dominates T-waves.[12] This filtered EGM enlarges the ratio of R- to T-wave amplitudes, enabling improved T-wave recognition and eliminating inappropriate tachytherapy for T-wave oversensing.

There has been much attention paid in recent years to the long term management of ICD leads, especially those under US Food and Drug Administration advisory for higher than expected mechanical failure. Inappropriate ICD shocks as a result of mechanical lead failure are a common problem encountered by all manufacturers.[11] Industry has responded with advanced monitoring of lead integrity as part of routine internal diagnostics. All manufacturers have trademarked names to this approach, but plainly put, this includes monitoring for fluctuating impedance levels plus or minus counting of nonphysiologic short V-V intervals. Variations from predefined thresholds will trigger any combination of audible patient alarms and clinician alerts, available at the time of interrogation or by remote viewing. In fact, these monitoring strategies have been to found to reduce all causes of inappropriate shocks when combined with remote monitoring.[13,14]

Some manufacturers also offer enhanced discrimination of lead noise, potentially causing oversensing. This is clinically relevant, as up to 10% of inappropriate shocks are due to right ventricular lead noise.[8] The algorithm, when employed, would require verification of short V-V intervals on the near field channel with simultaneous high amplitude signals on a far field electrogram. Lead noise due to make–break artifacts in the setting of fracture would be present in high amplitude only on the near field electrogram and not on the far field electrogram.

REMOTE MONITORING

Telemedicine in ICD management involves intermittent assessment of lead parameters and battery status in form of remote follow-up but can also represent continuous remote monitoring.[15] This consists of automatic, unscheduled remote transmissions for alert events (ie, arrhythmia onset or abnormal lead impedance), as well as initiated uploads for perceived or real clinical events. With modern devices, this can often be done wirelessly and without patient initiation in order to improve compliance.[16] The benefits of remote monitoring have been demonstrated in recent large randomized trials showing, among other things, reduction in clinic visits and cardiac resource utilization,

reduced capacitor charges (therefore improved battery longevity), and reduction in inappropriate shocks.[17,18]

The most studied technology is Biotronik Home Monitoring (Biotronik, Berlin, Germany), with 3 randomized clinical trials documenting efficacy. The largest trial was the The Lumos-T Safely Reduces Routine Office Device Follow-Up Trial (TRUST). This was a multicenter clinical trial with 2:1 randomization to standard in-office visits versus home monitoring. This trial reached its primary efficacy end point in reducing total in-hospital device evaluation by 45%[19] (visits per patient-year: 3.8 vs 2.1). No increase in adverse events was noted in the home monitoring group. The secondary efficacy endpoint was also met with a significant reduction in detection times of clinically relevant problems (symptomatic or silent). The median time from onset to physician evaluation of combined first atrial fibrillation (AF), ventricular tachycardia (VT), and ventricular fibrillation (VF) events was 1 day in the home monitoring group versus 35.5 days in the conventional care group.[19]

Biotronik Home Monitoring has also been shown to significantly reduce ICD shocks.[13] In the Effectiveness and Cost of ICD Follow-up with Telecardiology (ECOST) trial, 433 patients were followed for an average of 24.2 months. The group randomized to home monitoring was shown to have a significant reduction in all ICD shocks as well as a 52% reduction in inappropriate shocks. The potential increase in battery usage associated with remote monitoring was more than offset by a significant reduction in overall capacitor charges for the monitored group versus control (499 vs 2081). This resulted in improved battery longevity overall in the home monitoring group.

Remote monitoring also has a role in the ambulatory management of congestive heart failure (CHF). The potential for early intervention in at risk CHF patients is especially important given the prevalence and economic impact of CHF care.[20]

ICD devices are capable of monitoring several clinical diagnostic parameters. These vary by manufacturer but include thoracic impedance, atrial fibrillation burden, ventricular extrasystole burden, average day and night rate, heart rate variability, activity level, and VT/VF episodes. Intrathoracic impedance is a surrogate measure for blood volume or pulmonary capillary wedge pressure, with an increase in fluid volume leading to a reduction in intrathoracic impedence.[21] Heart rate variability is used as a surrogate for sympathetic tone, with declining variability in the presence of increased sympathetic tone.[22] Activity level can be a surrogate for functional status.

The potential of remote monitoring for earlier heart failure intervention was studied prospectively in the Program to Access and Review Trending Information and Evaluate Correlation to Symptoms in Patients with Heart Failure (PARTNERS-HF) trial.[23] This prospective, multicenter observational study analyzed data from 697 patients with an average follow-up of 11.7 months. All patients had a cardiac resynchronization therapy ICD, and 95% of them had New York Heart Association (NYHA) class 3 CHF. Patients received standard in-office follow-up, but their device's heart failure diagnostic data were saved for subsequent analysis. A combined heart failure device diagnostic algorithm was developed. The algorithm was considered positive if a patient had 2 of the following abnormal criteria during a 1-month period:

- Long atrial fibrillation duration
- Rapid ventricular rate during atrial fibrillation
- High fluid index (>60)
- Low patient activity
- Abnormal autonomics suggestive of elevated sympathetic tone (high night heart rate or low heart rate variability)
- Notable device therapy (low percentage of biventricular pacing or implantable cardioverter–defibrillator shocks)

OR

- If the patient had only had a very high fluid index (>100)

Patients with positive diagnostics using this algorithm were found to have a 5.5-fold increased risk of heart failure hospitalization due to congestion within the next 30 days.[23]

Most of the data regarding remote monitoring have been based on prospective trials. The ALTITUDE project (launched in 2008) was formed to prospectively follow and monitor patients implanted with a Boston Scientific ICD or CRT-D and followed with their proprietary monitoring system, LATITUDE (Boston Scientific Corp., Natick, MA). Over 150,000 patients have been enrolled in this program. Several studies have been published to date using this data. Saxon and colleagues[24] found a 50% reduction in all-cause mortality for the patient with remote follow-up (average of 4 uploads/month) versus standard in-office follow-up. This finding was consistent for both ICD and CRT-D groups in this study.

The emergence of remote monitoring is associated with a new set of logistic problems not yet addressed. First, there will be engineering and application differences among each device manufacturer that may impact patient care. To illustrate, the Clinical Evaluation of Remote Notification to Reduce Time to Clinical Decision (CONNECT) trial utilizing 1 company's monitoring system, was unsuccessful at submitting automatic clinician alerts in 45% of device triggered alerts.[21] The most challenging problem associated with remote monitoring is data management. This requires proper infrastructure in place to ensure that actionable data will be used to care for patients in a timely manner. With the crossover in care that occurs for many patients between heart failure physician and rhythm specialist, it is often unclear who will assume responsibility for the remote follow-up. If there is shared responsibility among providers, this requires complex collaboration that may be difficult in some cases. Lastly, there have been liability concerns raised regarding failure to act on information gathered remotely.

SUBCUTANEOUS ICD

One cannot discuss new technology in ICD therapy without mentioning the totally subcutaneous ICD system (S-ICD) from Boston Scientific. Complications related to transvenous lead implantation can be seen as partly offsetting the clear mortality reduction seen with ICD technology.[25,26] The system is completely extrathoracic. It consists of a pulse generator and a single, sensing/shocking electrode. The generator is implanted above the left fifth and sixth intercostal spaces in the midaxillary line. The electrode is positioned parallel to the left sternal margin. In a safety and efficacy study, 100% of patients capable of undergoing defibrillation threshold testing had successful defibrillation with this device.[27] In the same study, the S-ICD had first shock success of 92.1% (35 of 38) with discrete episodes of VT or VF. For the 3 episodes that failed to convert, 2 required a second shock; 1 of them terminated spontaneously during device charging.[27]

This device should be considered in certain patient populations who either lack vascular access or in cases in which it seems beneficial to avoid transvenous lead placement. The device it is not capable of providing pacing support. Therefore, patients requiring bradytherapy support, and those with VT amendable to antitachycardia pacing and those with cardiac resynchronization therapy (CRT) indications, should not be considered. A screening electrocardiogram prior to implantation recorded from the chest wall in 3 potential sensing vector projections is required to ensure an adequate R- to T-wave ratio to diminish T-wave oversensing. Despite this, with early use, there has been a high incidence of inappropriate shocks due to T-wave oversensing, with a 10.8% annual incidence rate.[28] Some implanters have advocated early exercise stress testing after implantation to refine an individual patient's risk for T-wave oversensing with appropriate reprogramming accordingly.[28]

This technology is only discussed briefly, as this topic is covered elsewhere in this issue.

MRI-COMPATIBLE ICD AND CRT-D

MRI has become the gold standard for soft tissue imaging. It has been estimated that up to 75% of cardiac-implantable electronic device patients will need an MRI at some point in their life.[29] This suggests an obvious need for MRI-compatible pacing and ICD systems. Medtronic was the first to gain FDA approval for this with their Revo MRI Pure Scan Pacing System.[30] Biotronik has come to market in Europe with an approved MRI conditional ICD and CRT-D system. This was approved with a chest exclusion zone. This technology has not been tested in the United States to date. A human trial is ongoing, called the ProMRI PROVEN study and is estimated to be completed in late 2015.[30] This topic is covered in detail elsewhere in this issue.

REFERENCES

1. Mond HG, Helland JR, Fischer A. The evolution of the cardiac implantable device connectory. Pacing Clin Electrophysiol 2013;36(11):1434–46.
2. Scherschel JA. The next standard in ICD lead technology: the DF-4 ICD lead connector system. EP Lab Dig 2013;9:34–5.
3. Kim MH, Bruckman D, Sticherling C, et al. Diagnostic value of single- versus dual-chamber electrograms recorded from an implantable defibrillator. J Interv Card Electrophysiol 2003;9(1):49–53.
4. Dewland TA, Pellegrini CN, Wang Y, et al. Dual-chamber implantable cardioverter-defibrillator selection is associated with increased complication rates and mortality in the NCDR. J Am Coll Cardiol 2011;58(10):1007–13.
5. Safak E, Schmitz D, Konorza T, et al. Clinical efficacy and safety of an implantable cardioverter-defibrillator lead with a floating atrial sensing dipole. Pacing Clin Electrophysiol 2013;36(8):952–62.
6. Sood N, Ruwald AC, Solomon S, et al. Association between myocardial substrate, implantable cardioverter defibrillator shocks and mortality in MADIT-CRT. Eur Heart J 2014;35(2):106–15.
7. Moss AJ, Schuger C, Beck CA, et al. Reduction in inappropriate therapy and mortality through ICD programming. N Engl J Med 2012;367(24):2275–83.
8. Daubert JP, Zareba W, Cannom DS, et al. Inappropriate implantable cardioverter-defibrillator shocks in MADIT-II: frequency, mechanisms, predictors, and survival impact. J Am Coll Cardiol 2008;51(14):1357–65.
9. Wilkoff BL, Williamson BD, Stern RS, et al. Strategic programming of detection and therapy parameters in implantable cardioverter-defibrillators reduces shocks in primary prevention patients: results from the PREPARE (Primary Prevention Parameters Evaluation) study. J Am Coll Cardiol 2008;52(7):541–50.
10. Wathen MS, DeGroot PJ, Sweeney MO, et al. Prospective randomized multicenter trial of empirical antitachycardia pacing versus shocks for spontaneous rapid ventricular tachycardia in patients with implantable cardioverter-defibrillators: pacing fast ventricular tachycardia reduces shock therapies (PainFREE Rx II) trial results. Circulation 2004;110(17):2591–6.
11. Poole JE. Analysis of ICD shock electrograms in the SCD-HeFT trial. Presented at Heart Rhythm 2004, 25th Annual Scientific Session, May 19-22, 2004, San Francisco, CA.
12. Volosin KJ, Exner DV, Wathen MS, et al. Combining shock reduction strategies to enhance ICD therapy: a role for computer modeling. J Cardiovasc Electrophysiol 2011;22(3):280–9.
13. Guedon-Moreau L, Lacroix D, Sadoul N, et al. A randomized study of remote follow-up of implantable cardioverter defibrillators: safety and efficacy report of the ECOST trial. Eur Heart J 2013;34(8):605–14.
14. Spenker S, Coban N, Koch L, et al. Potential role of home monitoring to reduce inappropriate shocks in implantablecardioverter-defibrillator patients due to lead failure. Europace 2009;11(4):483–8.
15. Burri H. Remote follow-up and continuous remote monitoring, distinguished. Europace 2013;15:i14–6.
16. Varma N, Brugada P. Automatic remote monitoring: milestones reached, paths to pave. Europace 2013;15(Suppl 1):i69–71.
17. Guedon-Moreau L, Mabo P, Kacet S. Current clinical evidence for remote patient management. Europace 2013;15:i6–10.
18. Crossley GH, Boyle A, Vitense H, et al. The CONNECT (Clinical Evaluation of Remote Notification to Reduce Time to Clinical Decision) trial: the value of wireless remote monitoring with automatic clinician alerts. J Am Coll Cardiol 2011;57:1181–9.
19. Varma N, Epstein NE, Irimpen A, et al. Efficacy and safety of automatic remote monitoring for implantable cardioverter–defibrillator follow-up: the Lumos-T safely reduces routine office device follow-up (TRUST) trial. Circulation 2010;122:325–32.
20. Heidenreich PA, Albert NM, Allen LA, et al, on behalf of the American Heart Association Advocacy Coordinating Committee, Council on Arteriosclerosis,

Thrombosis and Vascular Biology, Council on Cardiovascular Radiology and Intervention, Council on Clinical Cardiology, Council on Epidemiology and Prevention, Stroke Council. Forecasting the impact of heart failure in the United States: a policy statement from the American Heart Association. Circ Heart Fail 2013;6:606–19.

21. Yu CM, Wang L, Chau E, et al. Intrathoracic impedance monitoring in patients with heart failure: correlation with fluid status and feasibility of early warning preceding hospitalization. Circulation 2005;112: 841–8 s wi.

22. Adamson PB, Smith AL, Abraham WL, et al. Continuous autonomic assessment in patients with symptomatic heart failure: prognostic value of heart rate variability measured by an implanted cardiac resynchronization device. Circulation 2004;110:2389–94.

23. Whellan DJ, Ousdigian KT, Al-Khatib SM, et al, PARTNERS Study Investigators. Combined heart failure device diagnostics identify patients at higher risk of subsequent heart failure hospitalizations: results from PARTNERS HF (Program to Access and Review Trending Information and Evaluate Correlation to Symptoms in Patients with Heart Failure) study. J Am Coll Cardiol 2010;55(17):1811–3.

24. Saxon LA, Hayes DL, Gilliam R, et al. Long-term outcome after ICD and CRT implantation and influence of remote device follow-up: the ALTITUDE survival study. Circulation 2010;122:2359–67.

25. Reynolds MR, Cohen DJ, Kugelmass AD, et al. The frequency and incremental cost of major complications among Medicare beneficiaries receiving implantable cardioverter–defibrillators. J Am Coll Cardiol 2006;47:2493–7.

26. Borleffs CJ, Lieselot VE, van Bommel RJ, et al. Risk of failure of transvenous implantable cardioverter–defibrillator leads. Circ Arrhythm Electrophysiol 2009;2:411–6.

27. Weiss R, Knight BP, Gold MR, et al. Safety and efficacy of a totally subcutaneous implantable-cardioverter defibrillator. Circulation 2013;128(9):944–53.

28. Kooiman KM, Knops RE, OldeNordkamp L, et al. Inappropriate subcutaneous implantable cardioverter defibrillator shocks due to T-wave oversensing can be prevented. Implications for management. Heart Rhythm 2013;11:426–34 pii:S1547-5271(13) 01394-5.

29. Available at: http://www.fda.gov/MedicalDevices/ ProductsandMedicalProcedures/DeviceApprovalsand Clearances/Recently-ApprovedDevices/ucm244469. htm. Accessed March 30, 2014.

30. Available at: http://clinicaltrials.gov/ct2/show/ NCT01809665?term=promri+Proven&rank=1. Accessed March 30, 2014.

MRI Conditionally Safe Pacemakers
Design and Technology Considerations

Omair Yousuf, MD*, Joseph E. Marine, MD,
Saman Nazarian, MD, PhD

KEYWORDS

- Magnetic resonance imaging • Safety • MRI-conditional • Pacemaker • ICD

KEY POINTS

- MRI scans of conventional (not MRI-conditional) pacemakers and implantable cardioverter-defibrillators (ICDs) can be performed safely under specific conditions in a controlled environment.
- MRI scanning of patients with pacemaker or ICD systems should be undertaken using a multidisciplinary approach that requires personnel trained in device management and advanced cardiac life support, availability of resuscitation equipment and facilities, and a thorough discussion of risk and benefits between patient and physician.
- MRI-conditional pacemaker systems have been redesigned to mitigate electromagnetic interference and heating.
- The safety of MRI in the setting of cardiac implantable electronic devices has been studied mainly using standard scanners with field strength of 1.5-T; therefore, the safety protocols should not be extrapolated to scanners with different field strengths or configurations, such as 3-T and open bore systems.

INTRODUCTION

The use of implantable cardiac electronic devices, including pacemakers, implantable cardioverter defibrillators (ICDs), and/or cardiac resynchronization therapy (CRT) devices, has increased dramatically, due in part to expanded indications for their use, their pivotal role in improving cardiovascular outcomes and mortality, and the aging of society. In parallel, use of MRI as a diagnostic modality has seen significant expansion, with more than 60 million scans performed annually worldwide.[1] This is, in large part, due to the unparalleled soft tissue resolution and lack of ionizing radiation with MRI. It is estimated that up to 75% of patients with implantable cardiac devices will develop an indication for MRI during their lifetime.[2,3] Moreover, the likelihood of needing an MRI doubles after 65 years of age—a demographic that is most likely to receive an implantable cardiac device.[4] Hence, the necessity for MRI is increasingly encountered in this cohort of patients.

Although MRI is a safe technology, implantable cardiac devices are subject to force and torque, heating, current induction, and/or electromagnetic interference in the MRI environment. As a result of reported fatalities, manufacturers of both conventional cardiac devices and MRI equipment consider the presence of an implanted cardiac device an absolute contraindication to MRI scanning. Accordingly, a scientific statement issued by the

Disclosures: None (O. Yousuf, J.E. Marine); Dr S. Nazarian is a scientific advisor to Biosense Webster Inc and Principal investigator for research support to Johns Hopkins University from Biosense Webster Inc. Dr S. Nazarian's research is also supported by grants from the National Institutes of Health (K23HL089333 and R01HL116280).
Johns Hopkins University, Baltimore, MD 21287, USA
* Corresponding author. 1800 N. Orleans Street, Zayed 7125, Baltimore, MD 21287.
E-mail address: OYousuf1@JHMI.edu

Card Electrophysiol Clin 6 (2014) 269–278
http://dx.doi.org/10.1016/j.ccep.2014.02.001
1877-9182/14/$ – see front matter © 2014 Elsevier Inc. All rights reserved.

cardiacEP.theclinics.com

American Heart Association, American College of Cardiology, and several radiological societies discourage the use of MRI in these patients.[3] They endorse a thorough and careful risk/benefit analysis and recommend performing MRIs only in compelling clinical circumstances.

Patients with an indication for MRI and no other acceptable alternative often must undergo MRI, particularly when the potential benefit of the diagnostic data obtained by MRI significantly outweighs the risk for device failure or other complications. Over the past decade, several studies have concluded that MRI can be performed safely in patients with implantable cardiac devices under specific clinical circumstances in a carefully selected environment with appropriately trained personnel.[5–10] Furthermore, given the increased need for MRI in patients with cardiac devices, there has been strong interest by device manufacturers in the development of pacemakers and lead systems specifically tested for safe but conditional use in the MRI environment.

SAFETY CONCERNS IN THE MRI ENVIRONMENT

The MRI environment has a wide range of potentially deleterious effects on implantable cardiac devices. Risks generally arise from the static and gradient magnetic fields and radiofrequency energy, which in isolation or in concert can cause device malfunction, localized tissue injury, loss of capture, inhibition of pacing, asynchronous pacing, current induction resulting in myocardial capture and arrhythmia, and delivery of inappropriate ICD therapies. The major MRI-induced cardiac device complications are discussed below and also listed in **Box 1**.

Despite the potential for these serious risks, some patients have a strong indication for MRI without an acceptable alternative. If a decision is made for a patient with an implanted cardiac device to undergo MRI scanning, a detailed discussion outlining the risks and benefits along with a documented informed consent should be undertaken between patient and treating physician. Furthermore, the study should be performed with rigorous safety standards, including the presence of personnel trained in device management and advanced cardiac life support, availability of a cardiac electrophysiologist and adequate emergency medical equipment, and appropriate monitoring throughout the study.

Force and Torque

The ferromagnetic components of cardiac devices are subjected to force and torque caused by the

---

Box 1
Potential cardiac implantable device complications from MRI

- Inappropriate defibrillator firing
- Asynchronous pacing
- Inhibition of pacing
- Battery depletion
- Induction of malignant tachyarrhythmias
- Power-on-reset
- Reed switch malfunction
- Image artifacts
- Device malfunction and damage
- Force and torque leading to device or lead dislodgement
- Thermal injury leading to myocardial necrosis or perforation
- Death

---

intense magnetic field. This situation can theoretically lead to movement of the device generator. The leads have little or no ferromagnetic materials and are unlikely to experience significant force and torque. Device generators implanted after the year 2000 seem to contain less ferromagnetic materials and experience lower force and torque levels. Overall, the risk of device dislodgement, even with acute implants, is exceedingly low. Most studies, however, have restricted MRI during the first 6 weeks after implantation.[11–13] This safety window has been implemented in studies not because of a high risk of MRI-induced dislodgement during the first 6 weeks but because of the high risk of spontaneous (not MRI-induced) dislodgement, which would bias the safety results. At the authors' institution, several MRI examinations have been performed safely with an absolute clinical necessity in the acute postimplant period.

Tissue Heating and Injury

Leads can act as antennas and may amplify local energy deposition at the lead tip or locations near the lead, thus resulting in heating of the surrounding myocardial tissue and edema or necrosis. Clinically, a temperature increase at the lead tip may result in increasing pacing thresholds, loss of capture, or myocardial perforation.[14] Troponin elevations have been reported in 4 of 113 MRI scans performed in a 1.5-T scanner in patients with a variety of cardiac implantable devices.[15] These enzyme elevations may reflect tissue necrosis from thermal injury.

Radiofrequency Noise

Electromagnetic interference often leads to inappropriate tracking in patients with pacemakers, due to preferential sensing of noise by the higher programmed sensitivity of the atrial lead. Noise reversion with asynchronous pacing, inappropriate detection of tachycardia, and battery depletion due to recording of multiple arrhythmia events also have been noted. Additionally, oversensing of noise and inhibition of demand pacing are serious concerns in pacemaker-dependent patients.

Power-On-Reset

Also known as electrical reset, power-on-reset is a backup programming mode to which implantable cardiac devices may revert after exposure to electromagnetic interference. After power-on-reset occurs, pacing is set to an inhibited mode and tachycardia therapies are enabled, which may increase the risk of inadequate shock therapies during MRI. Although older literature has reported a power-on-reset rate as high as 6% by MRI,[13] the authors recently reported experience in 438 patients, in which electrical reset events occurred in 1.5% of device patients.[16] If not recognized by appropriate monitoring of the patient in the scanner, the event may be life threatening in a patient who is pacemaker dependent. With proper recognition of electrical reset, however, pacing should resume on cessation of scanning.

Reed Switches

Older implantable cardiac devices were equipped with an electrical (reed) switch that responded to magnetic fields and was used for emergent asynchronous pacing, deactivation of ICD therapies, or assessment of battery longevity. The state (open or closed) of the switch is susceptible to the strong magnetic field of the MRI environment—the response of which is variable and inconsistent but may include asynchronous pacing or loss of pacing.[12,17] Modern systems have largely replaced the reed switch with Hall sensors.

MRI OF PATIENTS WITH CONVENTIONAL (NON–MRI-CONDITIONAL) IMPLANTABLE CARDIAC DEVICES

Although a majority of studies have not shown any harmful effects of MRI on cardiac devices, there have been isolated reports of asystole, ventricular fibrillation, and death.[9] These potentially adverse effects have been identified largely in older devices and leads. One study demonstrated that if a specific safety protocol was followed, MRI examinations could safely be performed in patients whose pacemakers were manufactured after the year 2000.[18] Furthermore, repeat MRIs in patients with pacemakers and ICDs have shown no clinically significant cumulative changes in lead impedance, battery voltage, or capture threshold.[19,20]

The authors' group reported on one of the largest experiences to date, in 555 MRI scans on 438 patients with non–MRI-conditional pacemakers (54%) or ICDs (46%) from various manufacturers.[16] Patients with leads implanted less than 6 weeks prior to MRI and those with epicardial or abandoned leads were excluded. Using the authors' specific clinical algorithm and safety protocol (Fig. 1), more than 1500 MRI examinations have been safely performed in patients with implantable cardiac devices. Pacemaker-dependent patients were programmed to asynchronous pacing to prevent inappropriate inhibition of pacing due to electromagnetic interference. Those without pacemaker dependence were programmed to a demand pacing mode to prevent inappropriate pacing from noise tracking. Tachycardia therapies and monitoring were disabled. Patients were rigorously monitored using telemetry, blood pressure, and pulse oximetry. Monitoring heart rate using the pulse oximetry signal is important because the ECG telemetry signal is often noisy and uninterpretable during MRI. After MRI, all devices are reinterrogated and programming is restored to original parameters. Of 438 patients reported in the authors' 2011 study, only 3 (1.5%) experienced electrical reset during scanning, but there was no long-term (up to 5 years) device malfunction. Small changes in lead impedances (<0.5%), sensing, and capture threshold were noted; however, these changes were clinically insignificant and did not require system revision or reprogramming.[16]

A recent retrospective review compared 109 patients with pacemakers and ICDs who underwent 125 MRI procedures with a cohort of 50 patients with implantable cardiac devices who did not undergo MRI. The MRI group did not have any deaths, device failures, induced arrhythmias, loss of capture, or power-on-reset episodes. In the MRI group, a small number of patients had decreases in battery voltage greater than or equal to 0.04 V (4%), increase of pacing threshold by greater than or equal to 0.5 V (3%), and changes in lead impedance of greater than or equal to 50 Ω (6%). Although there were statistically significant differences in the lead impedances and pacing thresholds between the control (non-MRI) and MRI group, the magnitude of changes was not clinically important.[5]

The MagnaSafe Registry is a multicenter prospective study designed to investigate device

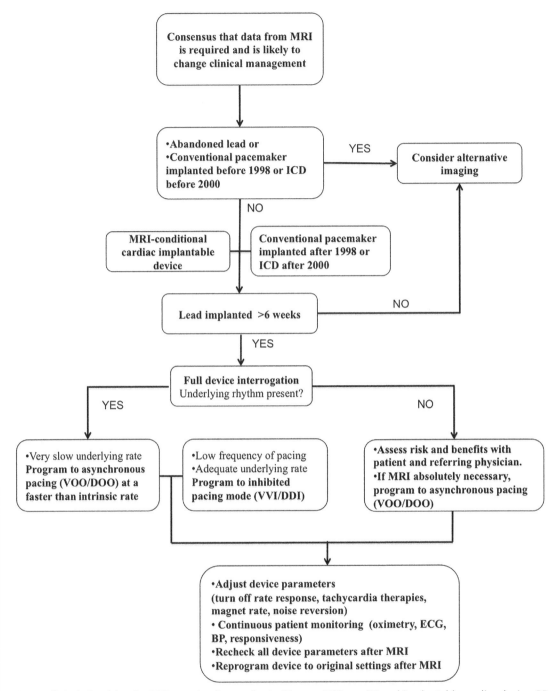

Fig. 1. Clinical algorithm for MRI scanning in a patient with non–MRI-conditional implantable cardiac device. BP, blood pressure; ECG, electrocardiogram.

parameter changes and adverse events in 1500 patients with implantable cardiac devices who undergo nonthoracic MRIs.[21] Preliminary findings as of late 2012 from the first 829 MRI studies (617 pacemakers, 212 ICDs, and 1620 leads) demonstrated no device failure, generator/lead replacement, loss of capture, induced arrhythmias, or death. A change in atrial and ventricular lead impedance of greater than or equal to 50 Ω occurred in 3% of pacemakers and 4% of ICDs. Impedance changes, however, were not associated with changes in atrial or ventricular pacing thresholds or measured electrogram amplitudes.[22]

MRI-CONDITIONAL DEVICES

Given the aforementioned challenges and risks of performing MRI examinations in patients with cardiac implantable devices, device manufacturers have devoted significant resources to the development of pacing systems acceptable for use under specific MRI conditions. The term, *MRI-conditional*, implies minimal hazards in a specified MRI environment under specific conditions of use. Despite the evidence of safety noted in the studies discussed previously, conventional pacemakers and ICDs are technically labeled *MRI-unsafe*.

MRI-conditional devices have redesigned components to minimize the potential for heating, dislodgement, current induction, and electromagnetic interference as a result of static, gradient, and combined field effects. MRI-conditional systems contain fewer ferromagnetic materials and incorporate lead design changes to mitigate heating. Additionally, MRI-conditional systems use a Hall sensor instead of a reed switch or incorporate magnet-detect sensors to prevent reed switch activation in MRI. The Hall sensor is a transducer that varies its output voltage in response to magnetic fields and has a more predictable behavior when exposed to MRI. Software changes include the incorporation of simple programming modes, including MRI pacing mode, that can be activated just before scanning.

In the first reported experience, Forleo and colleagues[23] compared the safety and efficacy between the Medtronic (Minneapolis, MN) EnRhythm MRI-compatible system and conventional dual-chamber pacemakers; 107 patients underwent nonrandomized implantation with either the MRI system (n = 50) or a dual-chamber, active-fixation lead (Medtronic 4076) non–MRI-conditional system (n = 57). At the time of implant and follow-up at 1, 3, 6, and 12 months, there were no cases of high pacing thresholds, inadequate sensing, or lead dislodgement in the 2 groups. The implantation success rate was 100% in both groups, and there were no differences in procedural or fluoroscopic times. There was a trend toward lower successful cephalic vein access (60% vs 68%) and higher rates of subclavian vein use (40% vs 31.6%) for at least 1 lead placement in patients with MRI-conditional leads. This trend may be due to the increased diameter and stiffness of the MRI-conditional leads.[23]

This study led to a prospective, randomized controlled clinical trial to evaluate the safety and effectiveness of an MRI-conditional dual-chamber pacemaker system in a 1.5-T MRI environment.[24] The study randomized 464 pacemaker-dependent and nondependent patients with an implanted Medtronic EnRhythm SureScan Pacemaker system to no MRI (control; n = 204) versus nonclinically indicated MRI examination 9 to 12 weeks after implantation (n = 258). Patients were monitored for arrhythmias, symptoms, and pacemaker system function. Pacemaker parameters were compared in both groups before and after MRI and 1 week and 1 month post-MRI. There were no MRI-related complications, including arrhythmias, loss of capture, pacemaker inhibition, or electrical resets. Changes in pacing capture threshold and sensing amplitude were minimal and did not differ between the 2 groups. This was the first randomized controlled trial that demonstrated patient and pacemaker system safety when exposed to a MRI environment. MRI was initially limited to nonthoracic imaging with anatomic exclusion between C1 and T12 vertebral levels.[24] This study led to the Food and Drug Administration (FDA) approval of the first MRI-conditional pacemaker—Revo MRI SureScan pacing system with CapSureFix MRI SureScan Lead, Model 5086 (Medtronic) and the SureScan software (Medtronic).

Most recently, the Advisa MRI study randomized 263 patients in a 2:1 ratio to chest and head MRI examinations between 9 and 12 weeks post-implant versus no MRI. No MRI-related complications were noted, and differences in pacing capture thresholds were minimal and similar between the MRI and control groups.[25] Based on this study, the FDA has lifted the thoracic restriction for MRI in patients with the SureScan pacing system.[26] This device has also received FDA approval.

NON–FDA-APPROVED DEVICES AND LEADS

All major device manufacturers have developed MRI-conditional devices that have Conformité Européenne (CE) designation for imaging in a 1.5-T MRI (**Table 1**). Thus far, Medtronic's Revo and Advisa MRI SureScan pacemakers are the only systems that have been approved by the FDA. This family of pacemakers is limited to dual-chamber pacemakers. Biotronik (Berlin-Neukölln, Germany) and St. Jude Medical (St. Paul, MN) have developed single-chamber MRI-conditional pacemakers. Medtronic's HF-T series is a CRT pacing (CRT-P) device that is CE approved for use in the MRI environment.

The ProMRI clinical study is a phase B study led by Biotronik that recently received FDA approval to evaluate the Entovis pacemaker system and leads in 245 patients at 35 clinical sites. The study is designed to test the safety and efficacy of

Table 1
Approved MRI-conditional cardiac implantable devices

Device	Manufacturer	Type	Thoracic Exclusion	Lead Fixation
Estella (ProMRI)	Biotronik	Pacemaker	No	Active and passive
Evia (ProMRI) Evia HF-T (ProMRI)	Biotronik	Pacemaker CRT-P	Yes	Active and passive
Advisa DR MRI SureScan[a]	Medtronic	Pacemaker	No	Active and passive
EnRhythm MRI SureScan	Medtronic	Pacemaker	Yes	Active and passive[b]
Ensura MRI SureScan	Medtronic	Pacemaker	No	Active and passive[b]
Revo MRI SureScan[a]	Medtronic	Pacemaker	No	Active and passive
Accent MRI	St. Jude Medical	Pacemaker	No	Active
Advantio MRI	Boston Scientific	Pacemaker	No	Active and passive
Ingenio MRI	Boston Scientific	Pacemaker	No	Active and passive
Reply MRI	Sorin	Pacemaker	No	Active
Lumax 740	Biotronik	ICD CRT-D	No	Active and passive

All devices except Advisa DR MRI SureScan and Revo MRI SureScan are CE approved.
[a] FDA-approved device.
[b] At the time of publication, passive leads are currently CE approved only.

single- and dual-chamber pacemaker systems in full-body MRI scans (without thoracic exclusion).[27] The recently completed phase A of the study evaluated the safety of the pacemaker system during nonthoracic MRI scans.

Currently, FDA-approved leads are specifically active-fixation leads that are silicone coated. They are relatively stiff, are larger in diameter, and have higher friction, making them potentially more challenging to implant. Medtronic has recently developed MRI-compatible polyurethane-coated leads that are thinner and may be easier to implant.[28]

MRI-CONDITIONAL ICD

MRI of patients with ICDs generally share the same risks as those previously discussed with pacemakers. ICDs have some unique features, however, that can affect safety in the MRI environment compared with pacemakers due to their larger size, more complex leads, and presence of capacitors for cardioversion and defibrillation. Additionally, it must be taken into consideration that a typical patient with an ICD has a different cardiac substrate from patients with pacemakers. ICD patients tend to have structural heart disease or history of malignant arrhythmias and, therefore, require continuous ECG monitoring while tachycardia therapies are disabled.

There is currently only 1 ICD and CRT-defibrillator (D) device that is marketed for safe use with MRI. The first MRI-conditional ICD and

CRT-D, Lumax 740 (Biotronik), recently received CE approval for use in an MRI environment under specific conditions.[29] The FDA has recently approved Biotronik's ProMRI technology to be investigated in ICD devices in the United States as part of Phase C of the ProMRI trial.[30] To the authors' knowledge, no published clinical trial has been undertaken with this device.

THORACIC IMAGING WITH MRI-CONDITIONAL DEVICES

Up to 40% of clinically indicated MRI scans include thoracic spinal imaging and cardiac MRI.[14] In the authors' study, thoracic examinations were associated with slightly greater change in capture thresholds and sensing amplitudes.[16] The changes were clinically insignificant, however, in all cases. The recent Advisa MRI study also demonstrated overall safety of thoracic MRI in patients with the SureScan MRI-conditional system.[25] Despite these reassuring results, more safety data are needed from larger registries regarding thoracic MRI examinations in the setting of standard and MRI-conditional pacemakers and ICDs.

Device (in particular ICD)-related artifacts significantly affect the image quality with thoracic MRI examinations. Image distortion and susceptibility artifacts occur within 15 cm of the generator. Device size and position, the imaging plane, and the scanning protocol all have an impact on the severity of image distortion. Steady-state free precession cine imaging is associated with more artifacts than gradient-echo imaging.[31] In the authors' study of conventional cardiac pacemakers and ICDs, it was possible to evaluate cardiac function by cine MRI in 85.5% of examinations in the setting of left-sided ICD/biventricular (BiV)-ICD systems and all MRI examinations in patients with left-sided pacemaker and right-sided pacemaker or ICD systems.[31] Late gadolinium-enhanced (scar) images, however, were significantly compromised. In patients with left-sided ICD/BiV-ICD systems, artifacts on late gadolinium-enhanced images were observed in 53.7% of short-axis image sectors. Future work is needed to reduce image artifacts, in particular the large artifact due to ICD transformers. A promising new study used a wideband inversion pulse for late gadolinium-enhanced MRI to improve image quality in the setting of ICD systems.[32]

PERFORMING 3-T MRI WITH CARDIAC DEVICES

The currently approved MRI-conditional devices (in Europe and the United States) are indicated for use only with 1.5-T MRI systems. Although cardiac and thoracic imaging is often performed at 1.5-T, 3-T scans are increasingly used for neurologic, musculoskeletal, and abdominal imaging. There is limited experience with the safety and efficacy of scanning patients with cardiac devices with 3-T MRI systems, and even less with scanning patients who are pacemaker dependent. In one study, 14 patients with conventional cardiac devices underwent 16 scans (9 pacemakers, 6 ICDs, and 1 loop recorder) at 3-T.[33] The investigators performed device interrogation immediately prior to and after MRI and 1 to 3 months post-MRI. There were no malignant arrhythmias. Furthermore, there were no changes in device parameters, including sensing, impedances, pacing thresholds, or battery parameters.[33] Similar findings were noted in another study of 44 patients with pacemakers undergoing 3-T brain MRI, with additional safety precautions taken using a transmit-receive head coil.[7]

Despite following safety precautions and protocols described previously, unexpected life-threatening events can occur during MRI examinations. Gimble[34,35] reported 2 cases of unexpected inhibition of pacing in a 3-T environment. The first case was a patient with a prior atrioventricular nodal ablation who was pacemaker dependent. The device was programmed to an asynchronous mode (VOO) at maximum output in a bipolar configuration. Immediately after initiation of scanning, the patient had asystole. The scan was discontinued. On further interrogation, it was recognized that the device had reverted to a sensing backup mode (VVI), leaving the patient susceptible to electromagnetic interference and without pacing support for nearly 10 seconds.[34]

In the second reported case, the patient had a previously implanted ICD with underlying sinus bradycardia.[35] The tachycardia therapies were disabled and the pacing mode was programmed to AAI. Pacing was inhibited immediately after the patient was moved to the MRI bore but prior to application of gradient magnetic fields. This phenomena was attributed to a magnetohydrodynamic effect or inhibition of pacing as a result of current induction from the back and forth motion of charged ions in the aortic lumen.[35] Neither patient had any long-term sequelae reported. Despite the lack of long-term effects in either patient, these cases highlight the paramount importance of adequate supervision, presence of well-trained personnel, and an informed, documented consent between patient and physician.

PATIENT SELECTION FOR MRI-CONDITIONAL DEVICES

Although it has been demonstrated that MRI scans of patients with conventional, non–MRI-conditional devices can be performed safely under specific conditions in a controlled environment (**Box 2**), unpredictable life-threatening events can occur, particularly in patients who are pacemaker dependent or have underlying structural heart disease. Rigorous demonstration of safety is of paramount importance, and the strong interest in research and development of MRI-conditional cardiac devices by industry is welcome. As device development continues, there will be an increasing number of MRI-conditional devices in the medical marketplace, and clinicians will be challenged to decide which patients are most likely to benefit from such devices.

To justify benefit, clinicians should be aware of the lifetime prevalence of requiring an MRI. It is estimated that the 1-year and lifetime risks of needing an MRI in patients between 75 and 79 years of age are 7.9% and 46%, respectively. Given the high-lifetime likelihood of MRI utilization, it may be argued that all implants should be MRI-conditional. There are several concerns related to this notion, however: (1) the likelihood of scenarios in which only an MRI suffices to obtain the necessary information for clinical decision making is much less common, (2) the increased cost of MRI-conditional devices is, at present, not trivial, and (3) many first-generation MRI-conditional

Box 2
Tools of the trade: issues to consider when performing an MRI scan on a patient with a cardiac device

- Have an algorithm (eg, see **Fig. 1**) and clinical protocol with trained personnel available during MRI scanning.
- Perform careful device interrogation with lead assessment before and after MRI scanning.
- Patients should be monitored throughout scanning with pulse oximetry, telemetry, and blood pressure. Verbal responsiveness should be assessed frequently.
- Advance cardiac life support–trained personnel and external defibrillator with external pacing capability must be present.
- Recognize device-related restrictions if scanning a conditional device (zonal, specific absorption rates).
- The device programmer should remain outside of the MRI scanner room.
- Recognize that retained leads may pose higher risk of heating.
- A thorough discussion of risk and benefit should be performed along with a documented signed consent between the physician and patient.
- Consider alternative imaging modality if risk outweighs potential benefit.

devices do not have the complex arrhythmia detection algorithms that conventional devices have. Thus, careful and individualized patient selection should be made when considering which device is most appropriate for implantation.

FUTURE IMPLICATIONS

Given the wide range of pacemakers and ICDs available in the market today and the expanding role of biomedical devices and technologies in the management and treatment of medical conditions, design and engineering processes will have a pivotal role in the future of many technologies as they relate to the MRI environment. In addition to pacemakers and ICDs, newer implantable devices that measure intracardiac pressures to manage heart failure and neuromodulation devices for vagus nerve and deep brain stimulation all have potential problematic interactions with the MRI environment and will need attention and design modifications. Furthermore, innovation will be necessary to modify implanted cardiac devices

as they are increasingly used in MRI-guided electrophysiology procedures and various surgical and chemotherapeutic interventions.[10]

Advances in engineering and innovation will be needed to address not only safety but also the impact of devices on MR image quality, cost-effectiveness, and the overall impact on patient care. Reduction in artifacts and image distortion for cardiothoracic imaging are of high importance and will require significant improvement for widespread application.

SUMMARY

The advancement of MRI-conditional cardiac device technology is a significant breakthrough, allowing safe scanning, even without zonal exclusion under specific conditions. MRI scanning of patients with cardiac devices should be undertaken with a multidisciplinary approach that requires trained personnel and equipment and a thorough discussion of risk and benefits between patient and physician.

This technology has led to greater diagnostic options for patients and also greater complexity of clinical issues. Although the clinical trials discussed provide strong evidence that the technology is safe and effective, postmarket data should be analyzed to assess long-term safety and function of these systems and the impact of this technology in real-world scenarios. MRI-conditional devices have mostly been tested and studied in 1.5-T field strength; hence, their use should be limited to that environment. In addition, the effects of multiple scans, abandoned or epicardial leads, and higher magnetic field strength on these devices are largely unknown.

The field of MRI-conditional pacemakers and ICDs is ripe for future investigation in innovation, device and design modification, and better understanding of the impact of this technology on the overall care of patients. Guidelines from professional societies should reflect this changing technological paradigm and provide consensus and guidance regarding MRI in patients with appropriate implantable cardiac devices.

REFERENCES

1. Sutton R, Kanal E, Wilkoff BL, et al. Safety of magnetic resonance imaging of patients with a new Medtronic EnRhythm MRI SureScan pacing system: clinical study design. Trials 2008;9:68.
2. Kalin R, Stanton MS. Current clinical issues for MRI scanning of pacemaker and defibrillator patients. Pacing Clin Electrophysiol 2005;28(4):326–8.

3. Levine GN, Gomes AS, Arai AE, et al. Safety of magnetic resonance imaging in patients with cardiovascular devices: an American Heart Association scientific statement from the Committee on Diagnostic and Interventional Cardiac Catheterization, Council on Clinical Cardiology, and the Council on Cardiovascular Radiology and Intervention: endorsed by the American College of Cardiology Foundation, the North American Society for Cardiac Imaging, and the Society for Cardiovascular Magnetic Resonance. Circulation 2007;116(24):2878–91.

4. Shinbane JS, Colletti PM, Shellock FG. MR in patients with pacemakers and ICDs: defining the issues. J Cardiovasc Magn Reson 2007;9(1):5–13.

5. Cohen JD, Costa HS, Russo RJ. Determining the risks of magnetic resonance imaging at 1.5 tesla for patients with pacemakers and implantable cardioverter defibrillators. Am J Cardiol 2012;110(11):1631–6.

6. Mollerus M, Albin G, Lipinski M, et al. Cardiac biomarkers in patients with permanent pacemakers and implantable cardioverter-defibrillators undergoing an MRI scan. Pacing Clin Electrophysiol 2008;31(10):1241–5.

7. Naehle CP, Meyer C, Thomas D, et al. Safety of brain 3-T MR imaging with transmit-receive head coil in patients with cardiac pacemakers: pilot prospective study with 51 examinations. Radiology 2008;249(3):991–1001.

8. Naehle CP, Strach K, Thomas D, et al. Magnetic resonance imaging at 1.5-T in patients with implantable cardioverter-defibrillators. Am J Cardiol 2009;54(6):549–55.

9. Roguin A, Schwitter J, Vahlhaus C, et al. Magnetic resonance imaging in individuals with cardiovascular implantable electronic devices. Europace 2008;10(3):336–46.

10. Shinbane JS, Colletti PM, Shellock FG. Magnetic resonance imaging in patients with cardiac pacemakers. era of "MR Conditional" designs. J Cardiovasc Magn Reson 2011;13:63.

11. Levine PA. Industry viewpoint: St. Jude Medical: pacemakers, ICDs and MRI. Pacing Clin Electrophysiol 2005;28(4):266–7.

12. Luechinger R, Duru F, Zeijlemaker VA, et al. Pacemaker reed switch behavior in 0.5, 1.5, and 3.0 Tesla magnetic resonance imaging units: are reed switches always closed in strong magnetic fields? Pacing Clin Electrophysiol 2002;25(10):1419–23.

13. Shellock FG, Tkach JA, Ruggieri PM, et al. Cardiac pacemakers, ICDs, and loop recorder: evaluation of translational attraction using conventional ("long-bore") and "short-bore" 1.5- and 3.0-Tesla MR systems. J Cardiovasc Magn Reson 2003;5(2):387–97.

14. Ainslie M, Miller C, Brown B, et al. Cardiac MRI of patients with implanted electrical cardiac devices. Heart 2014;100:363–9.

15. Sommer T, Naehle CP, Yang A, et al. Strategy for safe performance of extrathoracic magnetic resonance imaging at 1.5 tesla in the presence of cardiac pacemakers in non-pacemaker-dependent patients: a prospective study with 115 examinations. Circulation 2006;114(12):1285–92.

16. Nazarian S, Hansford R, Roguin A, et al. A prospective evaluation of a protocol for magnetic resonance imaging of patients with implanted cardiac devices. Ann Intern Med 2011;155(7):415–24.

17. Irnich W, Irnich B, Bartsch C, et al. Do we need pacemakers resistant to magnetic resonance imaging? Europace 2005;7(4):353–65.

18. Roguin A, Zviman MM, Meininger GR, et al. Modern pacemaker and implantable cardioverter/defibrillator systems can be magnetic resonance imaging safe: in vitro and in vivo assessment of safety and function at 1.5 T. Circulation 2004;110(5):475–82.

19. Junttila MJ, Fishman JE, Lopera GA, et al. Safety of serial MRI in patients with implantable cardioverter defibrillators. Heart 2011;97(22):1852–6.

20. Naehle CP, Zeijlemaker V, Thomas D, et al. Evaluation of cumulative effects of MR imaging on pacemaker systems at 1.5 Tesla. Pacing Clin Electrophysiol 2009;32(12):1526–35.

21. Russo RJ. Determining the risks of clinically indicated nonthoracic magnetic resonance imaging at 1.5 T for patients with pacemakers and implantable cardioverter-defibrillators: rationale and design of the MagnaSafe Registry. Am Heart J 2013;165(3):266–72.

22. Russo RJ. Is a change in cardiac device lead impedance after magnetic resonance imaging at 1.5 Tesla associated with other parameter changes?: preliminary results from the MagnaSafe Registry. Heart Rhythm Society 34th Annual Scientific Sessions. May 9, 2013. Denver, CO. (Lecture ID 75513).

23. Forleo GB, Santini L, Della Rocca DG, et al. Safety and efficacy of a new magnetic resonance imaging-compatible pacing system: early results of a prospective comparison with conventional dual-chamber implant outcomes. Heart Rhythm 2010;7(6):750–4.

24. Wilkoff BL, Bello D, Taborsky M, et al. Magnetic resonance imaging in patients with a pacemaker system designed for the magnetic resonance environment. Heart Rhythm 2011;8(1):65–73.

25. Gimbel JR, Bello D, Schmitt M, et al. Randomized trial of pacemaker and lead system for safe scanning at 1.5 Tesla. Heart Rhythm 2013;10(5):685–91.

26. Available at: http://newsroom.medtronic.com/phoenix. zhtml?c=251324&p=irol-newsArticle&ID=1771917&- highlight=. Accessed December 31, 2013.

27. Available at: http://www.biotronik.com/wps/wcm/ connect/int_web/biotronik/newsroom/press_re- leases?p=http://www.biotronik.com/wps/wcm/con- nect/int_web/biotronik/newsroom/press_releases/ press_release_expansion_of_promri&pw=770&pt=. Accessed December 31, 2013.

28. Santini L, Forleo GB, Santini M. Evaluating MRI- compatible pacemakers: patient data now paves the way to widespread clinical application? Pacing Clin Electrophysiol 2013;36(3):270–8.

29. Lobodzinski SS. Recent innovations in the develop- ment of magnetic resonance imaging conditional pacemakers and implantable cardioverter-defibrilla- tors. Cardiol J 2012;19(1):98–104.

30. Available at: http://biotronik.com/wps/wcm/connect/ int_web/biotronik/newsroom/press_releases?p5http:// www.biotronik.com/wps/wcm/connect/int_web/bio- tronik/newsroom/press_releases/press_release_ expansion_of_promri&pw5770&pt5. Accessed April 3, 2014.

31. Sasaki T, Hansford R, Zviman MM, et al. Quantitative assessment of artifacts on cardiac magnetic reso- nance imaging of patients with pacemakers and implantable cardioverter-defibrillators. Circ Cardio- vasc Imaging 2011;4(6):662–70.

32. Stevens SM, Tung R, Rashid S, et al. Device artifact reduction for magnetic resonance imag- ing of patients with implantable cardioverter- defibrillators and ventricular tachycardia: late gadolinium enhancement correlation with elec- troanatomic mapping. Heart Rhythm 2014;11: 289–98.

33. Gimbel JR. Magnetic resonance imaging of implant- able cardiac rhythm devices at 3.0 tesla. Pacing Clin Electrophysiol 2008;31(7):795–801.

34. Gimbel JR. Unexpected asystole during 3T magnetic resonance imaging of a pacemaker-dependent pa- tient with a 'modern' pacemaker. Europace 2009; 11(9):1241–2.

35. Gimbel JR. Unexpected pacing inhibition upon exposure to the 3T static magnetic field prior to im- aging acquisition: what is the mechanism? Heart Rhythm 2011;8(6):944–5.

New Approaches to Decrease Cardiac Implantable Electronic Device Infections

Matthew J. Kolek, MD[a], Christopher R. Ellis, MD[b],*

KEYWORDS

- Cardiac implantable electronic devices (CIEDs) • Pacemaker • Implantable cardioverter defibrillator
- Infection • Complication • Endocarditis

KEY POINTS

- Cardiac implantable electronic device (CIED) infections are becoming increasingly more common.
- CIED infections are associated with considerable morbidity, mortality, and cost.
- Rates of CIED infections are lowest when devices are implanted in high-volume centers by experienced operators.
- Careful antimicrobial stewardship at the time of CIED implantation is crucial to prevent infections.
- Evidence-based strategies to prevent CIED infections include the use of prophylactic antibiotics, chlorhexidine-alcohol skin preparation, and antibiotic-impregnated pulse generator envelopes.

INTRODUCTION

The number of cardiac implantable electronic devices (CIEDs) implanted in the United States has grown rapidly over the past 2 decades. This trend is due to expanding indications, based on findings from landmark clinical trials that have shown the benefits of cardiac resynchronization therapy (CRT) and prophylactic implantable cardioverter-defibrillators (ICDs), as well as the need for permanent pacing in our aging patient population.[1–3] As a result, CIEDs are implanted in increasingly complex patients with multiple comorbidities. Accordingly, CIED infections, defined broadly as infections involving the generator implant site (pocket) and/or intravascular hardware, have become increasingly common. In fact, the increase in incidence of CIED infections has outpaced the growth in device implantation, in large part due to the medical complexity of today's CIED patients.[2,4,5] The incidence in large registries and controlled trials ranges from 1.6% to 3%.[4,6–8] Infected patients present with a spectrum of signs and symptoms that might be localized to the device generator pocket or represent life-threatening systemic illness (**Box 1**).[9,10]

CIED infections are associated with increased morbidity, mortality, and health care expenditures.[1,4,7,11] As a result, the importance of preventing CIED infections cannot be overstated. Most CIED infections occur because of bacterial seeding at the time of implantation, revision, or generator replacement. Therefore, careful "antimicrobial stewardship" is crucial for prevention. Important methods include meticulous sterile technique; appropriate training and supervision of electrophysiology (EP) laboratory personnel, fellows,

Disclosures: Christopher R. Ellis: Speaker fees/honorarium (modest <$5000/yr) from TyRX Pharmaceuticals (now a subsidiary of Medtronic Inc.); Research funding from Boston Scientific (significant >$100,000).
[a] Department of Cardiovascular Medicine, Vanderbilt Heart and Vascular Institute, 1211 21st Avenue South, Nashville, TN 37232-8802, USA; [b] Cardiac Electrophysiology, Vanderbilt Heart and Vascular Institute, 5414 Medical Center East, Nashville, TN 37232-8802, USA
* Corresponding author.
E-mail address: Christopher.ellis@vanderbilt.edu

Card Electrophysiol Clin 6 (2014) 279–284
http://dx.doi.org/10.1016/j.ccep.2014.02.007
1877-9182/14/$ – see front matter © 2014 Elsevier Inc. All rights reserved.

and students; minimization of procedure times; implantation by board-certified electrophysiologists at high-volume centers; and timing of device implantation to occur just before discharge for inpatients. Recent controlled trials have identified additional methods for preventing CIED infections and are reviewed here.

RISK FACTORS FOR CIED INFECTIONS

The recent increase in CIED infections is likely due to implantation in younger patients with multiple comorbidities, who subsequently require serial device generator changes and lead revisions. Patient and procedural characteristics that are risk factors for infection have been described and are presented in **Table 1**. A recent review of device-related infections in Medicare patients by Arnold Greenspon and colleagues demonstrated an exponential rise in the odds of a CIED-related

infection with each subsequent pocket entry (ie, 3rd, 4th, 5th device pulse generator change associated with up to 16.9-fold increase in infection rate, **Table 2**).

PREVENTION OF CIED INFECTIONS

Optimal skin preparation is crucial for preventing surgical site infections. Chlorhexidine-alcohol scrub has been shown to be superior to povidone-iodine at preventing surgical infections (41% relative risk reduction).[12] In addition, perioperative antibiotics play an important role in the prevention of surgical site infection for many types of procedures.[13] de Oliveira and colleagues[14] conducted a randomized, placebo controlled trial of perioperative cefazolin at the time of CIED implantation or generator exchange. The trial was stopped early due to an 81% reduction in CIED infections in the cefazolin group. We routinely administer cefazolin (or vancomycin for penicillin-allergic patients) at the time of device implantation, revision, or generator exchange. However, some investigators have advocated the routine use of vancomycin for prophylaxis, given temporal trends in bacterial drug resistance (**Table 3**). Jan and colleagues[15] evaluated microbiological isolates in a large cohort of patients with confirmed CIED infections, showing that 86% of isolates were *Staphylococcus* species with a 30.5% rate of resistance to oxacillin. Conversely, 100% of Staph isolates were susceptible to vancomycin. In a separate single center study of patients who suffered from a CIED infection, 78% of culture-positive cases had *Staph* isolates, and the proportion of all

Table 1
Risk factors for cardiac implantable electronic device infection

Risk Factor	Odds Ratio	References
Diabetes	3.2–3.4	6,24
Renal insufficiency	4.6–6.3	6,24,25
Systemic anticoagulation	2.8–3.4	6,24
Chronic steroid therapy	13.9	26
Preimplant fever	8.7	27
Prior device infection	—	26
Three or more leads	5.4	26
Early pocket reentry	7–16.3	14,27
Device revision/generator change	1.7–3.1	6,14,24

Table 2
Risk of cardiac implantable electronic device infection as a function of the number of subsequent procedures (eg, pulse generator exchanges) after index procedure

Effect	Level	Hazard Ratio	P-value
Age	80–84 vs 65–69	0.766	.0172
	>85 vs 65–69	0.677	.0061
Renal failure	Yes vs No	1.56	<.0001
No. of operation	2 vs 1	2.886	<.0001
	3 vs 1	8.15	<.0001
	4 vs 1	14.4	<.0001
	5 vs 1	16.9	<.0001

Data from Patel JP, Kurtz SM, Lau E, et al. Removal/replacement procedures and deep infection risk for pacemakers and ICDs in the United States: Medicare Analysis from 1997 to 2010. Denver (CO): Heart Rhythm Scientific Sessions; 2013.

Table 3
Temporal trends in microbiological isolates from patients with cardiac implantable electronic device infection

Study	Nᵃ	S aureus (%)	MSSA (%)	MRSA (%)	CNS (%)	Other (%)
Chua et al,[22] 2000	99	24	—	—	68	8
Sohail et al,[26] 2007	26	43	35	8	35	22
Klug et al,[27] 2007	32	19	—	—	72	9
de Oliveira et al,[14] 2009	13	62	54	8	38	0
Tarakji et al,[10] 2010	414	36	20	16	44	20
Sohail et al,[16] 2011	63	51	37	14	27	22
Jan et al,[15] 2011	252	10	8	2	75	15
Athan et al,[23] 2012	149	42	24	17	38	20
Kolek et al,[8] 2012	13	31	15	15	31	38

Abbreviations: CNS, coagulase negative *Staphylococcus*; MRSA, methicillin resistant *S aureus*; MSSA, methicillin sensitive *S aureus*; *S aureus*, *Staphylococcus aureus*.
ᵃ Number of positive isolates from patients with cardiac implantable electronic device infection.

methicillin resistance among these was 53%. However, the use of cefazolin, as compared with vancomycin, for antimicrobial prophylaxis at implantation was not associated with early CIED infection (odds ratio 0.89, $P = .84$).[16] These studies highlight the evolving proportions of resistant CIED pathogens and the need for further randomized studies of prophylactic antibiotic regimens.

Most CIED infections occur as a result of bacterial seeding during device implantation or revision. Da Costa and colleagues[17] collected specimens for bacterial culture from patients at the time of pacemaker implantation and found that 37% of device pockets were colonized with bacteria (mostly *Staphylococcus* species) just before suturing. Factors such as implanting center volume, operator training and experience, and procedural time play an important role in prevention. Freeman and colleagues[10] analyzed the rates of complications (including CIED infections) after ICD implantation by hospital volume in 224,233 patients in the National Cardiovascular Data Registry. They found that patients who had their procedure at centers in the bottom quartile for volume were more likely to suffer a complication than those at centers in the top quartile (adjusted odds ratio 1.26). In centers within the lowest quartile, less than 50% of devices were implanted by a board-certified electrophysiologist, compared with more than 80% in the highest volume quartile. These findings highlight the importance of technical aspects of CIED implantations, including center volume, EP laboratory procedures, and operator training and experience, in the prevention of device infections.

The recently developed, Food and Drug Administration–approved AIGISRx antibacterial envelope (TyRX Inc, Monmouth Junction, NJ, USA) has shown great promise as a new tool in the authors' armamentarium to prevent CIED infections. This polypropylene envelope releases minocycline and rifampin from a bioresorbable polyarylate polymer over approximately 7 days, directly into the CIED generator pocket (**Fig. 1**). In an animal model of direct bacterial inoculation into the device pocket, the AIGISRx envelope showed excellent activity against *Staphylococcus epidermidis, Staphylococcus capitis, Escherichia coli,* and *Acinetobacter baumannii.*[19] Importantly, systemic levels of minocycline and rifampin were undetectable. In the Cooperative Multicenter study Monitoring a CIED Antimicrobial Device (COMMAND) study, implantation success rate was 99% and

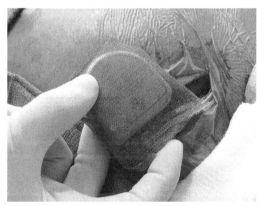

Fig. 1. ICD generator with an antibacterial envelope just before implantation.

use of the antibacterial envelope was associated with a very low 0.48% incidence of infection in 624 patients.[20]

The AIGISRx antibacterial envelope became available for use at the authors' institution in August 2009. Based on available clinical trials data and expert opinion, use of the device was indicated for patients with more than or equal to 2 CIED risk factors: diabetes mellitus, chronic kidney disease (serum creatinine ≥1.5 mg/dL), systemic anticoagulation, chronic systemic corticosteroid use, leukocytosis greater than or equal to 11,000 white blood cell/μL within 24 hours of implantation, prior CIED infection, greater than or equal to 3 leads, pacemaker dependence, and early pocket reentry (within 2 weeks). To date, the authors have implanted approximately 400 envelopes.

The AIGISRx envelope consists of 2 rectangular sheets of polypropylene mesh joined together on 3 sides by a 3-mm seam. The device pocket should be upsized by approximately 10% to 15% by volume to accommodate the envelope. Leaving the envelope submerged in saline or antibacterial solution should be avoided as some of the antibacterial granules might dissolve (as evidenced by orange discoloration of fluid). Likewise, aggressive irrigation and suctioning of the pocket with the pulse generator housed within the envelope should be avoided. The authors' practice has been to invert the envelope so that the seam is on the inside, moisten it in solution to reduce friction, and place the pulse generator within it once all leads are connected. This may not be advisable with the bioresorbable AIGISRx, as the seam is weaker the envelope may tear when inverted. The authors irrigate the pocket just before inserting the pulse generator and envelope (see **Fig. 1**).

Some electrophysiologists have expressed concerns about the difficulty of generator exchange or device revision after the AIGISRx envelope has been implanted for an extended period of time.[9] It has been found that removal of the envelope is best accomplished if it and the pulse generator are removed as a unit. Although this is feasible in most patients, it does require additional time for careful dissection, and care must be taken to avoid excessive heating in the pocket, which may damage lead insulation. A new, bioabsorbable version of the envelope is currently available, which should reduce some of these concerns. The authors have transitioned to its use over the prior generation AIGISRx; however, pricing concerns may affect widespread adoption.

A controlled study of the AIGISRx antibacterial envelope was conducted in 899 patients with at least 2 CIED infection risk factors. After a mean follow-up period of 18.7 ± 7.7 months (minimum 90 days), the incidence of CIED infection was 0.4% in AIGISRx recipients and 3% in controls. This difference persisted after full adjustment for covariates (odds ratio 0.09, 95% confidence interval 0.01 to 0.73, P = .02).[8] Given the absolute risk reduction of 2.6% seen in the authors' study, approximately 40 patients would need to be treated, on average, to prevent one CIED infection. At a unit cost of $895 for the larger, ICD version of the AIGISRx envelope, the cost savings from preventing one CIED infection would have to be $35,800 in order for the envelope to be cost neutral. Data from a recent analysis of the Nationwide Inpatient Sample of hospital discharge records indicated that the average inpatient charges for the treatment of a CIED infection were $146,000, well beyond this break-even point. Therefore, not even considering decreased morbidity, mortality, and the increase in quality-adjusted life years, use of the AIGISRx envelope in carefully selected patients at increased risk for CIED infections should be economically feasible. A formal multicenter prospective randomized controlled trial using the bioresorbable AIGISRx-R is being designed and will provide essential data on the size of its treatment effect.

TREATMENT OF CIED INFECTIONS

A comprehensive review of the management of CIED infections is beyond the scope of this article, but can be found in a recent review by Nof and Epstein.[9] The cornerstone of treatment of CIED infections is to remove all infected hardware whenever possible. At the authors' institution, they use a multidisciplinary approach including clinical experts in transvenous lead extraction, cardiovascular imaging, infectious diseases, and cardiac surgery. Once blood cultures are obtained, parenteral antibiotics targeting skin pathogens are administered. After careful planning with special consideration given to patients who are pacemaker dependent or at high risk for ventricular arrhythmias, hardware is explanted typically using laser-powered excimer sheaths and other contemporary methods. Sometimes bulky vegetations require surgical removal (**Fig. 2**), which is usually performed via a small lateral thoracotomy at their center. Other cases are best handled with a hybrid approach using transvenous and open surgical methods to accomplish full system removal while minimizing risks to the patient. The length of antibiotic therapy is individualized but is generally continued for 14 days after removal of infected hardware or a minimum of 6 weeks if hardware removal is not possible or if additional cardiac vegetations are present. Decisions regarding reimplantation must also be highly individualized, with

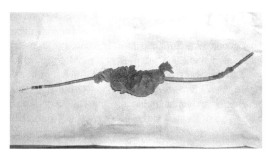

Fig. 2. Massive ICD lead vegetation adherent to the tricuspid valve and right atrial wall.

careful consideration of continued indication for a CIED, pacemaker dependence with requirement for temporary pacing, and the presence of cardiac vegetations and foreign materials such as dialysis shunts and prosthetic joint implants that might serve as a reservoir of infection. Early (<1 week) CIED device reimplantation is acceptable when there is no evidence of systemic infection (pocket infection/local erosion), and the device is reimplanted on the contralateral side.

OUTCOMES AND COMPLICATIONS

CIED infections are associated with increased morbidity, mortality, and health care expenditures. In a study of the National Hospital Discharge Survey from 1996 to 2003, Voigt and colleagues[1] reported that the adjusted odds ratio for mortality in patients who developed a CIED infection was 2.41. de Bie and colleagues[7] found a similar odds ratio for mortality of 2.4 for patients who suffered a CIED infection in a large, single center study. Importantly, among Medicare recipients with CIED infections, women were found to have a higher long-term mortality than men.[21] The clinical management of CIED infections frequently includes prolonged hospitalization; parenteral antibiotics; consultation with experts in cardiac EP, infectious diseases, and cardiac surgery; device explantation; and, if indicated, reimplantation.[22,23] In 2008, the average inpatient charges for a patient with a CIED infection were $146,000, although total costs of care can frequently exceed $1,000,000 per case.[2,4] Although techniques for extraction of infected CIED systems continue to evolve, evidence-based strategies for prevention are the mainstay of reducing the overall health care burden of this important complication.

SUMMARY AND RECOMMENDATIONS

The number of CIEDs implanted annually has risen rapidly over the past 2 decades, in large part because of expanded indications for primary

prevention ICDs and cardiac resynchronization therapy. Devices are being implanted in patients with multiple medical comorbidities. In addition, many patients, particularly those with primary prevention ICDs, are living longer with devices, necessitating multiple generator changes and device revisions. These factors have all contributed to a rising incidence of CIED infections. Strategies to prevent CIED infections that should be universally applied include meticulous sterile technique, appropriate training of EP laboratory personnel, and minimization of procedure times. Perioperative antibiotics and chlorhexidine-alcohol skin preparation have been shown to reduce infections in randomized studies and should be used routinely. In addition, several risk factors for CIED infection have been established, and patients with these should receive particular scrutiny. Because complications including CIED infections occur with the least frequency at high-volume centers where operators are most likely to be certified electrophysiologists, patients at high risk for infections should be considered for referral to these centers. Antibacterial envelopes (AIGISRx) have shown efficacy in preventing CIED infections in high-risk patients, although formal randomized controlled trial data are needed. Finally, if an infection is suspected, the patient should promptly be referred to an experienced center for comprehensive CIED management.

REFERENCES

1. Voigt A, Shalaby A, Saba S. Rising rates of cardiac rhythm management device infections in the United States: 1996 through 2003. J Am Coll Cardiol 2006; 48:590.
2. Ellis CR, Kolek MJ. Rising infection rate in cardiac electronic device implantation; the role of the AIGISRx® antibacterial envelope in prophylaxis. Comb Prod Ther 2011,1.1–9.
3. Kurtz SM, Ochoa JA, Lau E, et al. Implantation trends and patient profiles for pacemakers and implantable cardioverter defibrillators in the United States: 1993-2006. Pacing Clin Electrophysiol 2010;33:705–11.
4. Greenspon AJ, Patel JD, Lau E, et al. 16-year trends in the infection burden for pacemakers and implantable cardioverter-defibrillators in the United States 1993 to 2008. J Am Coll Cardiol 2011;58:1001–6.
5. Cabell CH, Heidenreich PA, Chu VH, et al. Increasing rates of cardiac device infections among medicare beneficiaries: 1990–1999. Am Heart J 2004;147:582–6.
6. Lekkerkerker JC, van Nieuwkoop C, Trines SA, et al. Risk factors and time delay associated with cardiac

device infections: Leiden device registry. Heart 2009;95:715–20.

7. de Bie MK, van Rees JB, Thijssen J, et al. Cardiac device infections are associated with a significant mortality risk. Heart Rhythm 2012;9:494–8.

8. Kolek MJ, Dresen WF, Wells QS, et al. Use of an antibacterial envelope is associated with reduced cardiac implantable electronic device infections in high-risk patients. Pacing Clin Electrophysiol 2012; 36:354–61.

9. Nof E, Epstein LM. Complications of cardiac implants: handling device infections. Eur Heart J 2013;34:229–36.

10. Tarakji KG, Chan EJ, Cantillon DJ, et al. Cardiac implantable electronic device infections: presentation, management, and patient outcomes. Heart Rhythm 2010;7:1043–7.

11. Sohail MR, Henrikson CA, Braid-Forbes MJ, et al. Mortality and cost associated with cardiovascular implantable electronic device infections. Arch Intern Med 2011;171:1821–8.

12. Darouiche RO, Wall MJ Jr, Itani KM, et al. Chlorhexidine–alcohol versus povidone–iodine for surgical-site antisepsis. N Engl J Med 2010;362:18–26.

13. Forbes SS, McLean RF. Review article: the anesthesiologist's role in the prevention of surgical site infections. Can J Anaesth 2013;60:176–83.

14. de Oliveira JC, Martinelli M, Nishioka SA, et al. Efficacy of antibiotic prophylaxis before the implantation of pacemakers and cardioverter-defibrillators. Circ Arrhythm Electrophysiol 2009;2:29.

15. Jan E, Camou F, Texier-maugein J, et al. Microbiologic characteristics and in vitro susceptibility to antimicrobials in a large population of patients with cardiovascular implantable electronic device infection. J Cardiovasc Electrophysiol 2011;23:375–81.

16. Sohail MR, Hussain S, Le KY, et al. Risk factors associated with early- versus late-onset implantable cardioverter-defibrillator infections. J Interv Card Electrophysiol 2011;31:171–83.

17. Da Costa A, Lelievre H, Kirkorian G, et al. Role of the preaxillary flora in pacemaker infections a prospective study. Circulation 1998;97(18):1791–5.

18. Freeman JV, Wang Y, Curtis JP, et al. The relation between hospital procedure volume and complications of cardioverter-defibrillator implantation from the Implantable Cardioverter-Defibrillator Registry. J Am Coll Cardiol 2010;56:1133–9.

19. Hansen LK, Brown M, Johnson D, et al. In vivo model of human pathogen infection and demonstration of efficacy by an antimicrobial pouch for pacing devices. Pacing Clin Electrophysiol 2009; 32:898–907.

20. Bloom HL, Constantin L, Dan D, et al, COoperative Multicenter study Monitoring a CIED ANtimicrobial Device Investigators. Implantation success and infection in cardiovascular implantable electronic device procedures utilizing an antibacterial envelope. Pacing Clin Electrophysiol 2011;34:133–42.

21. Sohail MR, Henrikson CA, Braid-Forbes MJ, et al. Comparison of mortality in women versus men with infections involving cardiovascular implantable electronic device. Am J Cardiol 2013;112:1403–9.

22. Chua JD, Wilkoff BL, Lee I, et al. Diagnosis and management of infections involving implantable electrophysiologic cardiac devices. Ann Intern Med 2000; 133:604–8.

23. Athan E, Chu VH, Tattevin P, et al. Clinical characteristics and outcome of infective endocarditis involving implantable cardiac devices. JAMA 2012; 307:1727–35.

24. Bloom H, Heeke B, Leon A, et al. Renal insufficiency and the risk of infection from pacemaker or defibrillator surgery. Pacing Clin Electrophysiol 2006;29: 142–5.

25. Dasgupta A, Montalvo J, Medendorp S, et al. Increased complication rates of cardiac rhythm management devices in ESRD patients. Am J Kidney Dis 2007;49:656–63.

26. Sohail MR, Uslan DZ, Khan AH, et al. Risk factor analysis of permanent pacemaker infection. Clin Infect Dis 2007;45:166–73.

27. Klug D, Balde M, Pavin D, et al. Risk factors related to infections of implanted pacemakers and cardioverter-defibrillators: results of a large prospective study. Circulation 2007;116:1349–55.

How the Subcutaneous Implantable Cardioverter Defibrillator Works

Indications/Limitations and Special Groups to Consider

Ian Crozier, MD*, Darren Hooks, PhD, MBChB,
Matthew Daly, MBChB, Iain Melton, MBChB

KEYWORDS

- Defibrillation • Implantable defibrillator • Subcutaneous • Transvenous • Ventricular fibrillation
- Ventricular tachycardia • Sudden cardiac death

KEY POINTS

- The subcutaneous implantable cardioverter defibrillator (S-ICD) is an important, recently introduced alternative to conventional transvenous defibrillators.
- The S-ICD has some theoretic advantages over transvenous defibrillators.
- The S-ICD is easily implanted without fluoroscopy.
- The S-ICD has minimal programmability.
- The S-ICD avoids the procedural risks and long-term hazards of transvenous lead implantation.
- The S-ICD effectively detects and terminates ventricular fibrillation.
- The S-ICD inappropriate shock rate is comparable with that of transvenous defibrillators.
- The S-ICD is not suitable for patients who require cardiac pacing but can be combined with a separate bipolar pacemaker.
- Long-term follow-up is awaited, and a randomized trial comparing the subcutaneous and transvenous defibrillators is under way.

INTRODUCTION

The subcutaneous implantable cardioverter defibrillator (S-ICD) (**Figs. 1–3**) has recently joined the growing ranks of cardiac implantable electronic devices (CIED). It is estimated that 3 million patients have CIEDs in North America, and that 120,000 implantable cardioverter defibrillators (ICDs) are implanted annually.[1] Approximately 3000 S-ICDs have been implanted worldwide, and we project that the proportion of patients with CIED who have S-ICDs will increase dramatically over the next decade.

CIEDs perform several functions: cardiac pacemakers, first introduced in 1958,[2] are the most commonly implanted and treat only bradycardia. ICDs terminate potentially life-threatening ventricular arrhythmias with shock therapy. ICDs were first introduced in 1980 and initially required epicardial components[3] but rapidly evolved to the transvenous ICD (T-ICD) with a prepectoral generator and right ventricular lead.[4] The addition

Disclosures: I. Crozier and I. Melton were investigators for Cameron Health. I. Crozier speaker's bureau for Cameron Health.
Department of Cardiology, Christchurch Hospital, PO Bag 4710, Christchurch 8140, New Zealand
* Corresponding author.
E-mail address: Ian.crozier@cdhb.govt.nz

Card Electrophysiol Clin 6 (2014) 285–295
http://dx.doi.org/10.1016/j.ccep.2014.02.005
1877-9182/14/$ – see front matter © 2014 Elsevier Inc. All rights reserved.

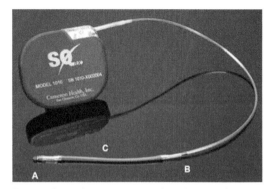

Fig. 1. The subcutaneous implantable cardioverter defibrillator (S-ICD) system. (A) Distal sense electrode. (B) Proximal sense electrode. (C) Shock coil electrode. (*Courtesy of* Boston Scientific, Natick, MA.)

of antitachycardia pacing[5] has reduced the need for shock therapy.[6] ICDs have been clearly shown to be lifesaving and superior to drug therapy in patients with resuscitated ventricular fibrillation or ventricular tachycardia with syncope or impaired left ventricular function.[7] ICDs have also been shown to improve survival in patients at increased risk of sudden cardiac death because of life-threatening ventricular arrhythmias, as marked by impaired cardiac function, either because of previous myocardial infarction[8] or associated with congestive heart failure.[9]

Despite their lifesaving ability, the clinical usefulness of T-ICDs has been compromised by complications, especially those related to the transvenous lead. Implanted into the right ventricle, the transvenous lead performs sensing,

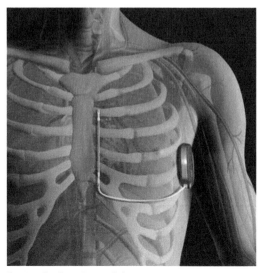

Fig. 2. The locations of the S-ICD system components in situ. (*Courtesy of* Boston Scientific, Natick, MA.)

pacing, and defibrillation functions. During shock application, current passes between a coil integrated into the lead and the defibrillator body, usually placed in the left infraclavicular region.

The transvenous lead is the major contributor to implantation complications with T-ICDs. This complication rate is as high as 10% and includes vascular injury, cardiac perforation and tamponade, arrhythmia induction, pneumothorax and hemothorax, and vascular obstruction.[10] Furthermore, transvenous leads have poor durability, with up to 40% failing by 8 years,[11] manifesting as inappropriate shock delivery caused by sensing of spurious signals misinterpreted as a malignant ventricular arrhythmia, or failure to deliver shock therapy because of shorting of high voltage components.

Reoperation for lead failure results in the need for lead extraction, with its associated risks. Alternatively, additional transvenous leads may be implanted, further increasing the risk of venous obstruction. Despite the overall advances in ICD design and features since 1980, lead failure rates remain high. In an attempt to reduce lead diameter, both the Medtronic Fidelis[12] and St Jude Riata[13] leads were produced and commonly implanted in the last decade and have experienced high failure rates, shaking the faith of both patients and physicians in ICDs.

A transvenous lead may not be able to be implanted in the right ventricle because of anatomic constraints. These patients include those with congenital heart disease with abnormal venous anatomy, and patients with venous obstruction, most commonly because of a previous CIED.

These lead-related issues provided the impetus for the development of the S-ICD, a defibrillator that can deliver lifesaving shock therapy for malignant ventricular arrhythmias, albeit at the cost of no antitachycardia pacing, and only limited post-shock backup pacing.[14]

DEFIBRILLATION IN TRANSVENOUS AND SUBCUTANEOUS DEFIBRILLATORS

Defibrillation requires the generation of a sufficient voltage gradient over enough of the myocardium to terminate fibrillation. The critical mass hypothesis postulates that a voltage gradient of ≈ 5 V per cm over $\approx 90\%$ of the myocardium is required for efficient defibrillation.[15,16] Although transvenous systems readily achieve this target, they result in areas with voltage gradients of more than 30 V per cm near the transvenous lead.[17] These high voltage gradients have been shown to damage myocytes in animal models, an effect known as electroporation, and clinically manifest by

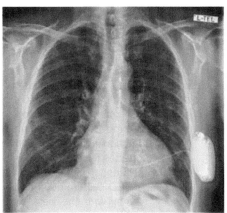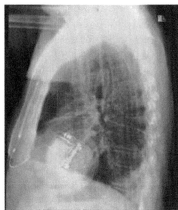

Fig. 3. Postoperative chest radiograph showing that the parasternal lead including the proximal electrode is adjacent to the midline and that the defibrillator is over the apex in the lateral view.

transient decreases in contractility and troponin release, and at voltage gradients greater than 50 V per cm electrical stunning and postshock ventricular arrhythmias.[18–22]

In contrast, the S-ICD more closely approximates an ideal model of defibrillation. By placing electrodes farther from the heart, myocardial voltage gradients are expected to be more spatially uniform. Although the S-ICD requires approximately 3 times greater energy delivery than a T-ICD to effect defibrillation (mean defibrillation threshold of 36.6 ± 19.8 J vs 11.1 ± 8.5 J[14]), only ≃10% of the energy is delivered to the heart,[23] and potentially damaging high voltage gradients are minimized.[17]

Table 1 shows a comparison of subcutaneous and T-ICDs.

PRECLINICAL DEVELOPMENT

Subcutaneous defibrillation was explored before the first human ICD implant[24] but was not pursued, presumably because of size and energy constraints. In the last decade, pediatric patients with congenital heart disease and no possibility of transvenous lead placement have forced the development of hybrid subcutaneous defibrillation systems. These systems used a combination of conventional T-ICDs connected to subcutaneous arrays but still required epicardial leads for cardiac

Table 1
Comparison of S-ICDs and T-ICDs

T-ICD	S-ICD
Established technology with proven benefits	Novel technology with limited experience and follow-up
Effectively detects and terminates ventricular fibrillation	Effectively detects and terminates ventricular fibrillation
Provides pacing for bradycardia, resynchronization, and tachycardia termination	Does not pace, apart from limited postshock pacing
Dependent on transvenous lead with documented reliability issues	Subcutaneous lead with potential but not proven long-term reliability
Implantation requires venous and right ventricular access	Can be implanted in patients without venous access or with complex cardiac anatomy
Device and lead explantation moderately risky	Explantation easy and low risk (initial experience only)
Highly programmable	Limited programmability
Lower shock strength	High shock strength (80 J)
High myocardial voltage gradients	Lower myocardial voltage gradients
Small device	Larger device

sensing and pacing.[25,26] Although these hybrid systems were shown to be effective in small case series,[25,26] they could not deliver the higher energies that would be required in most adult patients and are not suitable for routine implantation.

Simultaneously, the concept of a dedicated S-ICD was revisited.[27] The development of a purpose-built S-ICD that could reliably detect and terminate ventricular fibrillation required that several key technical challenges be overcome. These challenges included determining an effective and practical defibrillation vector and lead configuration, manufacturing a defibrillator with greater shock strength than a T-ICD, and developing a system that could reliably detect ventricular fibrillation without intracardiac or epicardial leads.

Early animal studies showed that, although defibrillation could be achieved in immature pigs, adult pigs required higher energies than are available in transvenous devices.[25] Canine studies confirmed that defibrillation could be achieved with 2 electrodes over the left parasternal region and apex, with a mean defibrillation threshold of 35 ± 16 J.[28]

To extend this concept to humans, several experimental studies were performed comparing a variety of electrode configurations in patients undergoing conventional defibrillator implants. Burke and colleagues[29] reported that defibrillation could be achieved in most patients with 50 J or less between a left pectoral pocket, and an apical cutaneous patch, whereas Lieberman and colleagues[30] showed that an anterior-posterior configuration resulted in lower defibrillation thresholds. Bardy and colleagues[14] investigated a range of left pectoral configurations for subcutaneous electrodes. Modeling studies suggested that defibrillation vectors using electrodes/generators placed on the right and left thorax resulted in lower predicted defibrillation thresholds than left-sided implants,[17] but to simplify the implantation and avoid the risks of leads crossing the midline, only unilateral left-sided placements were assessed. The lowest defibrillation threshold was obtained with defibrillation between an apical generator and an 8-cm left parasternal electrode. This strategy produced a mean defibrillation threshold of 36.6 ± 19.8 J, compared with 11.1 ± 8.5 J for transvenous defibrillation in the same patients.[14,31] Pectoral generators and shorter parasternal electrodes resulted in higher defibrillation thresholds.[14]

THE DEFIBRILLATOR SYSTEM

The only commercially available S-ICD is the Boston/Cameron Health system (Boston Scientific,

Natick, MA.). It consists of an electrically active pulse generator connected to a 3-mm-diameter tripolar parasternal lead positioned parallel to and 1 to 2 cm to the left of the sternal midline (see **Figs. 1–3**). The lead has an 8-cm shocking coil flanked by 2 sensing electrodes. The distal sensing electrode is positioned adjacent to the manubrial-sternal junction, and the proximal sensing electrode is positioned adjacent to the xiphoid. Detection signals are derived from the 2 sense electrodes (labeled A and B in **Fig. 1**) or between either sense electrode and the pulse generator. The S-ICD system automatically selects the sensing vector with the best signal for rhythm detection. Once signals are validated as free of noise and double detection, system beat discrimination, followed by rate detection, is used to determine rhythm type and the need for therapy. A conditional discrimination zone incorporating a feature extraction technique can be programmed between 170 and 240 bpm to avoid treating supraventricular tachycardia (SVT). Ventricular tachyarrhythmia reconfirmation follows capacitor charging to avoid shocking nonsustained ventricular tachyarrhythmias. All shocks are biphasic 80 J, with polarity reversal possible. In addition, 50-bpm demand pacing is available after shock for 30 seconds using a 200-mA biphasic transthoracic pulse. Pacing is activated only after 3.5 seconds of postshock asystole.

The S-ICD features automation of all parameters except 4: shock therapy (on/off), postshock pacing (on/off), conditional SVT discrimination zone (on/off), and upper rate cutoff for the conditional shock zone (between 170 and 240 bpm). Data storage includes pre-event electrograms and markers through to event termination. Up to 24 treated episodes can be stored, averaging 34 seconds of data per episode.

S-ICD SCREENING AND IMPLANTATION

The patient's surface electrocardiography in supine and standing positions should be screened using a proprietary screening tool before implantation to ensure satisfactory sensing. S-ICD implantation uses anatomic landmarks and does not require fluoroscopy and may be performed in an operating theater, cardiac laboratory, or any sterile procedure room. The procedure can be performed with local anesthesia and conscious sedation; however, in our experience, general anesthesia is preferable.

Placement of external defibrillation patches for rescue defibrillation is different from transvenous devices. One patch should be placed below the lower left costal margin in the midclavicular line, away from the surgical field. The other patch should be placed on the right posterior chest, over the area between the right scapula and the high thoracic spine.

The patient should be positioned supine, with the left arm abducted 15° to 30° to allow access to the left lateral chest.

Implantation of the S-ICD requires 3 incisions; we recommend that the incisions be marked before draping to ensure accurate placement. The first is a 6-cm left lateral incision made along the Langer lines over the sixth rib for pocket formation (**Fig. 4**A). The medial point of this incision should extend to the midclavicular line. The dissection should be carried down to fascia

overlying the rib cage, and then, the pocket formed over the rib cage laterally, inferiorly, and superiorly of the incision. Often, the lateral and superior portion of this pocket extends beyond the margin of the latissimus dorsi muscle, and the dissection should be continued below the latissimus dorsi if required to create a pocket of sufficient size. Care should be taken to visualize blood vessels and secure hemostasis during the dissection of the pocket.

The parasternal lead must be placed no more than 1 to 2 cm to the left of the midline to ensure optimal defibrillation efficiency (**Figs. 2** and **4**). Two horizontal incisions 2 to 3 cm long are

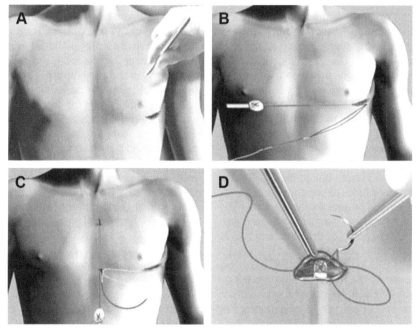

Fig. 4. The surgical steps required for implantation. (*A*) The 6-cm left lateral incision made along the Langer lines over the sixth rib for pocket formation. The medial point of this incision should extend to the midclavicular line. The dissection should be carried down to fascia overlying the rib cage, and then, the pocket formed over the rib cage laterally, inferiorly, and superiorly of the incision. Often, the lateral and superior portion of this pocket extends beyond the margin of the latissimus dorsi muscle, and the dissection should be continued below the latissimus dorsi if required to create a pocket of sufficient size. Care should be taken to visualize blood vessels and secure hemostasis during the dissection of the pocket. (*B*) Tunneling from the xiphoid incision, advancing the tool along the inferior margin of pectoralis major to the pocket. It is important to ensure that the tunneling is performed over the rib and the muscular fascia and not through the subcutaneous fat, to prevent the lead lying superficially. This procedure can be facilitated by feeling the tip of the tunneling tool through the overlying skin during the tunneling. As the tip of the tool approaches the pocket, the implanter can usually guide and feel the tunneling tool using blunt finger dissection from the pocket in the muscular fascial plane. The lead is then attached with a large loop of suture through the eyes of the tunneling tool and lead. (*C*) The lead pulled through and a small portion delivered out of the xiphoid incision. Leaving the suture intact, the tunneling tool is advanced from the inferior to superior parasternal incision, ensuring that the course remains adjacent to and parallel to the midline, and in the fascial plane. Once the tip of the tunneling tool is delivered through the superior incision, the lead can be pulled into place. (*D*) The lead must be securely attached to the fascia to prevent subsequent lead migration. We recommend 2 nonabsorbable sutures such as silk or monofilament at the 2 parasternal incisions. When anchoring the tip of the parasternal electrode, the more easily accessible subcutaneous fat is insufficient to secure the lead. Instead, it is recommended that the periosteal fascia above the sternum and ribs provides a better suture anchor site. (*Courtesy of* Boston Scientific, Natick, MA.)

placed: one at the xiphoid and the second at the sternal-manubrium junction at the second rib (see **Fig. 4**C). These incisions should be made large enough to ensure that both the underlying fascia is readily visible and sutures can be placed in the fascia for lead fixation. The incisions should be a minimum of 14 cm apart, to ensure that the defibrillating coil and the proximal and distal electrodes are all parasternal. The incision should extend from the midline to 2 to 3 cm to the left of the midline and be carried down to the abdominal fascia and fascia overlying the lateral border of the sternum, respectively. A tunneling tool is used to pull the parasternal lead into position from the generator pocket (see **Fig. 4**B, C). It is important to ensure that the tunneling is performed over the rib and the muscular fascia and not through the subcutaneous fat to prevent the lead lying superficially, which increases the risk of subsequent erosion. Commencing at the xiphoid incision, the tool is advanced along the inferior margin of pectoralis major to the lateral pocket (see **Fig. 4**B). The lead is then attached with a large loop of suture through the eyelets of the tunneling tool and distal electrode (see **Fig. 4**B) and the lead pulled through and a small portion delivered out of the xiphoid incision. Leaving the suture intact, the tunneling tool is advanced from the inferior to superior parasternal incision, ensuring the course remains adjacent to and parallel to the midline, and in the fascial plane (see **Fig. 4**C). Once the tip of the tunneling tool is delivered through the superior incision, the lead can be pulled into place. The lead must be securely attached to the fascia at both the superior and xiphoid incision to prevent subsequent lead migration. We recommend 2 nonabsorbable sutures such as silk or monofilament at each incision, with the xiphoid sutures placed securely through the abdominal fascia below the rib margin, and the lead secured with the anchoring sleeve provided, ensuring that the proximal electrode is not covered (see **Fig. 4**D).

In women, the pocket incision can usually be placed in the inframammary crease and the tunneling, and anchoring process is identical in men, because the proper path for tunneling of the lead is inferior to any breast tissue. Similarly, because of the midline location of the parasternal lead, breast tissue in women does not interfere with the parasternal incisions and lead placement. The subcutaneous defibrillator has the added benefit of not interfering with subsequent mammography.

Once the parasternal electrode is appropriately placed and secured, and after connecting the lead to the generator, a suture should be inserted through the connector block suture portal to anchor the S-ICD to the underlying fascia. Care should be taken to avoid anchoring the generator too tightly to the fascia, because it might lever or tent the generator up at the far end, putting upward pressure on the skin. We recommend that the wound is sutured with a minimum of 1 subcutaneous layer for the parasternal incisions and 2 subcutaneous layers for the pocket incision to avoid wound dehiscence.

Once the surgery is completed, defibrillator testing should be performed to confirm appropriate detection and termination of ventricular fibrillation with 65 J to give a 15-J safety margin. Ventricular fibrillation can be induced via the device and programmer using 50 Hz stimulation between the parasternal shock coil and pulse generator.

INDICATIONS, CONTRAINDICATIONS, AND SPECIAL GROUPS

The S-ICD effectively detects and treats ventricular fibrillation and tachycardia but does not have pacing capability, apart from 30 seconds of post-shock pacing. Therefore, the S-ICD is indicated in any patient at risk for these arrhythmias, including patients resuscitated from ventricular fibrillation or patients with a primary prevention indication for an ICD (**Table 2**). The S-ICD is

Table 2				
Indications and recommendations for T-ICDs and S-ICDs				
T-ICD Indicated	T-ICD Recommended	T-ICD and S-ICD Recommended	S-ICD Recommended	S-ICD Indicated
• Requirement for pacing, bradycardia, resynchronization or over-pacable ventricular tachycardia	• Hypertrophic cardiomyopathy	• Resuscitated ventricular fibrillation • Primary prevention patients	• Young patients • Previously infected T-ICD	• Venous access compromised or absent • Cardiac anatomy precludes T-ICD

especially suitable in patients with compromised venous access, often a complication of previous CIED implants, or in whom the cardiac anatomy precludes the placement of a right ventricular lead, such as the Fontan procedure. Previously, these patients could be offered only an epicardial ICD, which requires a thoracotomy and can be technically difficult because of previous cardiac surgical procedures. A few pediatric cases have received hybrid subcutaneous defibrillation systems[26]; however, the defibrillation energy is unlikely to be sufficient for many patients, especially as they become adults, and they still require an epicardial pace-sense lead. These hybrid systems are now redundant because of the availability of purpose-built S-ICDs, which offer greater certainty of defibrillation.

We recommend that the S-ICD be considered in young patients in whom an ICD is indicated. Many such patients, particularly those with preserved left ventricular function, can be expected to live with their defibrillator for decades. Implanting a T-ICD commits them to a high risk for future lead failure and the associated risks of lead revision or lead extraction.

The S-ICD is not suitable for patients who require cardiac pacing, including patients with bradycardia, patients requiring cardiac resynchronization pacing, and those with pace terminated ventricular tachycardia.

The S-ICD has been designed to be compatible with a separate bipolar pacemaker. Therefore, in patients with a previously implanted pacemaker, an S-ICD can be implanted. In patients in whom a transvenous ICD cannot be implanted for vascular or anatomic constraints, but who require pacing, both an S-ICD and epicardial bipolar pacemaker could be considered. However, the current experience of the combination of an S-ICD and a separate pacemaker is limited to isolated case reports.[32]

CLINICAL TRIALS

The first implants were performed in 2008 in a pilot of 6 patients in New Zealand.[14] All devices were implanted successfully without procedural complications and detected and terminated induced ventricular fibrillation. Subsequently, 55 patients were implanted in a European trial in 2008 to 2009.[14] In the 53 evaluable patients, all 137 episodes of induced ventricular fibrillation were detected, and 52 had 2 consecutive episodes of ventricular fibrillation terminated by a 65-J shock, giving a 15-J safety margin. Two patients had revisions for device infections, and 4 for lead migration. The patients were followed up for a mean of 10 months,

and a total of 12 spontaneous ventricular tachycardia episodes were detected and treated. Oversensing and inappropriate shocks were caused by inadequate lead placement in the generator in 1 patient, muscle noise in 3 patients, and double sensing of a rate-related bundle branch block in 1 patient. In response to these oversensing issues, the detection algorithm was revised, and no further episodes of inappropriate shock occurred in this small group.[14]

Subsequently, a larger US-based trial of 321 patients was reported.[33] In this study, 304 patients successfully completed the implant defibrillation protocol at 65 J, although 17% required shock polarity reversal to achieve success. The remaining 17 patients did not successfully complete the induction/defibrillation protocol, for various reasons, including hemodynamic instability, for a 95% overall defibrillation success rate, and 314 patients were discharged with the device. During follow-up for a mean of 11 months, 119 spontaneous episodes in 21 patients were treated successfully, 92% on the first shock, with no arrhythmic deaths. The rate of inappropriate shocks over this period was 13.1%, predominantly because of SVT in the high rate zone or T-wave oversensing. Device-related and implantation-related complications occurred in 8% by 180 days, including 4 device infections requiring explantation. In this study, 78 patients underwent repeat defibrillation testing at greater than 150 days after implantation. Of the 75 evaluable patients, 72 reverted with 65 J, and 3 failed at 65 J but reverted at 80 J.

In a case-controlled study of 69 patients with S-ICDs, procedural time and procedural complication rate were not significantly different from T-ICDs, and conversion rates for ventricular fibrillation of 89.5% increasing to 95.5% with polarity reversal for the S-ICD compared well with 90.8% for 10-J safety margin testing in the T-ICD. With 217 days mean follow up, both S-ICD and T-ICD effectively treated events. Three patients in each group received inappropriate shocks, all caused by T-wave oversensing in the S-ICD group.[34]

COMPLICATIONS AND CONCERNS

In the Weiss study, complications occurred in 8% by 180 days, no more than would be expected with T-ICDs; however, 6 of the 382 (1.6%) patients in the initial studies developed device infections requiring revision,[14,33] suggesting that device infection may be more common than with T-ICDs, perhaps because of the larger device, and multiple incisions. After the initial implants, several cases of lead migration occurred[14,35]; however, with the modification of the implantation technique with a secure second suture at the xiphoid, this issue has not recurred.

Inappropriate shocks are important adverse events in ICD recipients, resulting in psychological morbidity[36]; they are associated with increased mortality[37] and reduce patient acceptance of ICD therapy. The current absence of large controlled studies makes it difficult to compare the rates of inappropriate shocks between S-ICD and T-ICDs. The detection algorithm in the S-ICD is more morphology based than with T-ICDs. In comparative testing of ICD algorithms against a library of induced arrhythmias, the S-ICD showed excellent sensitivity for ventricular arrhythmia detection and was more specific than T-ICDs.[38] In practice, the inappropriate therapy rate was the same as T-ICDs in the small comparative trial.[34] In the largest published experience,[33] inappropriate shocks occurred in 13.1% over 11 months, higher than the inappropriate shock rate of 11.5% over 20 months with T-ICDs in the MADIT II (Multicenter Automatic Defibrillator Implantation Trial II) trial,[39] and the 1-year inappropriate shock rates of 3.6% and 7.5% with T-ICDs in the interventional and control limbs of the PREPARE (Primary Prevention Parameters Evaluation) study.[40] T-wave oversensing has been the predominant cause of inappropriate detections in the S-ICD and seems more common in patients with congenital heart disease, hypertrophic cardiomyopathy, long QT syndrome, and catecholaminergic polymorphic ventricular tachycardia.[41] Patients with a large T/QRS ratio are at greater risk of T-wave oversensing and have a relative contraindication to an S-ICD.

Time to therapy is longer than with transvenous devices, with average times of 14 ± 2.5 seconds[14] and 14.6 ± 2.9 and up to 29 seconds.[33] Although this time to detection has caused concern,[41] longer time to therapy safely reduces shocks by avoiding treating events that would otherwise terminate spontaneously[40] and is consistent with recent programming trends for T-ICDs.

Perhaps the greatest expressed concern is the lack of antitachycardia pacing. However, although antitachycardia pacing reduces the needs for shocks, and is important in patients with slow ventricular tachycardia, only a few patients in ICD trials develop a pace terminable ventricular tachycardia.[6] Furthermore, antitachycardia pacing may be delivered to an episode that would have otherwise reverted spontaneously and may accelerate the ventricular tachycardia.[6] Antitachycardia pacing has not been shown to reduce mortality,[6] and the largest trial confirming the mortality benefit of primary prevention ICD therapy used shock-only ICDs.[9] Therefore, we believe that a shock-only ICD such as the S-ICD is appropriate in most ICD candidates.

THEORETIC BENEFITS

In addition to avoiding short-term and long-term complications of transvenous leads, the S-ICD may prove to have other benefits over the T-ICD. Ventricular pacing is essential in only a few patients with defibrillators and may be harmful in others. Unnecessary ventricular pacing has been shown to increase mortality by exacerbating cardiac dysfunction and heart failure.[42] Furthermore, ventricular pacing may contribute to arrhythmia burden. In a sophisticated analysis of ventricular arrhythmia events in patients with ICDs from the PainFREE Rx II (Pacing Fast Ventricular Tachycardia Reduces Shock Therapies) and EnTrust trials, Sweeney and colleagues[43] showed that 30% of ventricular tachycardias were pacing associated, and Himmrich and colleagues[44] had previously shown that these events could be prevented only by disabling pacing. This proarrhythmic effect of ventricular pacing may in part explain why the event rate of treated life-threatening arrhythmias is greater than the mortality benefit seen in many ICD trials.[7,45,46]

An even greater concern is that shocks may contribute to mortality in patients with T-ICDs. Shocks were clearly associated with increased mortality in the SCD-HeFT (Sudden Cardiac Death in Heart Failure Trial) trial, with most deaths being caused by progressive heart failure.[37] This observation is at least in part because shock therapy is a marker of more advanced underlying disease. However, the observation that excess mortality persisted when baseline prognostic factors were corrected for, and was also present for inappropriate shocks,[37] suggests that shocks contributed to the mortality. If transvenous shocks do increase mortality, this is likely to be related to myocardial damage from high voltage gradients during defibrillation.[18–22]

The S-ICD is predicted to generate fewer of these damaging high voltage gradients,[17] and in a small animal study,[47] subcutaneous defibrillation avoided the cardiac troponin release seen with transvenous defibrillation.

FUTURE PERSPECTIVES

The currently available S-ICD is a first-generation device. It has performed well and is becoming an established therapy. Evolution of this device is inevitable. The first step is a modest size reduction and improvement in battery longevity, which should improve patient acceptability.

A reduction in inappropriate therapy because of T-wave oversensing is equally important. In the short-term, the problem of T-wave oversensing in the S-ICD could be reduced by requiring patients to have a satisfactory R-wave/T-wave ratio in at least 2 of the 3 vectors, and by assessing for T-wave oversensing during exercise.[48] In the longer-term, improved sensing through enhanced signal processing, T-wave oversensing detection algorithms, or automatic integration of data from more than 1 of the 3 potential sensing vectors of the device should address this issue.

The greatest limitation of the current S-ICD is the lack of ventricular pacing, apart from limited post-shock pacing. It is possible to implant a separate pacemaker with the current S-ICD if it is bipolar, but this is appropriate only in isolated cases.

It would be technically possible to develop a hybrid device with a transvenous pacing lead and subcutaneous defibrillation; however, this approach carries similar vascular risks to a transvenous device but has the theoretic advantage of subcutaneous over transvenous defibrillation. In addition, because of the absence of any transvenous component, magnetic resonance imaging scanning is hypothesized to be safer.

The most logical development is the marriage of the S-ICD with leadless pacing. We envisage that in the future, the S-ICD will be leadless pacing compatible. If the patient subsequently required pacing, a leadless pacemaker would be implanted, which would communicate with the S-ICD and could provide both bradycardia and tachycardia pacing capabilities.

SUMMARY

The S-ICD has recently been developed as an alternative to conventional T-ICDs. It avoids both the short-term and long-term hazards of the transvenous lead. The first-generation device effectively detects and terminates malignant ventricular arrhythmias but has only limited post-shock pacing. The overall rate of inappropriate shocks seems comparable with T-ICDs. It has theoretic advantages over transvenous devices, with no risk of pacing-induced arrhythmias, and avoids high myocardial defibrillation voltage gradients. It is suitable for candidates for an implantable defibrillator who do not require pacing and is recommended in patients with compromised vascular or cardiac access. It should be considered in younger patients and those who need a shock-only device.

With the current state of knowledge, it is not possible to determine if the real-life performance of S-ICD is comparable, superior, or inferior to the T-ICD. This subject can be addressed only by accumulated experience, as will be obtained by the EFFORTLESS (Evaluation oF FactORs ImpacTing CLinical Outcome and Cost EffectiveneSS of the S-ICD) registry,[49] and, more importantly, by direct randomized comparison in the PRAETORIAN (A Prospective, Randomized comparison of subcutaneous and tRansvenous ImpLANtable cardioverter-defibrillator therapy) trial.[50]

ACKNOWLEDGMENTS

We wish to thank all our patients who consented to implantation of an S-ICD as an investigational device.

REFERENCES

1. Schulman PM, Rozner MA, Sera V, et al. Patients with pacemaker or implantable cardioverter-defibrillator. Med Clin North Am 2013;97:1051–75.
2. Elmqvist R. Review of early pacemaker development. Pacing Clin Electrophysiol 1978;1:535–6.
3. Mirowski M, Reid PR, Mower MM, et al. Termination of malignant ventricular arrhythmias with an implanted automatic defibrillator in human beings. N Engl J Med 1980;303:322–4.
4. Bardy GH, Johnson G, Poole JE, et al. A simplified, single-lead unipolar transvenous cardioverter-defibrillator system. Circulation 1993;88:543–7.
5. Greve H, Koch T, Gulker H, et al. Termination of malignant ventricular tachycardias by use of an automatic defibrillator in combination with an artificial antitachycardia pacemaker. Pacing Clin Electrophysiol 1988;11:2040–4.
6. Wathen MS, DeGroot PJ, Sweeney MO, et al. Prospective randomized multicenter trial of empirical antitachycardia pacing versus shocks for spontaneous rapid ventricular tachycardia in patients with implantable cardiovertor defibrillators: pacing fast ventricular tachycardia reduces shock therapies (PainFREE Rx II) trial results. Circulation 2004;110:2591–6.
7. The AVID Investigators. A comparison of antiarrhythmic drug therapy with implantable defibrillators in patients resuscitated from near-fatal ventricular arrhythmias. N Engl J Med 1997;337: 1576–83.
8. Moss AJ, Zareba W, Hall WJ, et al. Prophylactic implantation of a defibrillator in patients with myocardial infarction and reduced ejection fraction. N Engl J Med 2002;346:877–83.
9. Bardy GH, Lee KL, Mark DB, et al. Amiodarone or an implantable cardioverter-defibrillator for congestive heart failure. N Engl J Med 2005;352: 225–37.

10. Alter P, Waldhans S, Plachta E, et al. Complications of implantable cardioverter defibrillator therapy in 440 consecutive patients. Pacing Clin Electrophysiol 2005;28:926–32.

11. Maisal W, Kramer D. Implantable cardioverter-defibrillator lead performance. Circulation 2008; 117:2721–3.

12. Hauser RG, Kallinen LM, Almquist AK, et al. Early failure of a small-diameter high-voltage implantable cardioverter-defibrillator lead. Heart Rhythm 2007; 4:892–6.

13. Parkash R, Exner D, Champagne J, et al. Failure rate of the Riata lead under advisory: a report from the CHRS device committee. Heart Rhythm 2013;10:692–5.

14. Bardy GH, Smith WM, Hood MA, et al. An entirely subcutaneous implantable cardioverter-defibrillator. N Engl J Med 2010;363:36–44.

15. Zipes DP, Fisher J, King RM, et al. Termination of ventricular fibrillation in dogs by depolarising a critical amount of myocardium. Am J Cardiol 1975;36: 37–44.

16. Zhou X, Daubert JP, Wolf PD, et al. Epicardial mapping of ventricular defibrillation with monophasic and biphasic shocks in dogs. Circ Res 1993;72: 145–60.

17. Jolley M, Stinstra J, Pieper S, et al. A computer modeling tool for comparing novel ICD electrode orientations in children and adults. Heart Rhythm 2008;5:565–72.

18. Tung L, Tovar O, Neunlist M, et al. Effects of strong electrical shock on cardiac muscle tissue. Ann N Y Acad Sci 1994;720:160–75.

19. Walcott G, Killingsworth C, Ideker R. Do clinically relevant transthoracic defibrillation energies cause myocardial damage and dysfunction? Resuscitation 2003;59:59–70.

20. Hasdemir C, Shan N, Rao A, et al. Analysis of troponin I levels after spontaneous implantable cardioverter defibrillator shocks. J Cardiovasc Electrophysiol 2002;13:144–50.

21. Tokano T, Bach D, Chang J, et al. Effect of ventricular shock strength on cardiac hemodynamics. J Cardiovasc Electrophysiol 1998;9:791–7.

22. Zivin A, Souza J, Pelosi F, et al. Relationship between shock energy and postdefibrillation ventricular arrhythmias in patients with implantable defibrillators. J Cardiovasc Electrophysiol 1999;10:370–7.

23. Lerman B, Deale O. Relation between transcardiac and transthoracic current during defibrillation in humans. Circ Res 1990;67:1420–6.

24. Schuder JC, Stoeckle H, Gold JH, et al. Experimental ventricular defibrillation with an automatic and completely implanted system. Trans Am Soc Artif Intern Organs 1970;16:207–12.

25. Berul CI, Triedman JK, Forbess J, et al. Minimally invasive cardioverter defibrillator implantation for children: an animal model and pediatric case report. Pacing Clin Electrophysiol 2001;24: 1789–94.

26. Stephenson EA, Batra AS, Knilans TK, et al. A multicenter experience with novel implantable cardioverter defibrillator configurations in the pediatric and congenital heart disease population. J Cardiovasc Electrophysiol 2006;17:41–6.

27. Bardy GH, Cappato R, Smith WM, et al. The totally subcutaneous ICD system (the S-ICD). Pacing Clin Electrophysiol 2002;25. II-578.

28. Cappato R, Castelvecchio S, Erlinger P, et al. Feasibility of defibrillation and automatic arrhythmia detection using an exclusively subcutaneous defibrillator system in canines. J Cardiovasc Electrophysiol 2013;24:77–83.

29. Burke MC, Coman JA, Cates AW, et al. Defibrillation energy requirements using a left anterior chest cutaneous to subcutaneous shocking vector: implications for a total subcutaneous implantable defibrillator. Heart Rhythm 2005;2:1332–8.

30. Lieberman R, Havel WJ, Rashba E, et al. Acute defibrillation performance of a novel, non-transvenous shock pathway in adult ICD indicated patients. Heart Rhythm 2008;5:28–34.

31. Grace AA, Smith WM, Hood MA, et al. A prospective randomized comparison in humans of defibrillation efficacy of a standard transvenous ICD system with a totally subcutaneous system (the S-ICD system). Heart Rhythm 2005;2:1036.

32. Van Opstal J, Geskes G, Debie L. A completely subcutaneous implantable cardioverter defibrillator system functioning simultaneously with an endocardial implantable cardioverter defibrillator programmed as a pacemaker. Europace 2011;13:141–2.

33. Weiss R, Knight BP, Gold MR, et al. Safety and efficacy of a totally subcutaneous implantable-cardioverter defibrillator. Circulation 2013;128: 944–53.

34. Kobe J, Reinke F, Meyer C, et al. Implantation and follow-up of totally subcutaneous versus conventional implantable cardioverter-defibrillator: a multicenter case-control study. Heart Rhythm 2013;10: 29–36.

35. Abkenari LD, Theuns DA, Valk SD, et al. Clinical experience with a novel subcutaneous implantable defibrillator system in a single center. Clin Res Cardiol 2011;100:737–44.

36. Raitt MH. Implantable cardioverter defibrillator shocks. A double-edged sword? J Am Coll Cardiol 2008;51:1366–8.

37. Poole JE, Johnson GW, Hellkamp AS, et al. Prognostic importance of defibrillator shocks in patients with heart failure. N Engl J Med 2008;359:1009–17.

38. Gold MR, Theuns DA, Knight BP, et al. Head-to-head comparison of arrhythmia discrimination performance of subcutaneous and transvenous ICD

arrhythmia detection algorithms: the START study. J Cardiovasc Electrophysiol 2012;23:359–66.

39. Daubert JP, Zareba W, Cannom DS, et al. Inappropriate implantable cardioverter defibrillator shocks in MADIT II. J Am Coll Cardiol 2008;51:1357–65.

40. Wilkoff BL, Williamson BD, Stern RS, et al. Strategic programming of detection and therapy parameters in implantable cardioverter-defibrillators reduces shocks in primary prevention patients. J Am Coll Cardiol 2008;52:541–50.

41. Jarman JW, Todd DM. United Kingdom national experience of entirely subcutaneous implantable cardioverter-defibrillator technology: important lessons to learn. Europace 2013;15:1158–65.

42. The DAVID trial Investigators. Dual-chamber pacing or ventricular backup pacing in patients with an implantable defibrillator. The dual chamber and VVI implantable defibrillator (DAVID) trial. J Am Med Assoc 2002;288:3115–23.

43. Sweeney MO, Ruetz LL, Belk P, et al. Bradycardia pacing-induced short-long-short sequences at the onset of ventricular tachycardias. A possible mechanism of proarrhythmia? J Am Coll Cardiol 2007;50:614–22.

44. Himmrich E, Przibille O, Zellerhoff C, et al. Proarrhythmic effect of pacemaker stimulation in patients with implanted cardioverter-defibrillators. Circulation 2003;108:192–7.

45. Moss AJ, Hall WJ, Cannom DS, et al. Improved survival with an implanted defibrillator in patients with coronary disease at high risk for ventricular arrhythmias. N Engl J Med 1996;335:1933–40.

46. Bigger JT, for the Coronary Artery Bypass Graft (CABG) Patch Trial Investigators. Prophylactic use of implanted cardiac defibrillators in patients at high risk for ventricular arrhythmias after coronary artery bypass surgery. N Engl J Med 1997; 337:1569–75.

47. Killingworth CR, Melnick SB, Livotsky SH, et al. Evaluation of acute cardiac and chest wall damage after shocks with a subcutaneous implantable cardioverter defibrillator in swine. Pacing Clin Electrophysiol 2013;36:1265–72.

48. Kooiman KM, Knops RE, Olde Nordkamp L, et al. Inappropriate subcutaneous implantable cardioverter defibrillator shocks due to T-wave oversensing can be prevented. Implications for management. Heart Rhythm 2014;11(3):426–34. http://dx.doi.org/10.1016/j.hrthm.2013.12.007.

49. Pedersen SS, Lambiase P, Boersma LV, et al. Evaluation of factors impacting clinical outcomes and cost effectiveness of the S-ICD: design rationale of the EFFORTLESS S-ICD registry. Pacing Clin Electrophysiol 2012;35:574–9.

50. Olde Nordkamp LR, Knops RE, Bardy GH, et al. Rationale and design of the PRAETORIAN trial: a prospective, randomized comparison of subcutaneous and transvenous implantable cardioverter-defibrillator therapy. Am Heart J 2012; 163:753–60.

Mechanisms of Malfunction and Complications of the Subcutaneous ICD

Martin C. Burke, DO

KEYWORDS

- Sudden cardiac death • Subcutaneous implantable cardioverter defibrillator • Implant
- Xiphoid process

KEY POINTS

- The entirely subcutaneous implantable cardioverter defibrillator (S-ICD) is a simple implant platform designed for safety and efficacy.
- The malfunctions and complications have largely been managed noninvasively through programming and software upgrades.
- The preimplant screening process is linked to the S-ICD sensing algorithm and improves the safety of the long-term implant.
- Infections and inappropriate shocks have been identified as the predominant clinical complications and have decreased as the experience with the device procedure has grown.

The entirely subcutaneous implantable cardioverter defibrillator (S-ICD) is a new implant platform to prevent sudden cardiac death.[1–3] The largest published cohort to date is the pivotal investigational device exemption trial.[2] The S-ICD concept has pursued a simpler ICD implant and device in an effort to combat the problems seen with transvenous high-voltage lead systems.[4–7] The S-ICD detects and treats ventricular tachyarrhythmias and presents both common and unique mechanisms of malfunction and complication in comparison to the traditional transvenous ICD implant procedure. In contrast and procedurally based, the S-ICD procedure platform, as opposed to the transvenous, does not carry the risk of pneumothorax, pericardial tamponade, or myocardial perforation. The early experience with the S-ICD procedure platform and the worldwide experience with the S-ICD have taught important lessons as the procedure advanced into multiple operators' hands. The prospective data evaluating this device and implant platform have been evaluated and regulated by the United States and outside US device agencies. The agencies have categorized complications as device, labeling, and/or procedurally –related.[2] The device regulatory bodies further stipulate that major complications result in invasive action needed. This article endeavors to specifically detail the function and possible malfunctions as well as complications related to patient selection, the implant procedure, and programming of the device for follow-up as well as the steps taken to solve them since the first human implant in 2008.

Disclosures: Dr M.C. Burke has received honoraria, consulting fees, and research grants from Cameron Health, Inc and Boston Scientific, Inc, specifically related to the entirely subcutaneous ICD. Boston Scientific has supported the clinical cardiac electrophysiology fellowship at the University of Chicago.
Section of Cardiology, Department of Medicine, Heart Rhythm Center, University of Chicago Medicine, University of Chicago, 5758 South Maryland, MC 9024, Chicago, IL 60637, USA
E-mail address: mburke@bsd.uchicago.edu

Card Electrophysiol Clin 6 (2014) 297–306
http://dx.doi.org/10.1016/j.ccep.2014.03.006

BRIEF OVERVIEW OF DEVICE AND IMPLANT
Device Hardware

The S-ICD System (Boston Scientific, Inc, Natick, MA) is similar to a single coil transvenous ICD system but the lead does not have to be placed into the heart. It has 2 components that are implanted completely subcutaneously: a 69 cc pulse generator and a single 45-cm, 9 French subcutaneous electrode (Q-TRAK, Boston Scientific, Inc., Natick, MA) that comprises 1 high-voltage defibrillation coil and 2 sensing electrodes, electrically insulated from the defibrillation high-voltage cable using a sturdy durometer polyurethane. It has been designed to be subcutaneously tunneled from the pulse generator pocket along the left lateral chest wall to an incision near the xiphoid process and then superiorly from the xiphoid process such that the distal tip is approximately 14 cm above the xiphoid incision, roughly at the *Angle of Louis*. The battery is projected to survive for 5 years with 3 capacitor reforms per year.

There are 3 programmable features in the device (**Fig. 1**): (1) defibrillation therapies on or off; (2) two detection cutoff rates (shock only and conditional zones); and (3) post-shock pacing on or off. The pulse generator is programmable as a single or dual detection zone device (dual zone is recommended), with supraventricular arrhythmia discrimination algorithms in the lower or conditional rate zone. Ambulatory shocks are delivered at a nonprogrammable maximum of 80 J × 5 shocks per cycle. A single high-voltage discharge from the device will lead to a months' accelerated depletion in battery life.

Sensing Electrodes and Vectors

The S-ICD System uses 1 of 3, nearly orthogonal and unique, sensing vectors to distinguish sinus rhythm from ventricular and supraventricular tachyarrhythmias. The 3 vectors (**Fig. 2**) are designated as A to Can (AC or secondary); B to Can (BC or primary); or A to B (AB or alternate). The 3 electrograms ("A" electrode at the parasternal angle of Louis, "B" electrode at the parasternal xiphoid, and Can or "C" electrode at the left lateral mid

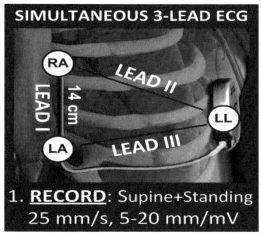

1. **RECORD**: Supine+Standing 25 mm/s, 5-20 mm/mV

Fig. 2. Trichannel ECG setup represents S-ICD vectors. The screening electrocardiogram orientation showing Einthoven's triangle on its side. Lead I represents the A to B vector (alternate). Lead II represents the A to Can vector (secondary). Lead III represents the B to Can vector (primary). The RA is the right arm electrode that is measured 14 cm from the xiphoid process at about the angle of Louis and is a surrogate for the S-ICD "A" sensing electrode. The LA is the left arm electrode placed adjacent to the xiphoid process on the left parasternal chest. It is a surrogate for the S-ICD "B" electrode. The LL is the left leg electrode placed at the midaxillary line adjacent to the left ventricular apex. It is a surrogate for the S-ICD can or "C" electrode. The primary vector (B to Can) is the most common vector auto-selected. The screening is performed in both the supine and standing positions and must pass in both positions in the selected vector. ECG, electrocardiogram; LA, left arm electrode; LL, left leg electrode; RA, right arm electrode; S-ICD, entirely subcutaneous implantable cardioverter defibrillator. (Copyright © 2014 Boston Scientific Corporation or its affiliates. All rights reserved. Used with permission of Boston Scientific Corporation.)

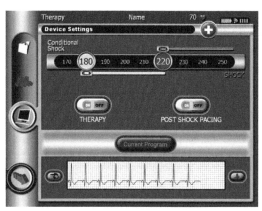

Fig. 1. The S-ICD programmer screen. The main programming screen for the S-ICD system. Device settings presented are the red shock-only detection rate selection at 220 bpm and the yellow conditional zone at 180 bpm. Therapy setting is switched on or off. Post-shock pacing setting is switched on or off. The electrocardiogram rhythm strip at the bottom represents the current programmed vector out of 3 possibilities selected. These represent the only programmable features for clinicians to consider. S-ICD, entirely subcutaneous implantable cardioverter defibrillator. (Copyright © 2014 Boston Scientific Corporation or its affiliates. All rights reserved. Used with permission of Boston Scientific Corporation.)

axillary chest wall) are verified for adequacy and positioned before the implant procedure by recording the electrograms cutaneously and applying a screening tool[2] to identify appropriate patients for implant before any incision. The electrodes combine to encompass most of the left ventricle to provide the largest R wave to T wave ratio.[8–10]

Current Implant Technique

The S-ICD System represents a new implant technique that requires a wide area sterile preparation. A great deal of preliminary research and development has placed this device from the apical midaxillary line to the sternum to have the best in defibrillation threshold, sensing to distinguish sinus rhythm from ventricular tachyarrhythmia and a position that has placed the smallest stress on the hardware. Anatomic orientation to the chest is needed to understand the implant of the S-ICD system. There are 3 anatomic regions of interest, including the midaxillary line, the xiphoid process, and the left to right parasternum at the second intercostal space (angle of Louis). The evaluation of the surface electrocardiogram in all 3 sensing vectors has been shown to be a significant correlate to the subcutaneous electrograms[8–10]; this has allowed for the creation of a screening tool (**Fig. 3**) to select patients for implantation before the actual surgery. It is essential to match the "A" and "B" electrode positions along the left

parasternum to the positions screened cutaneously before surgery. The xiphoid process is essentially the fiduciary anatomic point and important as it essentially provides a landmark to identify the inferior boarder of the heart with the exception of patients with pectus excavatum or unique congenital heart disease. After careful and wide area prep with the arm at 45°, the initial incision is made to form a pocket adjacent to the left ventricular apex in a posterior direction ending just beyond the midaxillary line. Once the pocket is an adequate size with hemostasis assured, then your attention is turned to the xiphoid incision, which is made vertical along the left parasternum. Then a tunneling tool is advanced from the xiphoid, while carefully staying on the fascial plane, to the left lateral pocket. Next, a silk tie is attached to the lead tip and the tunneling tools with an adequate slack are pulled to the xiphoid. The lead is then secured to the xiphoid fascia to allow for inferior to superior tunneling along the left parasternum to the Angle of Louis. Before tunneling superiorly along the parasternum, the lead can be measured along the chest. Laying the lead cutaneously along the targeted path to be used allows for an appropriate placement of the "A" electrode and an accurate superior parasternal incision. The lead is then tunneled superior with specific attention to maintaining the correct fascial plane. Once in position, the lead tip is sewn down to the fascia. All 3 incisions are then closed in preparation for defibrillation threshold testing.

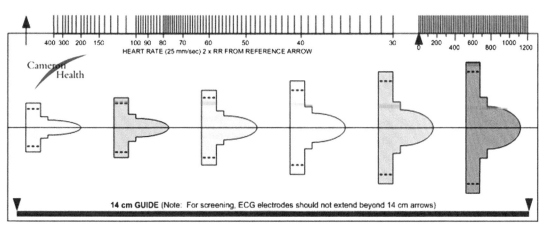

Fig. 3. The S-ICD screening tool. The screening tool is an essential contributor to the safety of the S-ICD system. The ability to identify a group of patients that will respond or not to the sensing algorithm before surgical implant is setup by the ratiometric R wave to T wave colorgrams. As the R wave amplitude changes so does the T-wave duration and amplitude. The tool has a measured 14-cm ruler for accurate measuring from the B electrode to the A electrode that is set to the actual real-time lead distance of the electrodes. The tool demonstrates a solid line that bisects the colorgrams to allow for the biphasic nature of the electrocardiogram and changes in position. The tool has been developed based on the functional engineering of the S-ICD device's sensing algorithm. S-ICD, entirely subcutaneous implantable cardioverter defibrillator. (Copyright © 2014 Boston Scientific Corporation or its affiliates. All rights reserved. Used with permission of Boston Scientific Corporation.)

Effectiveness Data

The primary effectiveness endpoint during the regulatory (United States and Outside United States) analysis of the S-ICD was the acute induced ventricular fibrillation (VF) conversion rate at the time of device implantation compared to a historically calculated performance goal of 88% as set by the Food and Drug Administration (FDA) using prior investigational ICD trial results. VF was induced using 50-Hz transthoracic stimulation under moderate to deep sedation or general anesthesia.[1,2] Detection was performed automatically by the device. Successful protocol-defined conversion testing required 2 consecutive VF conversions at 65 J in either shock vector (initial or reversed); up to a maximum of 4 VF conversion attempts using the same polarity was allowed. A sensitivity analysis was performed in which incomplete effectiveness testing attempts during acute implant were imputed as failures to assess the potential impact of missing endpoint observations. These incomplete effectiveness data resulted from failure to complete the full testing protocol due to clinical concerns or inability to induce VF. The efficacy data of the Investigational Device Exemption (IDE) trial[2] even with the sensitivity analysis met the objective performance endpoint at just above 92% effectiveness.

The safety analysis of the S-ICD has been reported.[1–3,11] The IDE study has used objective performance criteria calculated by the FDA from safety and efficacy data of investigational device studies in previous first-generation ICD clinical trials. The objective performance criterion target set by the FDA for *safety* was greater than 79% complication free rate. There has been mostly short-term data[3] detailing spontaneous episode conversion, and early limited center experience reports are mixed.[2,3,12,13]

The initial pilot study and CE mark trial reported by Bardy and colleagues[1] describes the initial experience in approximately 60 patients, a small study at a few centers, with a 6-month safety and effectiveness dataset. The initial complication free rate reported in the New England Journal of Medicine combined clinical trials is 82% with most of the events related to the operator handling of the device and implantation procedure. Consequently, alterations to the implant procedure and labeling ensued after the initial 60 patient enrollment. Changes to the procedural approach addressed staying true to the anatomic landmarks and securing the lead to the fascia at the xiphoid process. Many lessons have been learned since the device hardware began human implants in 2008 and has led to fewer and less morbid complications or malfunctions (**Fig. 4**).

DEVICE SYSTEM–RELATED MALFUNCTIONS

For a first-generation device, the pulse generator and lead system have been remarkably sturdy as evidenced by the device-related complication free rate of 99% seen in the IDE trial.[2] Device-related complications comprised the major analysis of the complication free rate. The hardware is comprised of battery, capacitor, and semiconductor. There were no malfunctions related to the capacitor or semiconductor in the device. The battery function and malfunction were monitored closely since the first human implant. During the early clinical studies, the manufacturer of the device issued an advisory[14] to implanting centers relating instances of early battery depletion among devices manufactured with a particular lot of batteries. Clinically, this hardware-related advisory affected only a small number of patients. Although, for a new device platform, it was taken seriously by

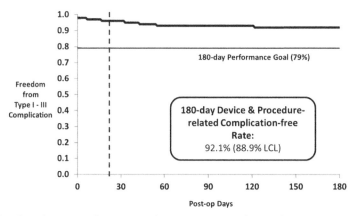

Fig. 4. S-ICD IDE freedom from complication Kaplan-Meier curve. The Kaplan-Meier curve for survival from complication in the IDE study. The evaluation demonstrates the 1-year complication-free rate for device, labeling- and procedure-related complications. (*From* Weiss R, Knight BP, Gold MR, et al. Safety and efficacy of a totally subcutaneous implantable cardioverter defibrillator. Circulation 2013;128:944–53; with permission.)

the manufacturer, implanting electrophysiologists, and regulatory bodies. Patients with devices containing the identified lot of batteries were monitored at the usual intervals. A rapid depletion of battery of more than 3% in a 3-month follow-up triggered an alert at follow-up and more frequent monitoring. The device has a battery depletion patient alert system typical of human implant ICDs. No untoward patient morbidity or mortality was realized as a consequence of the advisory.

The S-ICD battery is made of 3 cell blocks and, simply put, a batch of battery cells depleted early due to misalignment of cells within a block. On clinical reports of early battery depletion, manufacturer quality assurance (QA) analysis was performed using the clinical and engineering evaluation of devices and identified the misalignment. The company (Cameron Health, Inc., San Clemente, CA) quickly instituted fluoroscopic analysis of all batteries on arrival from the third-party vendor. This rapid QA process allowed for no further issues with most S-ICD hardware implanted worldwide. The battery longevity of the device has been projected at 5 years with 3 recaps per year and constant sensing of the patient's heart rhythm. For each shock, the device's battery is depleted by a month of longevity. The clinical follow-up of the S-ICD hardware including the battery has to date maintained its projected longevity based on the entire functioning of the S-ICD.

Software-related Malfunctions

The S-ICD software or operating system has been very reliable as it has been built using the standard guidance for therapeutic devices. Software or operating system malfunctions or resets have not had a clinical effect to date. The clinical performance of the software in the device has been monitored closely by the manufacturer and regulatory bodies interested in the safety and efficacy of the device. The complication free rate of 99% seen in the pivotal IDE study[2] did not include any software complication requiring reoperation. In the case of the IDE trial no software malfunctions led to reoperation. Random software resets have been seen during follow-up of the device without clinical circumstance. Six software revisions/upgrades or hardware uploads (routine for new operating system platforms) have been performed via the programmer to improve software reliability, battery longevity, and system efficiency.

SCREENING AND SENSING MALFUNCTION

Site investigators/operators have been responsible for screening all prospective patients who met the selection criteria and were appropriate for inclusion in the study. Patients were required to pass a preoperative surface electrocardiogram (ECG) screening test. The FDA-approved device requires the prescreen ECG in both supine and standing or seated positions.[10] The screening ECG is a modified trichannel surface ECG (see **Fig. 2**) that mimics the 3 sensing vectors of the S-ICD system as a surrogate on the surface of the chest. Once the 3 vector ECG tracings were obtained, a template tool (see **Fig. 3**) was used to assess the R wave to T wave ratio for appropriateness before device implantation. Despite this preimplant sensing screen, 2 patients who passed the screen in the IDE trial required device removal for inappropriate double counting of a wide QRS electrocardiogram.[2] These lessons learned led to revisions in the prescreen recommendations and the final labeling in the User's Manual designed to improve the accuracy of the screening tool. The data analysis from the Multicenter Automatic Defibrillator Implantation Trial to Reduce Inappropriate Therapy (MADIT-RIT)[15] has postulated a zero tolerance for inappropriate shocks—a compelling goal. The inappropriate shock rate in the IDE trial[2] was similar to TV-ICD rates pre–MADIT-RIT[16–18] and has been comprised of T-wave oversensing, electromagnetic interference from intensive electric fields and supraventricular tachycardia (SVT) shocks in the shock-only sensing zone.

Detection of Ventricular Tachycardia/VF

The S-ICD has been sensitive to both induced and spontaneous ventricular tachyarrhythmias.[1–3] During the IDE study,[2] there was one incident of delay to detect induced ventricular fibrillation that resulted in an external rescue shock at the operator's discretion before delivery by the S-ICD. Certainly, induced VF defibrillation testing has been considered to be nonrepresentative of conditions found during spontaneous events. There has *not* been an adjudicated spontaneous event of failure to detect ventricular tachyarrhythmias in a programmed zone or failure to deliver an appropriate shock (**Fig. 5**). The time to therapy is deliberate and consistent with treatment times seen in the MADIT-RIT[15] and has not led to worse clinical morbidity or mortality.[1–3,11]

T Wave Oversensing, Double Counting, and Electromagnetic Interference

T wave oversensing (TWOS) has become the most common inappropriate shock mechanism of the S-ICD system during both clinical trials and commercial use (**Fig. 6**). Oversensing caused inappropriate shocks in 25 patients (8%) in the IDE study[2] and has occurred at a 5% annual rate in the

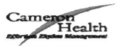

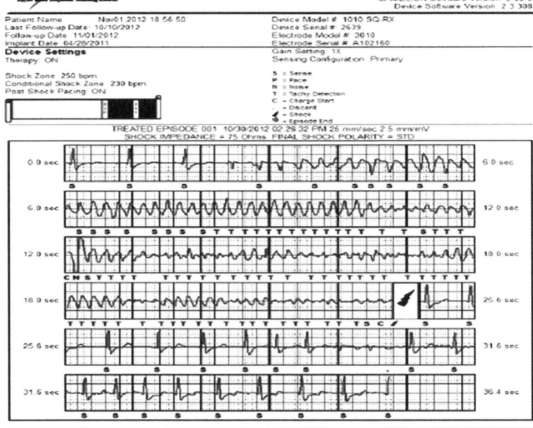

Fig. 5. Spontaneous ventricular fibrillation shock event. A stored spontaneous shock event from an S-ICD patient. The stored event shows a treated event and stored electrograms. The device identifies the shock polarity as standard and the shock lead impedance measurement for the event of 75 Ω. The event starting at the top left shows normal rate and rhythm with an abrupt change in morphology that is polymorphic and degenerates to VF and after approximately 18 seconds receives a shock (marked with the lightning bolt). The marker channel demonstrates a more deliberate sensing algorithm where the initial tachycardia is not an arrhythmia until it sustains its polymorphism. The marker channel is not as sensitive as an implanter might be accustomed. Not every electrogram of VF is marked with a "T" for tachycardia. The patient converts back to baseline morphology, marked by "S" for normal sensed beat. Also noted are premature atrial beats (marked as morphologically normal with an "S") and nonsustained ventricular tachycardia that is ignored without detriment to the patient. (Copyright © 2014 Boston Scientific Corporation or its affiliates. All rights reserved. Used with permission of Boston Scientific Corporation.) S, normal sensed beat; S-ICD, entirely subcutaneous implantable cardioverter defibrillator; T, tachycardia; VF, ventricular fibrillation.

EFFORTLESS Registry.[11] In the IDE, 22 patients experienced oversensing of T-waves or, more rarely, broad QRS complexes leading to double counting, whereas 3 patients experienced oversensing as a result of external noise while working with electrical equipment. The dynamic nature of repolarization and less often QRS duration has created challenges to the S-ICD sensing algorithm regarding double counting and T wave oversensing. The screening tool has helped to identify these patients before device procedure and implantation in the IDE study as well as since commercial release. Experience with the tool has led to adjustments in the prescreen method for specificity to qualify the patient for implant. Clinically, most oversensing leading to inappropriate shock events have been prevented by reprogramming a different sensing vector or amplitude, whereas less often a revision of sensing electrode position or removal of the device system has been required. The current screening protocol should help and, if it had been used during the IDE study,[2] then it

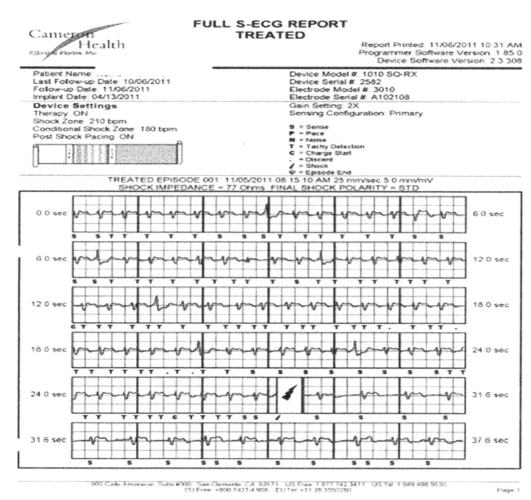

Fig. 6. Spontaneous T-wave oversensing shock event. A stored spontaneous shock event from an S-ICD patient. The stored event shows a treated event and stored electrograms. The device identifies the shock polarity as standard and the shock impedance of 77 Ω. The event starting at the top left shows a problem with a normal rate and morphologic rhythm with "T" marks where the T wave of repolarization would be expected. This continues for a much more deliberate time than the VF event presented in **Fig. 5** but eventually delivers a shock after nearly 30 seconds. There was little change in morphology but double counting or overcounting of the T wave led to a shock (marked with the lightning bolt). The marker channel demonstrates a more deliberate sensing algorithm where the initial tachycardia is not an arrhythmia until it sustains a very high rate over time. The marker channel is not as sensitive as an implanter might be accustomed to. The post-shock electrogram is not any different and the algorithm is even more deliberate. (Copyright © 2014 Boston Scientific Corporation or its affiliates. All rights reserved. Used with permission of Boston Scientific Corporation.) S, normal sensed beat; S-ICD, entirely subcutaneous implantable cardioverter defibrillator; T, tachycardia; VF, ventricular fibrillation.

would have excluded the 2 patients explanted for QRS double counting. Finally, programming dual zone detection and treatment rates (including a conditional zone [rate + discriminators]) have reduced the rate of inappropriate shocks for TWOS (56% relative reduction) and SVT (70% relative reduction).[2]

Supraventricular Tachycardia Inappropriate Shocks

Supraventricular tachycardia in the high-rate zone (no discriminators on), where rate alone determines whether a shock is delivered, was the cause of inappropriate shocks in 16 IDE patients (5.1%) and as selection screening and programming improved, this incidence moved down to an annual rate of 2% in the EFFORTLESS Registry.[2,11] These types of inappropriate shocks, so far, have been representative of normal sensing behavior by the *S-ICD System* at rates above the high-rate or shock-only zone (no discriminators). There are no reports of patients with an S-ICD having experienced an inappropriate shock within the conditional zone due to a discrimination error.

This bolsters the importance of dual chamber pacing as predicted by the START study data analysis[19] and the reported decrease in inappropriate shocks in the pivotal IDE study.[2]

The pivotal IDE study reported that 32 of the 41 patients who experienced an inappropriate shock were managed noninvasively with system reprogramming and/or medication changes.[2] Resolution of inappropriate shocks was associated with an invasive procedure in 9 patients: 2 devices were explanted because of QRS morphology changes that affected detection, 2 devices were turned off for reasons unrelated to inappropriate shocks, 1 electrode was repositioned, 1 pulse generator was repositioned, a MAZE surgery was performed, a radiofrequency ablation was performed, and an electrophysiology study was performed without ablation.[2]

PROCEDURE- AND LABELING-RELATED COMPLICATIONS

The S-ICD implant platform and device materials, including the programmer, have been designed for simplicity and ease of use in a well indicated population. As stated earlier, there are 3 well-defined worldwide complication categories that have been populated if invasive action has been taken to resolve the complication.[2] Device-related complications have been discussed. The remaining 2 categories include *procedure-* and *labeling*-related complications. Procedure-related complications include adverse clinical events that occur as a direct result of the procedure. The labeling has been set forth in the User's Manual[20] for handling of the device in and around the implant procedure to prevent procedural complication. The User's Manual since the regulatory studies began in 2008 has been very specific as to the human factor handling of the device. The pre-IDE strategies took into account many different device and procedural handling factors. Despite the many preimplant risk management features included in the User's Manual, human factor and procedural issues, although low in incidence, have been experienced.

Human Factor Complications

Being inattentive to the labeling in the User's Manual has led to complications requiring invasive action. In the case of the IDE and CE mark trials (prospective, multicenter), 3 specific instances of labeling-related complications included *failure to place the lead pin deep enough into the header* (n = 1) [ref] and *failure to suture the lead at the xiphoid process causing lead dislodgement* (n = 2).[1,2] Failure to place the pin deep enough leads to poor alignment of the "B" pin electrode

to the auto clamp interface in the device header, which has led to inappropriate sensing and need for operative revision. A demarcated landing zone for the lead pin into the header of the device allows for better alignment of the "A" and "B" electrodes in the header. Likewise, placement of the suture sleeve at the xiphoid process will keep the lead and the actual "B" electrode in the correct left parasternal position and stable from a sensing perspective. An operator could easily avoid these complications by carefully following the labeling clearly defined in the User's Manual.

Infection

There were 18 infections in the pivotal IDE study where 13 were managed noninvasively, whereas 5 infections required extraction (n = 4) or surgical revision (n = 1). Most of the invasive actions taken occurred early in the trial.[2] Steps were taken after identification of these complications to decrease this infection rate by better standardizing and emphasizing unique aspects of patient preparation through physician training materials and education. True device/pocket infection would not resolve with the use of oral antibiotics without extraction. The rate of TV-ICD–related infection has been on the rise.[21] The total number of infections in this study compares favorably with currently published data on ICD infections, which range from 0.13% to 19.9%.[22,23] Interestingly, the S-ICD has been used in patients whose TV-ICD was explanted due to infection without report of reinfection throughout the follow-up period. Most notably, there have been no reports of S-ICD–related endocarditis, a complication reported in 22% to 54% of cardiac device infections and associated with a 2-fold increase in mortality.[23,24] The S-ICD has seen early procedural complications requiring explantation for infection that were markedly decreased by expanding the chest wall prep area and sterile technique.

S-ICD Programming

The programmer interface (see **Fig. 2**) has been designed most simply in an effort to decrease the morbidity with both failures to program and/or overprogramming an ICD. Research and development of the sensing algorithm before human implant rendered many automatic functions within the device to simplify the end-user interaction post-implantation. The Start Study[19] has provided bench validation testing in comparison to industry standard TV-ICDs and demonstrated a significantly improved specificity for sensing with the addition of dual detection zone programming. Leaving the device programmed to a single shock-only zone has produced 56% to 74%[2] more inappropriate shocks and is not recommended. Programming the detection zones is 1 of 3 programmable features. The other 2 programming features are therapy "on" or "off" and post-shock pacing "on" and "off". Failure to program the device on has not been reported. Programming post-shock pacing "on" should lead to a thoughtful analysis of the A to B sensing vector as it becomes the default sensing vector during post-shock pacing, and if it is not a stout sensing vector having post-shock pacing "on" and active, post-therapy may lead to undersensing of VF during postshock reconfirmation. This is a theoretical concern and has not been reported to date.

SUMMARY

The S-ICD is a safe and effective defibrillator system that is an enticing addition to the electrophysiologist's toolbox in preventing sudden cardiac death. Early experience with the S-ICD has seen improvements in the device hardware and software as well as lessons learned that have decreased the incidence of human factor complications with the device and procedure. The low morbidity with the S-ICD system has been a good starting point for a new implant platform for cardiac arrest prevention that hopefully will be even lower as the experience broadens.

REFERENCES

1. Bardy GH, Smith WM, Hood MA, et al. An entirely subcutaneous implantable cardioverter-defibrillator. N Engl J Med 2010;363:36–44.
2. Weiss R, Knight BP, Gold MR, et al. Safety and efficacy of a totally subcutaneous implantable cardioverter defibrillator. Circulation 2013;128:944–53.
3. Olde Nordkamp LR, Dabiri Abkenari L, Boersma LV, et al. The entirely subcutaneous Implantable cardioverter-defibrillator: initial clinical experience in a large dutch cohort. J Am Coll Cardiol 2012; 60(19):1933–9.
4. Reynolds MR, Cohen DJ, Kugelmass DJ, et al. The frequency and incremental cost of major complications among medicare beneficiaries receiving implantable cardioverter defibrillators. J Am Coll Cardiol 2006;47:2493–7.
5. Alter P, Waldhans S, Plachta E, et al. Complications of implantable cardioverter defibrillator therapy in 440 consecutive patients. Pacing Clin Electrophysiol 2005;28:926–32.
6. Borleffs CJ, van Erven L, van Bommel RJ, et al. Risk of failure of transvenous implantable cardioverter defibrillator leads. Circ Arrhythm Electrophysiol 2009;2:411–6.
7. Kleemann T, Becker T, Doenges K, et al. Annual rate of transvenous lead defects in implantable cardioverter-defibrillators over a period of >10 yrs. Circulation 2007;115:2474–80.
8. Bellardine-Black CL, Stromberg K, Van Balen GP, et al. Is surface ECG a useful surrogate for subcutaneous ECG? Pacing Clin Electrophysiol 2010;33: 135–45.
9. Burke MC, Song Z, Jenkins J, et al. Analysis of electrocardiograms for subcutaneous monitors. J Electrocardiol 2003;36(Suppl):227–32.
10. Burke MC, Toff WD, Ludmer PL, et al. Comparisons during multiple postures of resting ECG's (COMPARE) study [abstract]. Heart Rhythm 2009; 6(Suppl 5):S126.
11. Lambiase PD, Theuns DA, Barr C, et al. International experience with a subcutaneous ICD: preliminary results of the effortless S-ICD registry [abstract]. Heart Rhythm 2012;9(5 Suppl 1):S15.
12. Aydin A, Hartel F, Schluter M, et al. Shock efficacy of the the subcutaneous ICD for prevention of sudden cardiac death: initial multicenter experience. Circ Arrhythm Electrophysiol 2012;5:913–9.
13. Jarman JW, Todd DM. United Kingdom national experience of entirely subcutaneous implantable cardioverter-defibrillator technology: important lessons to learn. Europace 2013;15:1158–65.
14. Saxon LA. The subcutaneous implantable defibrillator: a new technology that raises an existential question for the implantable cardioverter defibrillator. Circulation 2013;128:935–7.
15. Moss AJ, Shuger C, Beck CA, et al, for the MADIT –RIT Trial Investigators. Reduction in inappropriate therapy and mortality through ICD programming. N Engl J Med 2012;367:2275–83.
16. Saxon LA, Hayes DL, Gilliam FR, et al. Long term outcome after ICD and CRT implantation and influence of remote device follow up: the ALTITUDE survival study. Circulation 2010;122:2359–67.
17. Wilkoff BL, Williams BD, Stern SL, et al, PREPARE Study Investigators. Strategic programming of detection and therapy parameters in implantable cardioverter-defibrillators reduces shocks in primary prevention patients: results from the PREPARE (Primary Prevention Parameters Evaluation) study. J Am Coll Cardiol 2008;52:541–50.
18. Gasparini M, Menozzi C, Proclemer A, et al. A simplified biventricular defibrillator with fixed long detection intervals implantable cardioverter defibrillator(ICD) interventions and hear failure hospitalizations in patients with non-ischemic cardiomyopathy implanted for primary prevention: the RELEVENT [Role of long dEtection window programming in patients with left ventricular dysfunction, Non-ischemic etiology in primary prevention treated with a biventricular ICD] study. Eur Heart J 2009;30:2758–67.

19. Gold MR, Theuns DA, Knight BP, et al. Head-to-head comparison of arrhythmia discrimination performance of subcutaneous and transvenous ICD arrhythmia detection algorithms: the START Study. J Cardiovasc Electrophysiol 2012;23:359–66.
20. Available at: http://physician.cameronhealth.com/product-manuals.htm. Accessed April 2012.
21. Epstein AE, Kay GN, Plumb VJ, et al, ACT Investigators. Implantable cardioverter-defibrillator prescription in the elderly. Heart Rhythm 2009;6:1136–43.
22. Wilkoff BL. How to treat and identify device infections. Heart Rhythm 2007;4:1467–70.
23. Le KY, Sohail MR, Friedman PA, et al, Mayo Cardiovascular Infections Study Group. Clinical predictors of cardiovascular implantable electronic device-related infective endocarditis. Pacing Clin Electrophysiol 2011;34:450–9.
24. Athen E, Chu VH, Tattevin P, et al, ICE-PCS Investigators. Clinical characteristics and outcome of infective endocarditis involving implantable cardiac devices. JAMA 2012;307:1727–35.

Analysis of Pacing and Defibrillation Lead Malfunction

Ernest W. Lau, MD

KEYWORDS

- Lead malfunction • Conduction fracture • Insulation breaches

KEY POINTS

- Conductor failure is by fracture through fatigue.
- Insulation failure is by abrasion through relative movements under cyclic stresses or by creep with no relative movement under constant stress.
- Significant damage can be done to the existent leads during device system revision, causing malfunction.
- Lead malfunction includes damage to biologic tissues (tricuspid stenosis or regurgitation, cardiac perforation, pericardial effusion without perforation) or of a biologic nature (thrombosis, vegetations).
- Lead design should allow for extractability as well as reliability.

INTRODUCTION

Lead malfunction is the most common cause of cardiac implantable electronic device therapy failure. A lead is fundamentally an insulated conductor cord for transmitting electrical impulses. A standard pacing or defibrillation (DF) lead (ie, excluding those containing extra components like sensors and microcircuits[1]) has 4 basic types of components: conductor elements, insulations, electrodes (bores, rings, dots, coils), and connector pieces (**Fig. 1**). The conductor elements are made of multiple metal wires (fila) wound into interweaving helices (coils) or braided into wire ropes (cables).[2] The insulations are made of polymers: silicone (polydimethylsiloxane), poly(ether) urethane, fluoropolymers such as ethylene tetrafluoroethylene (ETFE) and polytetrafluoroethylene (PTFE), and silicone-polyurethane copolymers such as Optim (St Jude Medical, Sylmar, CA).

The electrodes are made of inert metals (eg, iridium, tungsten, platinum). The components are assembled by bonding, crimping, welding, and other processes.

Lead malfunction has been defined as not performing according to specifications or intentions.[3] Whether structural compromises without electrical anomalies[4,5] constitute malfunctions by that definition is open to interpretation. Even when all the electrical parameters are within normal limits, structural compromises in a lead may still pose dangers to the patient through cardiac perforation,[6] thrombogenesis,[7] bacterial infection,[8] interference with adjacent leads,[9] and difficulty in extraction.[10–12] The analysis of lead malfunctions is largely (but not exclusively) the study of lead structural compromises or failures. The pulse generator is both a cause[13] and a potential source of solutions for lead structural compromises and malfunctions.[14–16]

Disclosures: Consultancy St Jude Medical.
Department of Cardiology, Royal Victoria Hospital, Grosvenor Road, Belfast BT12 6BA, UK
E-mail address: ernest.lau@btinternet.com

Card Electrophysiol Clin 6 (2014) 307–326
http://dx.doi.org/10.1016/j.ccep.2014.02.006
1877-9182/14/$ – see front matter © 2014 Elsevier Inc. All rights reserved.

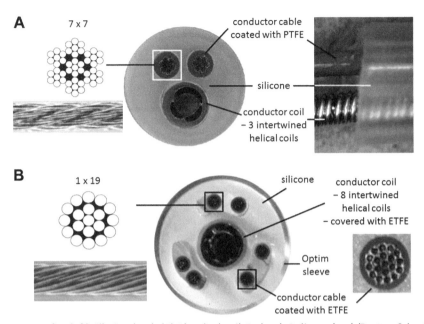

Fig. 1. Components of a defibrillation lead. (*A*) The dual-coil Endotak Reliance lead (Boston Scientific, St Paul, MN) has a trifilar conductor coil and two 7 × 7 configuration conductor cables coated with polytetrafluoroethylene (PTFE). (*B*) The dual-coil Durata lead (St Jude Medical, Sylmar, CA) has an octafilar conductor coil and six 1 × 19 configuration conductor cables coated with ethylene tetrafluoroethylene (ETFE). The lead has an extra outer insulation layer made of Optim, a silicone-polyurethane copolymer (St Jude Medical). (*Courtesy of [A] Boston Scientific, St Paul, MN; and [B] St Jude Medical, Sylmar, CA.*)

LEAD COURSE IN VIVO

Structural compromises are unevenly distributed along the length of a lead but are clustered in certain segments, suggesting their occurrences are related to its course in vivo.[15,17–20]

The Basic Course

The basic course of a lead in vivo (ie, in the absence of cardiorespiratory and musculoskeletal movements) depends on patient anatomy, implantation techniques, and lead design. The basic lead course contains a series of bends crossing multiple planes and requires 2 or more views to appreciate (**Figs. 2–5**). A lead implanted through cephalic cut-down bends caudomedially by approximately 80° over the medial border of the pectoralis minor and craniomedially by approximately 60° at the cephaloaxillary junction in the coronal plane (see **Fig. 3**). A lead implanted through axillosubclavian venous puncture can bend dorsomedially by 70° to 90° at the pectoralis major fixation and ventromedially by 70° to 90° at the venous entry in the transverse plane (see **Fig. 4**). Regardless of the venous access, the lead bends caudomedially by approximately 50° around the base of the lung apex before descending caudally toward the midline, and bends dorsally by approximately another 40° in the transverse plane as it wraps around the aorta if coming from the left. The lead bends caudally and dorsally by approximately 50° in the coronal and sagittal planes respectively at the superior vena cava (SVC) origin. The lead has a variable amount of slack in the right atrium (RA). If the lead tip is positioned inside the right ventricle (RV), the lead may have an extra bend over the tricuspid valve (TV). A left ventricular lead has some extra bends in the coronary sinus. The basic lead course can change significantly over time (such as with pulse generator migration), with concomitant lead length redistribution from one part of the course to another (see **Fig. 4**).

Side of Implantation

The right brachiocephalic vein (BCV) is shorter than the left BCV and does not wrap around the aorta, but this does not greatly affect the bends in the course of a lead implanted from the right (see **Figs. 2, 4** and **5**). However, the lead has more redundant lengths in the pocket and an SVC coil in a DF lead may be closer to the shoulder, which may increase the risk of failure for right-sided implantation of certain lead models.[21]

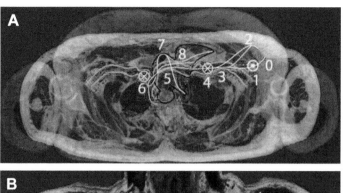

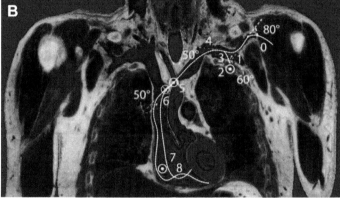

Fig. 2. Lead course based on anatomy. Sections of the thorax based on the Visible Human Project. (*A*) Superimposed transverse sections at the axillosubclavian-brachiocephalic vein and the midventricular cavity levels. (*B*) Coronal section at the midaxillary lines. A circle with a dot inside points out of the plane; a circle with a cross inside points into the plane. The lead course in vivo has a series of bends crossing multiple planes: the medial border of the pectoralis minor (0), the cephaloaxillary vein junction (1), the pectoralis major fixation (2), the axillosubclavian vein entry (3), the base of the lung apex (4), the aorta wrap (5), the superior vena cava origin (6), the right atrium (7), and the tricuspid valve (8).

Venous Access

Subclavian vein puncture has been associated with a higher risk of lead failure than cephalic cut-down,[22,23] even though leads implanted through cephalic cut-down still fail.[24] Because leads implanted through both accesses eventually follow the same intravenous course (see **Fig. 2**), the venous entry site, extra venous course, and pectoralis major fixation of subclavian vein puncture may compromise lead survival more than the acute bends over the medial border of the pectoralis minor and at the cephaloaxillary junction of cephalic cut-down. The term subclavian vein puncture may be a misnomer, because puncture by walking the needle down the clavicle until it passes beneath the bone[25,26] may enter the BCV or internal jugular vein, medial to the subclavian vein.[27] The needle track also often passes through the medial subclavicular musculotendinous complex comprising the subclavius, costoclavicular ligament, and costocoracoid ligament. Leads entrapped in the complex can experience high mechanical stresses during shoulder movement (despite the absence of direct contact between the clavicle and the first rib) and develop structural compromises over time (the subclavian crush).[27,28] Axillary or lateral subclavian vein puncture[29–35] should reduce the risks of lead entrapment within the complex and hence of lead malfunction, but clinical data on the adoption of axillary vein puncture and its impact on lead failure are lacking. In experiments, catheters placed in the costoclavicular angle through a medial subclavian vein puncture, a lateral subclavian vein puncture, and cephalic cut-down recorded pressure increases of 126 ± 26 mm Hg, 63 ± 15 mm Hg, and 38 ± 13 mm Hg respectively compared with baseline with caudal traction of the arm,[36] suggesting lower mechanical loading on leads with more lateral venous access.

Pocket

Most pulse generators are implanted in the pectoral region, in either a prepectoral or a subpectoral pocket. The subpectoral pocket requires more extensive dissection but offers more protection

A

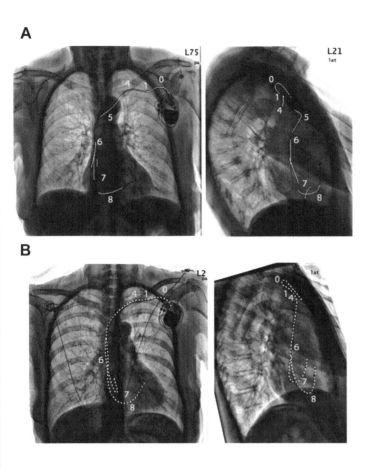

B

Fig. 3. The courses of leads implanted through the left cephalic cut-down. The courses of leads implanted through the left cephalic cut-down can be variable. Bend 0 around the medial border of the pectoralis minor is pronounced in (*A*) but subtle in (*B*). In the lateral view, bend 5 around the aorta is obvious in (*A*) but absent in (*B*). In the posteroanterior view, the aorta is caudal to the left brachiocephalic vein in (*B*). The medial border of the pectoralis minor (0), the cephaloaxillary vein junction (1), the pectoralis major fixation (2), the axillosubclavian vein entry (3), the base of the lung apex (4), the aorta wrap (5), the superior vena cava origin (6), the right atrium (7), and the tricuspid valve (8).

against erosion and better cosmetic appearance than the prepectoral pocket.[37,38] However, the leads and pulse generator inside a subpectoral pocket are subjected to stronger compressive forces from the pectoralis major than those inside a prepectoral pocket and may be more vulnerable to structural compromises as a result.[21,39]

Slack

Slack may be defined as the difference between the length of a lead body segment and its span (provided a straight course between its 2 end points is anatomically possible). Lead slack is difficult to quantify objectively and consistently, but a qualitative subjective grading system has been attempted.[40] In small quantities, slack is good and necessary to avoid lead tip displacement as the cardiac, thoracic, and pectoral dimensions and shapes change with cardiorespiratory and musculoskeletal movements. However, excessive slack creates tight bends in a lead segment, which can generate significant bending and compressive loads (especially when the lead segment struts the opposite walls of the anatomic space containing

it) and cause structural compromises over time. Excessive slack also predisposes to lead dislodgement.[41] Because of the size of the chambers compared with the lead diameter, the amount of slack in the RA and RV is highly variable.

Lead Design

The course adopted by a lead in vivo is likely to be controlled by both load and displacement. For the same load, a stiffer lead bends less but only has a straighter course in vivo if the course is controlled by load and not displacement.[42] For the same course (bends and slacks) in vivo, a stiffer lead contains more internal mechanical stresses, but the highest mechanical stresses may be caused by and contained within the insulation polymers and not the metal conductor elements (The Association for the Advancement of Medical Instrumentation, Cardiac Rhythm Management Device Committee, Leads Working Group is planning a study to quantify the use conditions for leads in vivo in order to develop better bench tests for their reliability.).

A

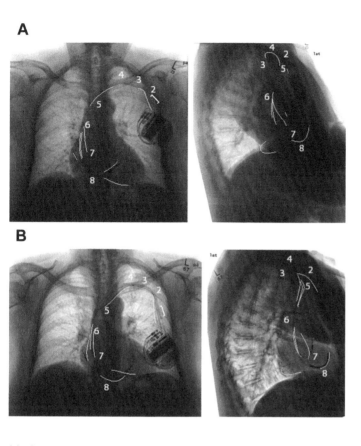

B

Fig. 4. The courses of leads implanted through the left axillary vein puncture. (A) One day after implantation. (B) Six weeks after implantation. The left ventricular lead has some additional bends in the coronary sinus. Bends 3, 5, and 6 are only obvious in the lateral projection. Bend 2 at the pectoralis major fixation was pronounced 1 day after implantation, but might not have been so during surgery with the patient in a supine position. Six weeks after implantation, the pulse generator had migrated caudally by about 2 rib spaces, dragging the pectoralis major fixation along (the distance between the suture sleeve and the pulse generator remained largely constant). Lead lengths were redistributed from the brachiocephalic vein and the axilla (between bends 2 and 5) to accommodate the migration, making bend 2 at the pectoralis major fixation less pronounced in the process. The basic courses of leads can change significantly over time. The medial border of the pectoralis minor (0), the cephaloaxillary vein junction (1), the pectoralis major fixation (2), the axillosubclavian vein entry (3), the base of the lung apex (4), the aorta wrap (5), the superior vena cava origin (6), the right atrium (7), and the tricuspid valve (8).

STRESS AND DEGRADATION

In vivo, a lead is exposed to a multitude of mechanical, chemical, and biological stresses, which, independently and synergistically, degrade its structural integrity. However, the degradation can be slow and may not become clinically significant during a lead's service life.

Mechanical Stresses

The mechanical loads to which a lead is exposed can be classified by their directions and periodicity. Axial loads are applied along the axis of the lead and cause it to displace, lengthen (extension), or shorten (compression, with the possibility of sideways buckling). Transverse loads are applied across the

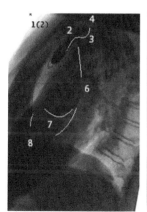
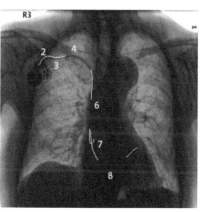

Fig. 5. The courses of leads implanted through right axillary vein puncture. The sharpest bends in the lead courses are at the pectoralis major fixation (bend 2) and venous entry (bend 3). The medial border of the pectoralis minor (0), the cephaloaxillary vein junction (1), the pectoralis major fixation (2), the axillosubclavian vein entry (3), the base of the lung apex (4), the aorta wrap (5), the superior vena cava origin (6), the right atrium (7), and the tricuspid valve (8).

axis of the lead and cause it to bend laterally or crush (uniform or nonuniform radial compression[36]). Torsional loads are applied around the axis of the lead and cause it to rotate or twist. Static loads vary little over time and come from the basic lead course (see **Figs. 2–5**). Low-amplitude high-frequency cyclic loads come from cardiorespiratory movements. High-amplitude low-frequency cyclic loads come from musculoskeletal movements.

Chemical Stresses

The inside of the body contains a variety of active chemical entities that attack any implanted foreign materials.[43] The passage of low-voltage and high-voltage currents between the electrodes of a lead may lead to the formation of additional active chemical entities (eg, hydrogen and oxygen molecules) capable of causing degradation.[44,45]

Biological Stresses

A lead may induce a local inflammatory response resulting in granulation or connective tissue encapsulation (with or without calcification),[46–48] cause thrombus formation,[48–51] or become colonized by bacteria.[52] Leads provide stable and nonhostile surfaces for bacteria to attach and form biofilms (complex communities of surface-associated cells enclosed in a polymer matrix containing open water channels).[53–55]

Fracture

In mechanical engineering, fracture is the physical separation of an object into 2 or more pieces under stress.[56] Fracture occurs in a single overstress event if the stress is higher than the ultimate strength of the material, or as the culmination of structural defects that have accumulated from cycles of stress over time (fatigue). A ductile material can deform both elastically and plastically, and its yield strength is less than its ultimate strength. A brittle material can only deform elastically but not plastically, and its yield strength is the same as its ultimate strength. A brittle material is prone to fracture because cracks propagate rapidly across it. The metal alloys used to make the conductor elements in a lead are ductile materials chosen specifically for their mechanical strength and resistance against chemical corrosion. In vivo, except in the context of extraction, a lead is unlikely to be exposed to mechanical stresses that are greater than the ultimate tensile strengths of the conductor elements. Conductor fractures in a lead generally occur as a result of fatigue.

Fatigue

In materials science, fatigue is the progressive structural damage in an object subjected to cyclic stresses caused by the initiation and propagation of cracks that may culminate in overload and abrupt fracture of the object (**Fig. 6**).[57] Cracks in an object can be caused by defects acquired during manufacturing or subsequent handling, or initiated during normal use if it involves cyclic loading. A crystalline material under mechanical stress (formally defined as force per unit area) can develop slip bands (shear lines between the crystalline planes) caused by dislocation (defect or irregularity within the crystal structure) movement or localized yielding at a stress concentration point, even when the nominal stresses are less than its yield strength. Over cycles of stress, more slip bands form and coalesce into microcracks. The tip of a crack forms a large stress concentration point, and extends in length (propagates) with each cycle of loading and unloading as long as the local stress exceeds the yield strength of the material and creates an adjacent plastic zone during loading. Defects (holes, inclusions) within the plastic zone are incorporated into the crack at its tip, accelerating its growth. Overload occurs when the local stress around the crack exceeds the ultimate strength of the material, resulting in abrupt fracture of the object. Fatigue fracture can be caused by compression, extension, bending, and torsion.

In practice, cyclic stresses follow a spectrum of temporal patterns. For theoretic considerations, cyclic stresses are modeled as an alternating stress following a sinusoidal pattern superimposed on a mean background stress (**Fig. 7**A). When the mean stress is 0, the cyclic stress is symmetric and reversed. When the mean stress is not 0 and in 1 direction but the minimum stress is in the opposite direction, the cyclic stress is asymmetric but still reversed. When the mean stress is not 0 and the minimum stress is 0, the cyclic stress is repeated with no reversal. When the means stress is not 0 and the minimum stress is in the same direction, the cyclic stress is fluctuating with no reversal. Cracks propagate when the local stress exceeds the yield strength of a material. The more the local stress exceeds the yield strength in a cycle, the faster cracks propagate and the shorter the fatigue life (number of cycles to fracture) of an object. Both the mean stress and the alternating stress affect the fatigue life. For symmetric reversed cyclic stress (mean stress 0), the fatigue life is inversely and nonlinearly related to the amplitude of the alternating stress (see **Fig. 7**B). For high-amplitude alternating

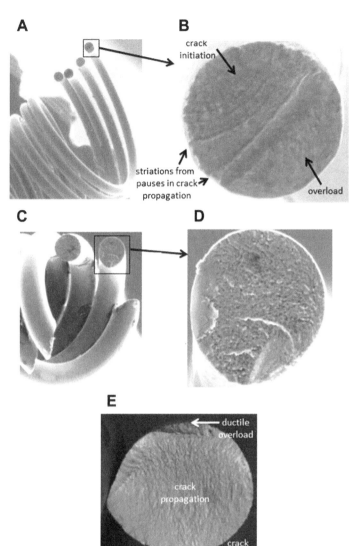

Fig. 6. Fatigue fracture of conductor coil wires. Scanning electron micrographs of conductor coil wire fracture caused by fatigue. (*A*, *B*) Bending fatigue with striations spreading from the initial crack to the final overload area. (*C*, *D*) Ductile overload with no clear fatigue crack. (*E*) Fatigue fracture caused by torsional stress on a conductor wire from a bending load on the coil. (*Courtesy of* St Jude Medical, Sylmar, CA; and Boston Scientific, St Paul, MN.)

stress, the fatigue life can be short ($<10^3$ or a thousand). For low-amplitude alternating stress, the fatigue life can be long (up to 10^8 or 100 million). For some materials, the fatigue life graph plateaus as the number of cycles increases, which means the object has an infinite fatigue life as long as the alternating stress is less than a certain amplitude (the endurance limit). For the same alternating stress, the higher the mean stress, the shorter the fatigue life (see **Fig. 7C**).

Creep

In materials science, creep is the spontaneous increase in strain (change in dimension per unit of the original dimension), even if the stress (which may be less than the yield strength) stays

constant, over time (**Fig. 8A**) [58] (A related concept is stress relaxation, which is the spontaneous decrease in stress, even if the strain stays constant, over time.) Creep becomes more pronounced as stress or temperature increases. For metals, creep only becomes noticeable when temperature reaches 30% of the absolute melting point (unlikely for the conductor elements in a lead in vivo). For polymers, creep can be significant even at normal body temperature. [19] Creep can lead to permanent deformation (ie, the strain remains even after the stress has been removed). Because the deformation occurs at less than the (crystalline) melting point of the material (metals and polymers), creep is also referred to cold flow, in contradistinction with hot flow, in which the deformation occurs at or greater than the

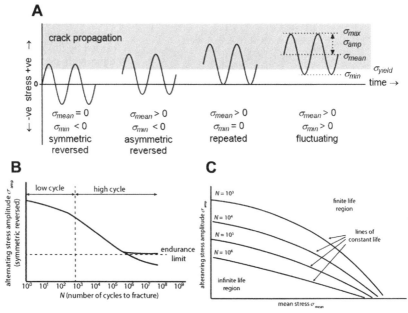

Fig. 7. Cyclic stress patterns and their impact on fatigue life. (*A*) A cyclic stress can be modeled as a sinusoidal alternating stress superimposed on a mean stress. Cracks propagate whenever the local stress exceeds the yield strength of the material. (*B*) For symmetric reversed cyclic stress (mean stress 0), the fatigue life (number of cycles to fracture) of an object is inversely and nonlinearly related to the alternating stress. High-amplitude alternating stress causes fatigue failure in few cycles (<10^3), whereas low-amplitude alternating stress allows a longer (even effectively infinite if the alternating stress is less than an endurance limit for some materials) fatigue life. (*C*) For the same alternating stress, the mean stress reduces the fatigue life of an object. (*Adapted from* Benham PP, Crawford RJ, Armstrong CG. Fracture mechanics. In: Benham PP, Crawford RJ, Armstrong CG, editors. Mechanics of engineering materials. 2nd edition. Essex, England: Pearson Education, Ltd.; 1996; with permission.)

melting point. Although metals become permanently deformed with creep, polymers may display some degree of recovery (disappearance of, or decrease in, strain after stress has been removed; see **Fig. 8**B) and memory (subsequent creep-relaxation behaviors affected by the past history of stress and strain).

Polymers are generally amorphous (ie, lacking the long-range ordered structure of a crystal) and consist of interpenetrating random coils of long molecular chains with possible short-range structures from crystallites, cross-linking (creating a network), and fillers (eg, silica particles in silicone).[59] Polymers display viscoelasticity and achieve creep through spatial reorganization of the molecular chains. A lead extracted intact often retains its shape in vivo, suggesting that the insulation materials have become permanently deformed (molded by the lead's anatomic course) at normal body temperature over a long period of time. Creep can cause polymer failure (cracking, crazing, necking, whitening, fracture; see **Fig. 8**C). For the insulation of a lead, creep causes redistribution (but not loss) of material, with thinning in one area matched by thickening in an adjacent area (like a crater; **Fig. 9**A). The thinned area becomes more

vulnerable to breach from abrasion or fracture under tension (see **Fig. 9**B).

Abrasion

In materials science, abrasion is the wearing down of the material of one surface because of movement relative to another under pressure. The wear (volume loss) rate is generally positively related to the normal force pressing the two surfaces into contact, the distance of relative movement between them, the hardness of the materials, and the roughness (size of asperities) of their surfaces.[60,61] Even though clinically significant abrasion damage to a lead mostly occurs to the insulations, the conductor elements can also be severely affected (from flattening of the fila to complete fracture of the conductor element).[8]

Environmental Stress Cracking

Environmental stress cracking (ESC) occurs to a polymer under the synergistic actions of chemical and mechanical stresses.[62] For a lead, ESC occurs mostly to polyurethane and requires exposure to cellular and extracellular body constituents (**Table 1**).[63,64] The cracks in the outer insulation

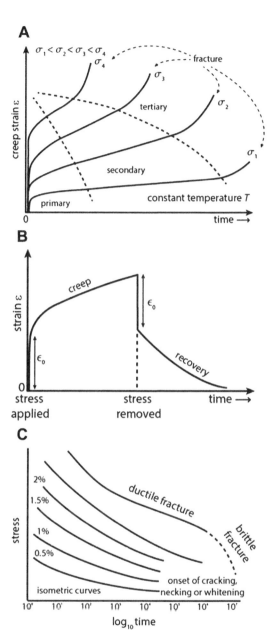

Fig. 8. Creep, recovery, and failure. (*A*) Creep is the spontaneous increase in strain at constant stress over time, and becomes more pronounced as stress increases. (*B*) Unlike metals, polymers recover from strain caused by creep over time once stress is removed. (*C*) Creep can cause failure other than fracture for polymers. Some polymers have an abrupt transition from ductile fracture to brittle fracture. (*Adapted from* Benham PP, Crawford RJ, Armstrong CG. Creep and viscoelasticity. In: Benham PP, Crawford RJ, Armstrong CG, editors. Mechanics of engineering materials. 2nd edition. Essex, England: Pearson Education, Ltd.; 1996. p. 573–97; with permission.)

under ESC may allow body chemicals to come into contact with the metal components, setting up a similar process called environmental stress fracture or stress corrosion cracking.[45]

ESC of polyurethane in vivo may be a 2-stage process: (1) oxidation of the ether soft segments by body chemicals weakens the polymer surface, allowing shallow, brittle microcracks to form under mechanical stresses of less than the ordinary yield strength; (2) body fluid components widen and deepen the formed cracks without inducing major detectable bulk chemical reactions (**Fig. 10**).[65] ESC of polyurethane is directly related to residual processing or applied mechanical stresses and the ether content in the polymer.[65,66] ESC of polyurethane in leads has been reduced but not eliminated by changes in polymer design and manufacturing.[47,67]

Metal Ion–induced Oxidation

Metal ion–induced oxidation (MIO) is a degradation process that affects only polyurethane in a lead and requires exposure to metal ions (principally cobalt) released from the conductor elements by solvation, galvanic or electrolytic corrosion, or chemical oxidation (eg, by hydrogen peroxide) in vivo (see **Table 1**).[65,68–70] The metal ions induce oxidation of the ether soft segment of polyurethane directly, or indirectly by acting as catalysts, even in the absence of mechanical stress. The polyurethane becomes brittle and cracks (**Fig. 11**), exposing the metal conductor elements to more body fluids, setting up a positive chain reaction.[70] MIO can be reduced by physically separating polyurethane from the conductor elements in a lead, such as by coating the conductor elements with a thin layer of a fluoropolymer.[67]

Chain Scission

The chemical bonds in the backbone (rather than just the cross-links between the chains) of a polymer (other than polyurethane) can break down over time (by hydrolysis, oxidation, or a combination of the two processes acting in tandem), leading to a reduction in the size of the molecular chain and molar mass of the polymer.[71–73] Such changes at a molecular level can lead to corresponding changes (reduction in tensile strength and abrasion/fatigue resistance) at a material level.

LEAD MALFUNCTION: MECHANISMS, MANIFESTATIONS, AND MITIGATING MEASURES

The degradation processes, malfunction mechanisms, manifestations, and mitigation measures

A

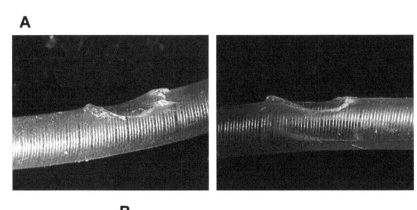

B

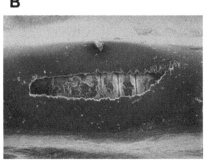

Fig. 9. Creep and associated insulation breach. (*A*) For the insulation of a lead, creep can cause redistribution (but not loss) of material, with thinning in one area (by direct local pressure or stretching) matched by thickening in an adjacent area, resulting in a crater shape. (*B*) The oval-shaped impression on the insulation is likely to be permanent deformation caused by creep. The thinned central area becomes more vulnerable to breach from abrasion. Note spalls of insulation material around the defect. (*Courtesy of* Medtronic, Minneapolis, MN.)

Table 1
Comparison of ESC and metal ion–induced oxidation of poly(ether)urethane in a lead

	ESC	Metal Ion–induced Oxidation
Conditions	Residual processing ± applied mechanical stresses Exposure to cellular/extracellular body constituents	Physical proximity to metal conductor elements
Crack	—	—
Surface	External (exposed to cells and body fluids)	Internal (exposed to entrapped metal ions released from corroded metal conductor elements)
Wall	Rough (ductile fracture)	Smooth (brittle fracture)
Orientation	Perpendicular to the mechanical stress (disorganized if multidirectional mechanical stresses)	Random
Distribution	Sites of mechanical stresses	Along metal conductor configuration

Data from Coury AJ. Chemical and biochemical degradation of polymers intended to be biostable. In: Ratner BD, Hoffman AS, Schoen FJ, editors. Biomaterials science - an introduction of materials in medicine. 3rd edition. Waltham (MA): Academic Press; 2013. p. 696–715.

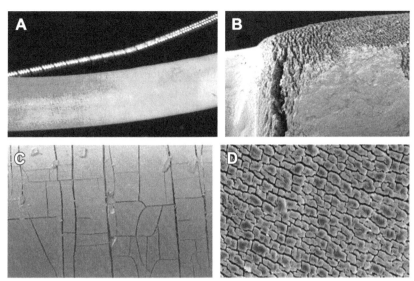

Fig. 10. ESC of polyurethane. Degradation of polyurethane by ESC starts from the outer surface exposed to chemical attacks under mechanical stresses. Cracking of polyurethane and the associated insulation breach can be macroscopically visible (*A*). The cracking can be highly localized (*B*), appear organized (perpendicular to the main stress vector; *C*), or disorganized (multidirectional stress vectors; *D*). (*Courtesy of* Medtronic, Minneapolis, MN.)

for the different components in a lead are listed in **Table 2**. Insulation breach is probably the most important cause of lead malfunction (4–5 times more common than conductor fracture).[74] The fluoropolymer layers around conductor elements serve multiple purposes in addition to providing extra insulation (**Box 1**).

Manifestations

The manifestations of lead malfunction are limited, and comprise failure to sense, pace, or shock: change in impedance; sensing nonexistent signals (noise); or delivering electrical impulses to the wrong place (short circuit, which may cause failure of shock therapy or electrical overstress damage to the pulse generator[75]). When the conductor elements or their joints (welding, crimps) are

compromised, the impedance typically increases. When the insulations are compromised, the impedance typically decreases. The manifestations may be only intermittent, making their ascertainment difficult. Because the degradation processes and malfunction mechanisms are generally irreversible, in the absence of other clearly reversible causes (eg, exposure to strong electromagnetic interference), the lead should be regarded as compromised even if the manifestation has only been observed once.

Conductor Fractures

The fila in the conductor elements of a lead are made of metal alloys (for mechanical strength and resistance against chemical corrosion; eg, MP35N), either as a solid wire or as the outer

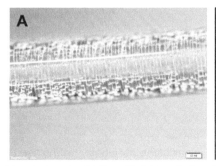
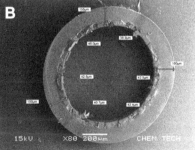

Fig. 11. Metal ion–induced oxidation. Metal ion–induced oxidation degrades polyurethane from its internal surface, which is in contact with the conductor elements and the source of metal ions. Note that the brickwork pattern of cracks in the insulation follows the turns in the underlying metal conductor coil (*A*) and the sharp, smooth-walled cracks indicate brittle fracture (*B*). (*Courtesy of* Medtronic, Minneapolis, MN.)

Table 2
Lead malfunction: mechanisms, manifestations, and mitigating measures

Component	Degradation Processes	Malfunction Mechanisms	Manifestations	Mitigating Measures
Conductor coil	Fatigue	Fracture	Failure to pace or sense Lead noise High impedance	↓ sharp bends in lead course Stagger static bends and flexion points Better conductor coil design
Conductor cable	Fatigue	Fracture	Failure to pace, sense or shock Lead noise High impedance	↓ sharp bends in lead course Stagger static bends and flexion points Better conductor coil design
Insulation	Abrasion Creep Chain scission	Breach	Failure to pace or sense Lead noise Low impedance Failure to shock Electrical overstress of pulse generator Stimulation of the pectoralis major	↑ thickness of insulation More slippery or abrasion-resistant materials Prepectoral pocket Avoid sharp bends in lead course Avoid close contact with other leads inside the cardiac chambers Possibly cover pulse generator with a slippery coating (eg, Parylene) Possibly ↓ spare space around conductor cables
Polyurethane insulation	ESC MIO	Breach		↑ polymer chain cross-links Coating metal conductors with fluoropolymers
Connection with electrode	Fatigue	Fracture	Failure to pace or sense Lead noise High impedance	Crimping (±welding) Stress-relieving design
Connector piece	Fatigue	Fracture	Failure to pace, sense, or shock Lead noise High impedance	Possibly shorter rigid crimp zone Possibly central arrangement of cables (no spiraling) Possibly spiral arrangement of cables Possibly splice joints inside the header Stress-relieving design

cladding of a drawn filled tube (or brazed strand) with a silver core (for improving electrical conductivity). The conductor coil is like a series of interweaving helical springs and possesses intrinsic axial, lateral, and torsional flexibility. The conductor cables are like wire ropes, primarily designed for tensile strength and they are unable to extend significantly in length.[76] Whether the conductor element is stretched, bent, or torqued, the fila are subject to both bending and torsional loads (the balance depends on the orientation of the fila to the direction of the load, which in turn depends on the structure of the conductor element[2,77]. When exposed to sufficient tension, the fila may break in a single overstress event if their tensile strengths are exceeded. Such breakage is unlikely to happen in vivo unless the fila have been weakened by fatigue or crushing. Most conductor element fractures probably come from fatigue caused by cyclic stresses.

For a lead in vivo, the anatomic course imposes a static mean stress at various points along its length. Cardiorespiratory movements impose low-amplitude high-frequency alternating stresses regularly. Musculoskeletal movements impose high-amplitude low-frequency alternating stresses sporadically. The points along a lead most vulnerable to fatigue fracture should be where a high-amplitude alternating stress meets a high mean stress. The 2 sharp bends (high mean stresses) at the pectoralis major fixation (bend 2) and venous entry (bend 3) for a lead inserted through axillosubclavian venous puncture (see **Fig. 2**) have no anatomic bases and may be subjected to severe bending, twisting, and pulling (high alternating stresses) during shoulder movements (**Fig. 12**). In contrast, the 2 sharp bends (high mean stresses) at the medial border of the pectoralis minor (bend 0) and the cephaloaxillary junction (bend 1) for a lead inserted through cephalic cut-down (see **Fig. 2**) have anatomic bases and are protected from severe deformation and displacement by the axillary soft tissues (low alternating stresses) during shoulder movements. These differences may explain why leads implanted through axillosubclavian venous puncture are more prone to conductor fatigue fracture than leads implanted through cephalic cut-down, especially around the suture sleeve.[78,79] A lead that bends more at rest

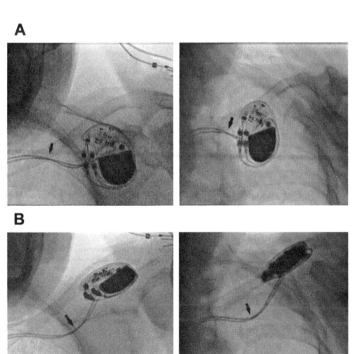

A

B

Fig. 12. Lead excursion with shoulder movements. (*A*) The shoulder is in neutral position. (*B*) The shoulder is in full abduction. The posteroanterior view is on the left and the left anterior oblique view is on the right. The 2 leads were inserted through left axillary vein puncture. Where the atrial and ventricular leads crossed corresponds with their pectoralis major fixations (*marked by arrows*). The pectoralis major fixations moved laterally and bent acutely with abduction of the shoulder, imposing severe axial (pulling) and traverse (bending) stresses on the two leads.

and during shoulder movements may be more prone to conductor fatigue fracture from both higher mean and alternating stresses.[42] However, a flexible conductor element in a lead with a higher curvature may still experience lower mean and/or alternating stresses than a stiffer conductor element in a lead with a lower curvature. A lead entrapped in the subclavicular musculotendinous complex may be exposed to mechanical stresses sufficient to cause conductor fracture in a few cycles, or create cracks for propagation by subsequent lower amplitude cyclic stresses, providing a materials science explanation for the subclavian crush (**Fig. 13**).

Insulation Breaches

Abrasion is probably the most significant insulation degradation process in vivo. However, even outright insulation breaches (including to the ETFE coating of conductor cables) may not cause electrical anomalies.[5,80]

External-origin (outside-in) abrasion of insulations occurs when another object rubs against a lead from the outside anywhere along its course. The device pocket can produce severe external-origin insulation abrasion. The pulse generator (both the can and the header) are made of hard materials compared with lead insulations. The fibrous tissues encapsulating the leads within the pocket or forming the pocket capsule can be dense and tough or even calcified (as experienced during lead extraction or pulse generator change).[47]

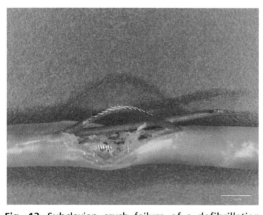

Fig. 13. Subclavian crush failure of a defibrillation lead. The silicone insulating the conductor elements from the outside and from one another is completely disrupted. The conductor cable to the right ventricular shock coil is severed. The conductor coil and the cable to the proximal superior vena cava shock coil remain in physical continuity, but are exposed because of abrasion of both the silicone and PTFE insulation. (*Courtesy of* Boston Scientific, St Paul, MN.)

The ribs form the deep surface of a subpectoral pocket. Significant pressure can be exerted on the pocket contents by the skin and subcutaneous tissues alone in a prepectoral pocket, and extra pressure is added by the pectoralis major (especially when it is contracting) in a subpectoral pocket. The relative movements of the contents can be large (centimeters rather than millimeters) as the pocket deforms with shoulder movements. A subpectoral pocket is generally more conducive to external abrasion of insulations than a prepectoral pocket.[39] Outer insulation damage in the pocket has generally been attributed to can-to-lead or lead-to-lead abrasion. Whether fibrous tissues cause significant external-origin insulation abrasion in the pocket is difficult to ascertain because they need to be disrupted and displaced during lead extraction and the extraction process can cause significant insulation damage. The BCV and SVC produce mainly mild to moderate linear external-origin insulation abrasion.[8,47] The cardiac chambers may produce severe external-origin insulation abrasion. The repetitive brushing movements by the TV leaflets with cardiac contractions can cause outer insulation breach for a lead traversing the valve into the RV.[81] Leads held in close proximity within the RA can develop outer insulation breach by lead-to-lead abrasion with cardiorespiratory movements.[8,9,82] Silicone is more susceptible to abrasion damage than the other polymers used for lead insulation.

Internal origin abrasion of insulations occurs when a lead segment deforms (compression, extension, bending, twisting), causing relative movements of the components within. The resulting insulation damage may be directed inwards (inside-in abrasion) or outwards (inside-out abrasion). Insulation breaches contained in the lead body (inside-in abrasion[83] or inside-out abrasion under the shock coil[19,84,85]) are likely to cause short circuits between the conductor elements because of the highly confined space available.

Conductor cable externalization with protrusion (CCE*) is a specific form of outer insulation breach affecting primarily the Riata and Riata ST family of DF leads and the QuickSite and QuickFlex family of left ventricular leads (St Jude Medical).[19,86] Differential lead component pulling with extension in one lead segment and conjugate reciprocal compression-bending in another mediated by fixed-length conductor cables has been proposed as a possible mechanism for the phenomenon.[76] The insulation defect of CCE* may appear as a slit rather than a scrape when inspected from the outside (**Fig. 14**), but it is wedge shaped with the wider edge on the inside pointing outwards (**Fig. 15**), suggesting that degradation is mainly

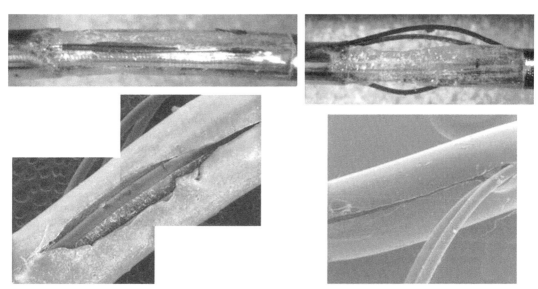

Fig. 14. Outside-in versus inside-out abrasion of defibrillation lead insulation. The left side shows outside-in abrasion: scrape wide and deep in center, tapering out at both ends, significant loss of material on the external surface. The right side shows inside-out abrasion: slit width and depth the same along the defect; little loss of material on the external surface. (*Courtesy of* St Jude Medical, Sylmar, CA.)

by inside-out abrasion (significant loss of material) and not creep (redistribution of material).[19]

Connection Failure

The lead body is generally flexible, which creates a potential problem where it joins more rigid segments like the tip or the connector piece(s) containing the pin(s).[87] Abrupt transition in stiffness can cause abrupt change in curvature,[88] which in turn may concentrate mechanical stresses and predispose to fracture. Crimping in addition to welding should strengthen the joint between the conductor elements and the lead tip.[89] A shorter crimp zone may reduce the concentration of mechanical stresses and hence may reduce conductor fatigue fracture in the connector piece.[90] The new DF4 header and associated connector pieces may bring extra benefits but may also pose unquantified failure risks.[91,92]

Biodegradation

An implanted lead is likely first to be covered by granulation tissues, which may take a long time (if ever) to convert into fibrous connective tissues.[47] Leads that are covered only by granulation tissues are easy to extract even after years of implantation. Calcium specks in the encapsulating tissue sheath[47] can act as abrasives when the lead moves relative to the sheath. Defects on the outer insulation surface by whatever degradation process facilitate adhesion by bacteria.[52] Release of active chemical entities by bacteria (eg, *Staphylococcus aureus*) and the reacting macrophages accelerate the biodegradation of silicone, leading to insulation breaches.[93] Clinically silent bacterial colonization occurs in up to 33% of device pockets.[94,95] Bacteria growing in biofilms adherent to implanted medical devices are highly resistant to antimicrobial agents, by several mechanisms.[53,54]

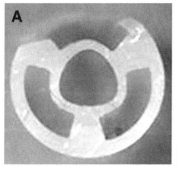
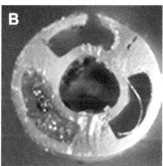

Fig. 15. Cross sections of outer insulation breaches of the Riata leads. The outer insulation breaches are wedge-shaped defects with significant loss but no redistribution of material, and hence are caused by abrasion rather than creep. For outside-in abrasion, the wedge-shaped defect has its wider edge on the outside pointing inwards (*A*). For inside-out abrasion, the wedge-shaped defect has its wider edge on the inside pointing outwards (*B*). (*Courtesy of* St Jude Medical, Sylmar, CA.)

Complications with Device System Revision

Device system revision is associated with a higher risk of complications than initial implantation, especially if lead modification (insertion and/or removal) and not just pulse generator change is involved. The most common complication is need for reoperation because of lead dislodgement or malfunction (1% of pulse generator changes only; 7.9% of lead modifications).[96] Infection may be up to 4 times more common for device system revision (2.1%) than for initial implantation (0.5%).[97]

A device system revision procedure can cause significant structural damage to the existent leads. Freeing enough lengths of leads for extracting the pulse generator out of the pocket alone may involve considerable manual handling (pulling, bending, and twisting) and dissection (blunt with a pair of arterial forceps, sharp with a scalpel blade, or thermal with electrocautery). The forces used in manual handling may be severe enough to cause outright overstress fractures of the conductor elements, especially if they are already compromised by previous crushing and fatigue.[98] Both blunt and sharp dissection can cause direct mechanical damage to the outer insulation. Electrocautery can cause thermal damage to the outer insulation, but the problem is less for silicone than for polyurethane or silicone-polyurethane copolymers.[99] Lead insertion almost always involves puncture of the subclavian vein or the BCV with an introducer needle. Lead removal often involves advancement of a sheath over the lead. Both processes may inflict direct mechanical damage to the insulations and conductor elements of the existent leads. Minute defects not enough to cause immediately obvious malfunction may still initiate or accelerate degradation processes that cause malfunction later (including infection). Using a blunt-tipped (eg, Tuohy) needle for venous puncture during lead insertion may reduce the risk of damage to the existent leads.

Lead Damage to Biological Tissues

The converse of biological damage to leads is lead damage to biological tissues. Leads can cause thrombosis, cardiac perforation, and clinically significant TV dysfunction (stenosis and regurgitation).[41,48,100–102] These biological consequences are not the intentions of lead design and hence can be regarded as instances of malfunction, or at least as collateral damage during the clinical use of leads. Lead design (eg, polyurethane may be less thrombogenic than silicone[103,104]) and implantation techniques (eg, prolapsing the lead body across the TV rather than crossing it directly

with the lead tip; minimum lead slack[100]) may help reduce the risk of such collateral damage to biological tissues.

SUMMARY

The survival of a lead in vivo is the result of long-term, dynamic interaction between the patient and the lead, mediated by one-off intervention from the implanter. Certain patient characteristics may predispose to lead malfunction,[40,105] but they may not be alterable. The reliability of the lead depends on both its design and manufacturing. Lead design is an iterative process incorporating previous experiences (especially from field performance[90]) and new experimental[61,71–73] and theoretic[76,88] insights to meet evolving clinical demands (eg, smaller caliber leads, quadripolar pacing leads), but it is slow (years to decades) and costly. Lead manufacturing is equally crucial; even an excellent design needs to be precisely manufactured according to specifications under stringent quality control. The implanter is theoretically the most changeable element but only has a single opportunity (short of reintervention) to affect the survival of a lead in vivo. Certain implantation techniques (eg, cephalic cut-down access, prepectoral pocket, minimum lead slack, not-too-tight sleeve suturing) may help reduce lead malfunction.

Leads are inanimate objects with no regenerative capabilities operating under a multitude of stresses in the harsh environment of the body. Design features that extend the longevity of a lead (eg, thicker insulation) may create other undesirable properties (eg, a larger lead caliber, higher perforation risk). Alongside efforts to enhance the longevity and reliability of leads, attention should also be directed toward making leads safer and easier to extract.[106] If leads are as safe and easy to replace as the pulse generator, dealing with lead malfunction may become more a financial than a clinical and technical issue.

ACKNOWLEDGMENTS

I am indebted to Dan Cooke and Dave Smith from Boston Scientific, Chris Jenney and John Helland from St Jude Medical, and Adam Himes and Jennifer Miller from Medtronic for their helpful comments and suggestions and for supplying photographs and scanning electron micrographs of leads and their components. This article contains a significant amount of materials science and engineering concepts, but reflects only a small portion of the work that has been conducted by these lead engineers and their colleagues over the years in developing better, more reliable, and safer leads for the benefit of patients and implanting physicians. For this continuous effort by the device industry, and the personal assistance toward enhancing this article rendered by the individuals mentioned, I am profoundly grateful.

REFERENCES

1. Gras D, Kubler L, Ritter P, et al. Recording of peak endocardial acceleration in the atrium. Pacing Clin Electrophysiol 2009;32(Suppl 1):S240–6.
2. Meagher JM, Altman P. Stresses from flexure in composite helical implantable leads. Med Eng Phys 1997;19:668–73.
3. Maisel WH, Hauser RG, Hammill SC, et al. Recommendations from the Heart Rhythm Society Task Force on Lead Performance Policies and Guidelines: developed in collaboration with the American College of Cardiology (ACC) and the American Heart Association (AHA). Heart Rhythm 2009;6: 869–85.
4. Maytin M, Epstein LM. Lead electrical parameters may not predict integrity of the Sprint Fidelis ICD lead. Heart Rhythm 2012;9:1446–51.
5. Theuns DA, Elvan A, de VW, et al. Prevalence and presentation of externalized conductors and electrical abnormalities in Riata defibrillator leads after fluoroscopic screening: report from the Netherlands Heart Rhythm Association Device Advisory Committee. Circ Arrhythm Electrophysiol 2012;5:1059–63.
6. Kay GN, Brinker JA, Kawanishi DT, et al. Risks of spontaneous injury and extraction of an active fixation pacemaker lead: report of the Accufix Multicenter Clinical Study and Worldwide Registry. Circulation 1999;100:2344–52.
7. Goyal SK, Ellis CR, Rottman JN, et al. Lead thrombi associated with externalized cables on Riata ICD leads: a case series. J Cardiovasc Electrophysiol 2013;24:1047–50.
8. Kolodzinska K, Kutarski A, Grabowski M, et al. Abrasions of the outer silicone insulation of endocardial leads in their intracardiac part: a new mechanism of lead-dependent endocarditis. Europace 2012;14:903–10.
9. Kutarski A, Malecka B, Kolodzinska A, et al. Mutual abrasion of endocardial leads: analysis of ex-planted leads. Pacing Clin Electrophysiol 2013; 36:1503–11.
10. Larsen JM, Theuns DA, Thogersen AM. Paradoxical thromboembolic stroke during extraction of a recalled St Jude Medical Riata defibrillator lead with conductor externalization. Europace 2014; 16(2):240.
11. Rubenstein DS, Weston LT, Kneller J, et al. Safe extraction of Riata looped extruding filler cables. J Cardiovasc Electrophysiol 2013;24:942–6.
12. Demirel F, Adiyaman A, Delnoy PP, et al. Extreme externalization of Riata intracardiac cardioverter defibrillator leads: a new peril of a troublesome lead. J Cardiovasc Electrophysiol 2013. http://dx. doi.org/10.1111/jce.12277.
13. Hauser RG, Abdelhadi RH, McGriff DM, et al. Failure of a novel silicone-polyurethane copolymer (Optim) to prevent implantable cardioverter-defibrillator lead insulation abrasions. Europace 2013;15:278–83.
14. Swerdlow CD, Gunderson BD, Ousdigian KT, et al. Downloadable software algorithm reduces inappropriate shocks caused by implantable cardioverter-defibrillator lead fractures: a prospective study. Circulation 2010;122:1449–55.
15. Swerdlow CD, Gunderson BD, Ousdigian KT, et al. Downloadable algorithm to reduce inappropriate shocks caused by fractures of implantable cardioverter-defibrillator leads. Circulation 2008; 118:2122–9.
16. Ellenbogen KA, Gunderson BD, Stromberg KD, et al. Performance of ICD lead integrity alert to assist in the clinical diagnosis of ICD lead failures: analysis of different ICD leads. Circ Arrhythm Electrophysiol 2013;6(6):1169–77.
17. Koneru JN, Gunderson BD, Sachanandani H, et al. Diagnosis of high-voltage conductor fractures in Sprint Fidelis leads. Heart Rhythm 2013; 10:813–8.
18. Erkapic D, Duray GZ, Bauernfeind T, et al. Insulation defects of thin high-voltage ICD leads: an underestimated problem? J Cardiovasc Electrophysiol 2011;22:1018–22.
19. Hauser RG, McGriff D, Retel LK. Riata implantable cardioverter-defibrillator lead failure: analysis of ex-planted leads with a unique insulation defect. Heart Rhythm 2012;9:742–9.
20. St Jude Medical. Riata lead evaluation study phase I results. 2012. Available at: http://professional.sjm.com/~/media/pro/resources/product-performance/riata/quality/SJM ICD Lead Design_and_Performance-July_2013.ashx.
21. Bernstein NE, Karam ET, Aizer A, et al. Right-sided implantation and subpectoral position are predisposing factors for fracture of a 6.6 French ICD lead. Pacing Clin Electrophysiol 2012;35:659–64.
22. Roelke M, O'Nunain SS, Osswald S, et al. Subclavian crush syndrome complicating transvenous cardioverter defibrillator systems. Pacing Clin Electrophysiol 1995;18:973–9.
23. Parsonnet V, Roelke M. The cephalic vein cutdown versus subclavian puncture for pacemaker/ICD lead implantation. Pacing Clin Electrophysiol 1999;22:695–7.
24. Bonney WJ, Spotnitz HM, Liberman L, et al. Survival of transvenous ICD leads in young patients. Pacing Clin Electrophysiol 2010;33:186–91.

25. Davidson JT, Ben-Hur N, Nathen H. Subclavian venepuncture. Lancet 1963;282:1139–40.

26. Mogil RA, DeLaurentis DA, Rosemond GP. The infraclavicular venipuncture. Value in various clinical situations including central venous pressure monitoring. Arch Surg 1967;95:320–4.

27. Magney JE, Flynn DM, Parsons JA, et al. Anatomical mechanisms explaining damage to pacemaker leads, defibrillator leads, and failure of central venous catheters adjacent to the sternoclavicular joint. Pacing Clin Electrophysiol 1993;16:445–57.

28. Magney JE, Parsons JA, Flynn DM, et al. Pacemaker and defibrillator lead entrapment: case studies. Pacing Clin Electrophysiol 1995;18:1509–17.

29. Magney JE, Staplin DH, Flynn DM, et al. A new approach to percutaneous subclavian venipuncture to avoid lead fracture or central venous catheter occlusion. Pacing Clin Electrophysiol 1993;16:2133–42.

30. Lau EW. Upper body venous access for transvenous lead placement - review of existent techniques. Pacing Clin Electrophysiol 2007;30:901–9.

31. Lau EW. Navigation by parallax in three dimensional space during fluoroscopy: application in guide wire-directed axillary/subclavian vein puncture. Pacing Clin Electrophysiol 2007;30:1054–66.

32. Lau EW. Axillary/subclavian vein puncture using navigation by parallax with an imaginary target. Pacing Clin Electrophysiol 2007;30:1531–41.

33. Nakata A, Harada T, Kontani K, et al. Extrathoracic subclavian venipuncture by using only the J-type guidewire for permanent pacemaker electrode placement. Int Heart J 2013;54:129–32.

34. Antonelli D, Feldman A, Freedberg NA, et al. Axillary vein puncture without contrast venography for pacemaker and defibrillator leads implantation. Pacing Clin Electrophysiol 2013;36:1107–10.

35. Seto AH, Jolly A, Salcedo J. Ultrasound-guided venous access for pacemakers and defibrillators. J Cardiovasc Electrophysiol 2013;24:370–4.

36. Jacobs DM, Fink AS, Miller RP, et al. Anatomical and morphological evaluation of pacemaker lead compression. Pacing Clin Electrophysiol 1993;16:434–44.

37. Kistler PM, Fynn SP, Mond HG, et al. The subpectoral pacemaker implant: it isn't what it seems! Pacing Clin Electrophysiol 2004;27:361–4.

38. Pena RE, Shepard RK, Ellenbogen KA. How to make a submuscular pocket. J Cardiovasc Electrophysiol 2006;17:1381–3.

39. Gilligan DM, Joyner CA, Gilliam FR. High incidence of atrial lead insulation failure in sub-pectoral defibrillator pockets. Heart Rhythm 2005;2:s6.

40. Ha AC, Vezi BZ, Keren A, et al. Predictors of fracture risk of a small caliber implantable cardioverter defibrillator lead. Pacing Clin Electrophysiol 2010;33:437–43.

41. Polewczyk A, Kutarski A, Tomaszewski A, et al. Late complications of electrotherapy - a clinical analysis of indications for transvenous removal of endocardial leads: a single centre experience. Kardiol Pol 2013;71:366–72.

42. Baxter W, Skadsberg N, Johnson WB, et al. New unanticipated insights on peak lead bending during pectoral flexure. Heart Rhythm 2010;7:S309.

43. Bundy KJ. Corrosion and other electrochemical aspects of biomaterials. Crit Rev Biomed Eng 1994;22:139–251.

44. Virtanen S, Milosev I, Gomez-Barrena E, et al. Special modes of corrosion under physiological and simulated physiological conditions. Acta Biomater 2008;4:468–76.

45. Bruck SD, Mueller EP. Materials aspects of implantable cardiac pacemaker leads. Med Prog Technol 1988;13:149–60.

46. Hunter LW, Lieske JC, Tran NV, et al. The association of matrix Gla protein isomers with calcification in capsules surrounding silicone breast implants. Biomaterials 2011;32:8364–73.

47. Kolodzinska A, Kutarski A, Koperski L, et al. Differences in encapsulating lead tissue in patients who underwent transvenous lead removal. Europace 2012;14:994–1001.

48. Novak M, Dvorak P, Kamaryt P, et al. Autopsy and clinical context in deceased patients with implanted pacemakers and defibrillators: intracardiac findings near their leads and electrodes. Europace 2009;11:1510–6.

49. Mandal S, Pande A, Mandal D, et al. Permanent pacemaker-related upper extremity deep vein thrombosis: a series of 20 cases. Pacing Clin Electrophysiol 2012;35:1194–8.

50. Ricciardi D, La MM, de AC, et al. A case of in vivo thrombogenicity of an externalized Riata ST lead. Europace 2013;15:428.

51. Tugcu A, Yildirimturk O, Tayyareci Y, et al. Right atrial pacemaker lead thrombosis causing tricuspid inflow obstruction. Pacing Clin Electrophysiol 2009;32:262–4.

52. Marrie TJ, Nelligan J, Costerton JW. A scanning and transmission electron microscopic study of an infected endocardial pacemaker lead. Circulation 1982;66:1339–41.

53. Costerton JW, Lewandowski Z, Caldwell DE, et al. Microbial biofilms. Annu Rev Microbiol 1995;49:711–45.

54. Donlan RM, Costerton JW. Biofilms: survival mechanisms of clinically relevant microorganisms. Clin Microbiol Rev 2002;15:167–93.

55. Stoodley P, Sauer K, Davies DG, et al. Biofilms as complex differentiated communities. Annu Rev Microbiol 2002;56:187–209.

56. Benham PP, Crawford RJ, Armstrong CG. Fracture mechanics. In: Benham PP, Crawford RJ, Armstrong CG, editors. Mechanics of engineering materials. 2nd edition. Essex, England: Pearson Education, Ltd; 1996. p. 514–43.

57. Benham PP, Crawford RJ, Armstrong CG. Fatigue. In: Benham PP, Crawford RJ, Armstrong CG, editors. Mechanics of engineering materials. 2nd edition. Essex, England: Pearson Education, Ltd; 1996. p. 544–72.

58. Benham PP, Crawford RJ, Armstrong CG. Creep and viscoelasticity. In: Benham PP, Crawford RJ, Armstrong CG, editors. Mechanics of engineering materials. 2nd edition. Essex, England: Pearson Education, Ltd; 1996. p. 573–97.

59. Heath DE, Cooper SL. Polymers: basic principles. In: Ratner BD, Hoffman AS, Schoen FJ, et al, editors. Biomaterials science - an introduction of materials in medicine. 3rd edition. Amsterdam, Boston, Heidelberg (German), London, New York, Oxford (United Kingdom), Paris, San Diego (CA), San Francisco (CA), Sydney (Australia), Tokyo: Academic Press; 2013. p. 64–79.

60. Archard JF, Hirst W. The wear of metals under unlubricated conditions. Proc R Soc Lond A 1956; 236:397–410.

61. Himes A, Wilson C. Wear of cardiac lead outer insulation due to internal cable motion. Tribol Int 2013;62:177–85.

62. Wright DC. Environmental stress cracking of plastics. Shawbury, Shrewsbury, Shropshire (United Kingdom): Rapra Technology; 1996.

63. Beyersdorf F, Kreuzer J, Schmidts L, et al. Examination of explanted polyurethane pacemaker leads using the scanning electron microscope. Pacing Clin Electrophysiol 1985;8:562–8.

64. Phillips R, Frey M, Martin RO. Long-term performance of polyurethane pacing leads: mechanisms of design-related failures. Pacing Clin Electrophysiol 1986;9:1166–72.

65. Coury AJ. Chemical and biochemical degradation of polymers intended to be biostable. In: Ratner BD, Hoffman AS, Schoen FJ, et al, editors. Biomaterials science - an introduction of materials in medicine. 3rd edition. Amsterdam, Boston, Heidelberg (Germany), London, New York, Oxford (United Kingdom), Paris, San Diego (CA), San Francisco (CA), Sydney (Australia), Tokyo: Academic Press; 2013. p. 696–715.

66. Martin DJ, Warren LA, Gunatillake PA, et al. New methods for the assessment of in vitro and in vivo stress cracking in biomedical polyurethanes. Biomaterials 2001;22:973–8.

67. Gradaus R, Breithardt G, Bocker D. ICD leads: design and chronic dysfunctions. Pacing Clin Electrophysiol 2003;26:649–57.

68. Stokes K, Coury A, Urbanski P. Autooxidative degradation of implanted polyether polyurethane devices. J Biomater Appl 1987;1:411–48.

69. Stokes K, Urbanski P, Upton J. The in vivo autooxidation of polyether polyurethane by metal ions. J Biomater Sci Polym Ed 1990;1:207–30.

70. Wiggins MJ, Wilkoff B, Anderson JM, et al. Biodegradation of polyether polyurethane inner insulation in bipolar pacemaker leads. J Biomed Mater Res 2001;58:302–7.

71. Simmons A, Hyvarinen J, Odell RA, et al. Long-term in vivo biostability of poly(dimethylsiloxane)/poly(hexa-methylene oxide) mixed macrodiol-based polyurethane elastomers. Biomaterials 2004;25:4887–900.

72. Chaffin KA, Buckalew AJ, Schley JL, et al. Influence of water on the structure and properties of PDMS-containing multi-block polyurethanes. Macromolecules 2012;45:9110–20.

73. Chaffin KA, Wilson CL, Himes AK, et al. Abrasion and fatigue resistance of PDMS containing multiblock polyurethanes after accelerated water exposure at elevated temperature. Biomaterials 2013; 34:8030–41.

74. Kleemann T, Becker T, Doenges K, et al. Annual rate of transvenous defibrillation lead defects in implantable cardioverter-defibrillators over a period of >10 years. Circulation 2007;115:2474–80.

75. Hauser RG, Hayes DL, Almquist AK, et al. Unexpected ICD pulse generator failure due to electronic circuit damage caused by electrical overstress. Pacing Clin Electrophysiol 2001;24: 1046–54.

76. Lau EW. Differential lead component pulling as a possible mechanism of inside-out abrasion and conductor cable externalization. Pacing Clin Electrophysiol 2013;36:1072–89.

77. Altman PA, Meagher JM, Walsh DW, et al. Rotary bending fatigue of coils and wires used in cardiac lead design. J Biomed Mater Res 1998;43: 21–37.

78. Smith DJ, Rajgarhia RK, Cooke DJ. Using field performance of marketed leads to develop a reliability test. Heart Rhythm 2012;9:S305–6.

79. Birnie DH, Parkash R, Exner DV, et al. Clinical predictors of Fidelis lead failure: report from the Canadian Heart Rhythm Society Device Committee. Circulation 2012;125:1217–25.

80. Fischer A, Klehn R. Contribution of ethylenetetrafluoroethylene (ETFE) insulation to the electrical performance of Riata® silicone leads having externalized conductors. J Interv Card Electrophysiol 2013;37:141–5.

81. Lau EW. External insulation breach near the tip of a single ventricular pacing lead. Journal of Innovations in Cardiac Rhythm Management 2012;3: 668–70.

82. Zabek A, Malecka B, Kolodzinska A, et al. Early abrasion of outer silicone insulation after intracardiac lead friction in a patient with cardiac device-related infective endocarditis. Pacing Clin Electrophysiol 2012;35:e156–8.

83. Arakawa M, Kambara K, Ito H, et al. Intermittent oversensing due to internal insulation damage of temperature sensing rate responsive pacemaker lead in subclavian venipuncture method. Pacing Clin Electrophysiol 1989;12:1312–6.

84. Swerdlow CD, Kass RM, Khoynezhad A, et al. Inside-out insulation failure of a defibrillator lead with abrasion-resistant coating. Heart Rhythm 2013;10:1063–6.

85. Goldstein MA, Badri M, Kocovic D, et al. Electrical failure of an ICD lead due to a presumed insulation defect only diagnosed by a maximum output shock. Pacing Clin Electrophysiol 2013; 36:1068–71.

86. Parvathaneni SV, Ellis CR, Rottman JN. High prevalence of insulation failure with externalized cables in St. Jude Medical Riata family ICD leads: fluoroscopic grading scale and correlation to extracted leads. Heart Rhythm 2012;9:1218–24.

87. Mera F, DeLurgio DB, Langberg JJ, et al. Transvenous cardioverter defibrillator lead malfunction due to terminal connector damage in pectoral implants. Pacing Clin Electrophysiol 1999;22:1797–801.

88. Lau EW. Compression-bending of multicomponent semi-rigid columns in response to axial loads and conjugate reciprocal extension-prediction of mechanical behaviours and implications for structural design. J Mech Behav Biomed Mater 2013;17:112–25.

89. Ananthakrishna R, Basavappa R. Uncommon site of pacemaker lead fracture. Pacing Clin Electrophysiol 2011;34:1576–7.

90. Hauser RG, Kallinen Retel LM. Early fatigue fractures in the IS-1 connector leg of a small-diameter ICD lead: value of returned product analysis for improving device safety. Heart Rhythm 2013;10:1462–8.

91. Sticherling C, Burri H. Introduction of new industry standards for cardiac implantable electronic devices: balancing benefits and unexpected risks. Europace 2012;14:1081–6.

92. Cassagneau R, Hanninen M, Ganiere V, et al. Failure of a spliced DF-4 ICD lead. Heart Rhythm 2013; 10:1829.

93. Kolodzinska A, Kutarski A, Kozlowska M, et al. Biodegradation of the outer silicone insulation of endocardial leads. Circ Arrhythm Electrophysiol 2013;6:279–86.

94. Kleemann T, Becker T, Strauss M, et al. Prevalence of bacterial colonization of generator pockets in implantable cardioverter defibrillator patients without signs of infection undergoing generator replacement or lead revision. Europace 2010;12:58–63.

95. Mason PK, Dimarco JP, Ferguson JD, et al. Sonication of explanted cardiac rhythm management devices for the diagnosis of pocket infections and asymptomatic bacterial colonization. Pacing Clin Electrophysiol 2011;34:143–9.

96. Poole JE, Gleva MJ, Mela T, et al. Complication rates associated with pacemaker or implantable cardioverter-defibrillator generator replacements and upgrade procedures: results from the REPLACE registry. Circulation 2010;122:1553–61.

97. Nery PB, Fernandes R, Nair GM, et al. Device-related infection among patients with pacemakers and implantable defibrillators: incidence, risk factors, and consequences. J Cardiovasc Electrophysiol 2010;21:786–90.

98. Lovelock JD, Patel A, Mengistu A, et al. Generator exchange is associated with an increased rate of Sprint Fidelis lead failure. Heart Rhythm 2012;9: 1615–8.

99. Lim KK, Reddy S, Desai S, et al. Effects of electrocautery on transvenous lead insulation materials. J Cardiovasc Electrophysiol 2009;20:429–35.

100. Polewczyk A, Kutarski A, Tomaszewski A, et al. Lead dependent tricuspid dysfunction: analysis of the mechanism and management in patients referred for transvenous lead extraction. Cardiol J 2013;20:402–10.

101. Baquero GA, Yadav P, Skibba JB, et al. Clinical significance of increased tricuspid valve incompetence following implantation of ventricular leads. J Interv Card Electrophysiol 2013;38:197–202.

102. Cassagneau R, Jacon P, Defaye P. Pacemaker lead-induced severe tricuspid valve stenosis: complete percutaneous extraction under extracorporeal life support. Europace 2013;15:1248.

103. Devanathan T, Sluetz JE, Young KA. In vivo thrombogenicity of implantable cardiac pacing leads. Biomater Med Devices Artif Organs 1980; 8:369–79.

104. Palatianos GM, Dewanjee MK, Panoutsopoulos G, et al. Comparative thrombogenicity of pacemaker leads. Pacing Clin Electrophysiol 1994;17:141–5.

105. Hauser RG, Maisel WH, Friedman PA, et al. Longevity of Sprint Fidelis implantable cardioverter-defibrillator leads and risk factors for failure: implications for patient management. Circulation 2011;123: 358–63.

106. Di CA, Bongiorni MG, Zucchelli G, et al. Transvenous extraction performance of expanded polytetrafluoroethylene covered ICD leads in comparison to traditional ICD leads in humans. Pacing Clin Electrophysiol 2010;33:1376–81.

The Canadian Experience with Device and Lead Advisories

Ciorsti J. MacIntyre, MD, FRCPC[a],
Andrew D. Krahn, MD, FRCPC, FHRS[b],
Ratika Parkash, MD, MS, FRCPC, FHRS[c],*

KEYWORDS

- Arrhythmias • Implantable cardioverter defibrillator • Device • Advisory • Complications

KEY POINTS

- Device/lead advisories have become increasingly common and pose significant management challenges.
- Complications caused by device/lead advisories can have serious effects on patient outcomes.
- A collaborative approach using a virtual network can provide an excellent mechanism to respond rapidly to advisories in a uniform manner.

INTRODUCTION

Cardiac implantable electrical devices (CIEDs) have undergone revolutionary changes in the last decade, linked to growth in both indications and capability. These changes have led to an increase in the use of both pacemakers and implantable cardioverter defibrillators (ICDs), collectively known as CIEDs.[1-3] It is projected that the population with heart failure will double by the year 2025, and the absolute number of patients eligible to receive an ICD for primary prevention or cardiac resynchronization therapy will likely increase accordingly.[4-6] These epidemiologic observations will translate into a significantly increased burden on the health care system, with fiscal pressures that will be hard pressed to cope with this projected demand.

THE CANADIAN EXPERIENCE WITH DEVICE AND LEAD RECALLS

Because of the recent increase in device and lead advisories,[7] the Canadian Heart Rhythm Society (CHRS) responded by establishing the Device Advisory Committee, now termed the Device Committee (DC). The purpose of this committee was to coordinate a network of Canadian arrhythmia device physicians to provide a system of device and lead surveillance, reporting, and uniform response to advisories in a timely and consistent manner.[8]

Establishment of the Canadian Device Advisory System

History has proved instructive in providing the basis of response to advisories before the last

The authors have nothing to disclose.
[a] Division of Cardiology, QE II Health Sciences Centre, 1796 Summer Street, Room 2134, Halifax, Nova Scotia B3H 3A7, Canada; [b] Division of Cardiology, Diamond Health Care Centre, University of British Columbia, 2775 Laurel Street, 9th Floor, Room 9173, Vancouver, British Columbia V5Z 1M9, Canada; [c] Division of Cardiology, QEII Health Sciences Centre, 1796 Summer Street, Room 2501D, Halifax, Nova Scotia B3H 3A7, Canada
* Corresponding author.
E-mail address: ratika.parkash@cdha.nshealth.ca

Card Electrophysiol Clin 6 (2014) 327–334
http://dx.doi.org/10.1016/j.ccep.2014.02.003
1877-9182/14/$ – see front matter © 2014 Elsevier Inc. All rights reserved.

decade. The Accufix lead advisory (Telectronics Pacing Systems, Englewood, CO) was a prime example of how intervention proved more dangerous than observation.[9] Using this concept of harm versus benefit in dealing with device advisories, the CHRS established a subcommittee dedicated to this issue. This committee was initially tasked with promoting a unified approach and providing guidelines for device follow-up centers in Canada for device advisories. Before the establishment of the CHRS-DC, response to advisories in Canada was handled in a varied fashion from center to center. Several ICD generator advisories were announced in 2005, including the Medtronic Marquis (Medtronic, Minneapolis, MN) and Ventak Prizm (Boston Scientific, Natick, MA).[10–12] The risk of generator failure in these advisories was from 1/1000 to 1/10,000 (Table 1),[12] yet many centers responded by replacing the pulse generator earlier than would otherwise occur, as dictated by battery replacement indicators. To provide evidence-based management in this regard, a group of investigators began a collaboration to collect and report a Canadian perspective on the outcome of generator replacement caused by an advisory ICD.[12] The results were remarkable in that the risk of early generator replacement outweighed any risk that may result from generator failure caused by the advisory (Table 2). At least as compelling was the variability in replacement rates across centers, ranging from 0% to 45%.[12] This situation resulted in a change in management of ICD generators under advisory. This format of using evidence to guide decision making provided the basis for further work carried out by the CHRS-DC.

Canadian Device Advisory Structure

The CHRS-DC consists of a Chair, appointed by the CHRS executive, and a member from each ICD implanting and follow-up center across Canada (Fig. 1). In addition, there is a working group that consists of the Chair, Deputy Chair (appointed by the Chair of the CHRS-DC), CHRS President, and a member at large. Advisories are considered by the committee when a greater degree of intervention beyond simple increased surveillance

Table 1
Current ICD advisories included in the survey and associated risk

Company/Device[a]	Date of Advisory	Advisory Issue[b]	Current Risk of Failure (%)[b]
Medtronic Marquis ICD	February, 2005	Accelerated battery depletion caused by internal battery short	0.001
Guidant Ventak Prizm 2 DR ICD	June, 2005	Short circuit caused by wire insulation problem within lead connector block	0.1
Guidant Ventak Prizm AVT, Vitality AVT, and Contak Renewal AVT ICDs	June, 2005	Random memory error, limiting delivery of therapies	0.0095
Guidant Contak Renewal 3, 4 Renewal 3, 4 AVT and Renewal RF ICDs	June, 2005	Magnetic switch faulty, impairing delivery of therapies	0.009
St Jude Photon DR, Photon Micro VR/DR, and Atlas VR/DR ICDs	October, 2005	Memory chip affected by atmospheric radiation, which can impair pacing and delivery of therapies	0.167
ELA Alto ICD	August, 2001	Migration of metal, which can impair pacing and delivery of therapies	2.6[c] 0.1[d]

[a] Predominantly subpopulation of listed devices affected by advisory.
[b] Data obtained from physician communications and public statement releases such as those from Medtronic and Guidant. The current risk of failure represents the number of failures divided by the number of devices implanted at the time of advisory disclosure.
[c] Manufactured between April and July, 2003.
[d] Manufactured between August, 2003 and August, 2004.
From Gould PA, Krahn AD. Complications associated with implantable cardioverter-defibrillator replacement in response to device advisories. JAMA 2006;295:1907–11; with permission.

Table 2
Complications with generators and lead advisories

| | Elective Advisory Device Replacements No. (%)[a] | Sprint Fidelis Lead Revision | | |
Severity and Complications		Lead Removed No. (%)[a]	Lead Abandoned No. (%)[a]	All Leads No. (%)[a]
Minor				
Infection not requiring system removal/incisional infection	9 (1.7)	16 (6.5)	3 (1.4)	19 (4.1)
Heart failure	1 (0.2)	0	1 (0.5)	2 (0.43)
Major				
Infection requiring extraction	10 (1.9)	7 (2.8)	2 (0.9)	9 (1.9)
Death	2 (0.4)	1 (0.4)	1 (0.5)	2 (0.43)
Hematoma requiring reoperation	12 (2.3)	4 (1.6)	0	4 (0.9)

[a] Number of patients with the complication.

Data from Gould PA, Krahn AD. Complications associated with implantable cardioverter-defibrillator replacement in response to device advisories. JAMA 2006;295:1910; and Parkash R, Crystal E, Bashir J, et al. Complications associated with revision of Sprint Fidelis leads: report from the Canadian Heart Rhythm Device Advisory Committee. Circulation 2010;121:2386.

with more frequent follow-up is required. The decision to intervene on a particular patient remains individualized, involving a discussion between the patient and their physician with the lead, device, and patient-specific factors in mind. In the current structure of the committee, the manufacturer contacts the working group of the committee to discuss the scope, risk, and suggested manufacturer response. Any points of clarification are raised by the working group, with response from the manufacturer. The Chair then crafts a response to the advisory based on the information provided from the manufacturer with an appropriate advisory classification (**Table 3**).[8] The response is circulated to the working group for refinement. The draft response is then circulated to the entire committee, concurrent with the public announcement of the advisory, so that sites have a draft to work from, with consensus established by email within 3 to 5 working days. Once approved, it is posted on the CHRS Web site and serves as a guideline for response to the advisory by each CIED follow-up center. In addition, the Chair serves as a method of communication between the CIED follow-up centers and the manufacturer. This system does not replace any individual relationship that each follow-up center may hold with clinical representatives appointed by the manufacturer in their region. Any follow-up information provided by the manufacturer or other data on an advisory may be reported in the form of an update, particularly if additional recommendations affecting patient management are required. This process has now been tested through several advisories with 3 different Chairs, and has worked well in providing a uniform and cohesive response to device advisories by the Canadian CIED centers.

THE SPRINT FIDELIS ADVISORY: EXAMPLE OF THE CHRS-DC PROCESS

The Sprint Fidelis lead advisory was issued in October, 2007 in response to an increasing concern regarding conductor fractures.[13] This advisory affected 6415 leads in Canada and 245,000 leads worldwide.[13,14] The estimated lead failure of 2.3% at 30 months was based on data from a remote monitoring database (CareLink), returned product analysis, a small chronic lead study, and 5 reported deaths worldwide in which the lead was considered a possible or likely contributing factor.[13]

The CHRS-DC Chair classified the advisory as semi-urgent and initiated a discussion via email

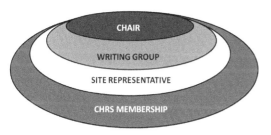

Fig. 1. Makeup of the CHRS-DC.

Table 3
Classification of device and lead advisories

Urgency	Description
Urgent	Risk of abrupt device/lead/system failure that may be life-threatening, without means to detect risk of failure during routine follow-up. This classification results in a preliminary response based on available data within 2 business days. This classification presumably stems from manufacturer notification of physicians of the advisory and may result in urgent notification of patients. An example is abrupt loss of pacing function or failed defibrillation
Semi-urgent	Risk of abrupt or rapid device/lead/system failure that may be life-threatening, with means to detect risk of failure during routine or increased follow-up, be it remote or in a device follow-up clinic setting. This classification results in a response based on available data within 5 business days. An example is abrupt loss of defibrillation function in patients with impedance or battery parameters within a certain measurable range, mandating rapid assessment and closer follow-up
Routine	Risk of device/lead/system malfunction that is not life-threatening, with or without means to detect risk of malfunction during routine follow-up. Most of these advisories are not expected to require a specific response from the CHRS-DC, but under certain circumstances (eg, highly prevalent system component in question), the committee may choose to generate or may be asked to generate a response. An example is premature battery depletion, which can be detected during follow-up, or increased risk of lead fracture, detectable with impedance monitoring. This classification is dependent on the number of patients and centers affected, to some degree

From Krahn AD, Simpson CS, Parkash R, et al. Utilization of a national network for rapid response to the Medronic Fidelis lead advisory: the Canadian Heart Rhythm Society Device Advisory Committee. Heart Rhythm 2009;6:474–7; with permission.

and survey of Canadian ICD centers within 3 hours of the advisory. Within 48 hours, a CHRS membership statement was issued including recommendations and preliminary lead failure rates for 60% of leads implanted across Canada. Within 5 working days, a letter to nonmember physicians and a patient letter were posted on the CHRS Web site for local adaptation and distribution. Data collection from all Canadian ICD centers regarding lead performance was completed within 8 weeks and subsequently published in *Heart Rhythm* (**Fig. 2**).[8]

This study comprised a formal survey sent to all ICD implant centers in Canada. A survey of 11 questions examining the frequency and presentation of lead failure, operator characteristics, and center response was circulated.[13] All 23 centers participated and provided complete survey data. The responses suggested a Fidelis lead failure rate of 1.29% at 21 months, with patients typically presenting with multiple inappropriate shocks without evidence of impending failure from routine lead follow-up. There was no association with specific operators or around high-volume or low-volume implant centers.[13]

Using the CHRS-DC network, the Fidelis advisory was further characterized in terms of predictors of lead failure, lead performance in a

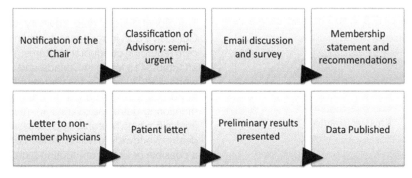

Fig. 2. Steps in the CHRS-DC process.

large population across many centers, and complications of lead revision. The overall rate of complications arising from lead revision caused by the Sprint Fidelis lead advisory has been significant (see **Table 2**). Complications were encountered in 14.5% of lead revisions. Of these complications, 7.25% were major, including 2 deaths (0.43%). The overall risk of complications (19.8%) was significantly higher in patients who underwent lead removal at the time of revision than in those in whom the lead was abandoned (8.6%).[15] The significant periprocedural risk, therefore, proved to be an important factor when deciding about lead revision in patients who had not yet developed issues with lead performance.

Using a subset of CHRS-DC centers, Birnie and colleagues[16] performed a comprehensive analysis of predictors of Fidelis fracture. This analysis showed that the rate of Fidelis fracture continued to increase over time. Factors conferring greatest risk included female gender, leads inserted via the subclavian or axillary vein, and history of previous lead fracture.

The studies performed by the CHRS-DC on the Sprint Fidelis lead advisory have provided a large body of evidence on which to plan future management of patients with this lead. Further data are emerging on technical aspects of lead placement within the heart, which may influence future implant techniques for all ICD leads.[17]

THE RIATA LEAD ADVISORY

The Riata and Riata ST lead advisory was announced on November 28, 2011 by St Jude Medical (Minneapolis, MN). This advisory was based on the possibility of externalization of ICD lead conductors via an inside-out abrasion mechanism.[18] Similar processes as reported with the Fidelis advisory were followed to deal with this advisory.

In a cross-country survey of 19 ICD implant and follow-up centers, data were obtained on 4358 leads (86.4% of the leads implanted in Canada). A total of 4.6% of studied leads were found to have confirmed or suspected electrical failure. Of these leads, there were significantly higher electrical failures in the 8-French models versus 7-French models (5.2% vs 3.3%, $P = .007$).[18] Several questions remain with respect to the Riata advisory, specifically, the electrical and mechanical manifestations of cable externalization within the vasculature. There is in effect a disconnect between mechanical failure, with externalization evident in as many as 25% of patients screened radiographically, and electrical failure, which is less common (approximately 2%–3% per year)

but seen more often than in ideal reference leads. This finding represents a novel mechanism of failure, with concerning theoretic risks unique to this advisory. In contrast to the decreased complication rate with lead abandonment versus lead extraction in the Sprint Fidelis lead advisory, the Riata lead poses a different problem. Lead abandonment has a potential risk for causing electrical arcing from lead-lead interaction, given the presence of cable externalization. However, the risk of extraction is not insignificant, given lead construction; many implanted leads are dual coil leads that have been implanted for up to 10 years, increasing the risk of lead extraction compared with the Fidelis leads, in which implant duration was significantly shorter.[19] Using the CHRS-DC network, prospective surveillance of the Riata leads under advisory is planned to assist with providing some guidance on these questions.

CURRENT SURVEILLANCE MECHANISMS

Implanted device and lead performance has traditionally been reported by individual health care professionals to manufacturers, in the form of verbal or written reports, or returned product analysis. The manufacturers, in turn, report system performance in their product performance reports. This process relies on the manufacturer to collect, process, and report the information in an unbiased fashion.[8]

There are several issues that are unique to CIEDs that require a focused surveillance system and that separate them from other medical devices. CIEDs in most instances provide lifesaving or life-sustaining therapy.[8,20–25] If a CIED malfunctions or if there is a complication, this can result in significant morbidity or mortality.

The goal of postmarket surveillance is to enhance public health by reducing the incidence of medical device adverse experiences.[26] Various mechanisms exist worldwide to provide some degree of postmarket surveillance. In Canada, there are currently 2 mechanisms for device postmarketing surveillance: the Canadian Medical Devices Sentinel Network Pilot Project and the Adverse Reaction Reporting for Specific Products.[27] The latter system has been long-standing and was the only form of postmarketing surveillance in Canada until the Sentinel system was established recently.

The Adverse Reaction Reporting is a mandatory system[28] that mandates manufacturers to report on issues including failure of the device, deterioration in its effectiveness, any inadequacy in its labeling or in its directions for use, or device malfunction that have led to or have the potential to lead to death or a serious deterioration in the state of health of a patient, user, or other person. Under this same system, a consumer is able to spontaneously report on device failure, which is then followed up by Health Canada through the manufacturer. Detection of potential problems is difficult under this system. Manufacturers as well as consumers report only issues that they are aware of but do not actively seek out device malfunctions, in effect leading to active summary reporting but at best passive surveillance.

The Canadian Medical Devices Sentinel Network pilot project has the potential to provide better postmarketing surveillance.[27] This system relies on a group of dedicated and trained representatives from 10 acute or community-based health care facilities within Canada to report high-quality data to the regulator about adverse events associated with medical devices. The detailed reports obtained will help to better characterize how organizations use devices, how problems are perceived and reported, and which aspects of the system contribute to a particular event, potentially mitigating risk at an earlier stage.

The Sentinel system is an improvement over the previous reporting system but is limited in scope and it may be several years before it is adopted as a standard reporting mechanism. The limited scope will not permit this mechanism to detect rare device performance issues that may lead to serious morbidity or mortality. In comparison, the CHRS-DC, in its limited capacity, has worked with device manufacturers to assist in defining the need for advisories and has made significant impacts on clinical management of device advisories. The need for groups such as the CHRS-DC to work in concert with governmental organizations is clear.

The United States has the most comprehensive postmarketing surveillance system. The current surveillance system relies on the Food and Drug Administration (FDA), medical device manufacturers, health care providers, hospitals and other medical care facilities, and patients to report device malfunctions. Postmarket surveillance, as it stands in the United States, is designed primarily to identify uncommon, but potentially serious, device-related adverse events. The FDA uses several different methods to conduct postmarket surveillance, including spontaneous reporting systems, analysis of large health care databases, scientific studies, registries, and field inspection of facilities. The FDA depends primarily on a passive adverse event reporting system, relying on patients and the health care industry to identify and report adverse events, including rare, serious occurrences. Manufacturers are required to report to the FDA any medical device–related event or malfunction that may have caused or could cause

a serious injury or death. Hospitals, nursing homes, and other medical facilities are required to report device-related serious injuries to the manufacturer and device-related deaths to both the manufacturer and the FDA. The FDA annually receives more than 160,000 adverse event reports regarding medical devices of all types, including some that involve pacemakers, ICDs, or leads. Manufacturers provide most reports. Fewer than 10,000 come directly from medical facilities. Postmortem device interrogation is rarely performed. The Manufacture and User Friendly Device Experience (MAUDE) database was established to assist with adverse event reporting and information dissemination for medical devices of all types. It contains hundreds of thousands of adverse event reports, including voluntary reports since June, 1993 and manufacturer reports since 1996. Selected information from this database is publicly searchable via the Internet. However, because submitted adverse event reports are often cryptic or incomplete, it is often difficult to determine if a true device malfunction or patient injury has occurred. Furthermore, updated information after manufacturer device analysis is often not included in the publicly available reports. In addition, multiple reporting (eg, by physician, manufacturer, and patient) could result in 3 reports for a single event. FDA analysts use the MAUDE database to detect patterns or events that may warrant further investigation. This surveillance method was never intended nor configured to be used for tracking device malfunction rates.[26] Even with this reporting system, there remains no active comprehensive surveillance mechanism in the United States to detect problems.[29–31]

England (http://www.ic.nhs.uk/), Denmark (http://www.pacemaker.dk/), Spain, and Germany have national registries.[32] These registries have permitted monitoring of the indications for CIED implantation, estimating the real-world benefit of using these devices, what the risks are associated with CIED use, and examination of cost-effectiveness. These registries have been successful but offer limited information with respect to active surveillance. The European Registry of Implantable Defibrillators was one of voluntary participation; a significant cohort was lost to follow-up.[33] The Spanish registry provided cross-sectional data but had no prolonged follow-up.[34] The Danish and UK registries are limited in the outcomes that they report. The Ontario ICD Database[35] has been running since 2008 but was established to investigate incidence of therapy and complications from ICDs alone and does not include information regarding pacemakers.[29,31] It also no longer tracks outcomes or enrolls new patients.

There have been several lead registries established by the various manufacturers using remote and in-person follow-up, including the CareLink registry, the System Longevity Study, and the St. Jude Medical Product Longevity and Performance (SCORE) Registry. They do provide comprehensive lead data, but their most significant disadvantage is the lack of correlation with clinical data. They also suffer from the same issue of incomplete data that arises with other surveillance systems. In addition, it is crucial that some aspect of device surveillance and reporting occurs independent of industry, to limit bias in data collection and interpretation.[26]

FUTURE DIRECTIONS

The frequency of device and lead advisories may continue to increase. There is no national or international standard addressing the appropriate management of advisory situations. In Canada, decisions regarding the need and nature of an advisory are made at a federal government level. Each advisory presents a unique set of circumstances, which makes the creation of universal guidelines beyond overarching principles a significant challenge.

The CHRS-DC has established a network with the capacity to rapidly gather data and in turn respond promptly to device and lead advisories. The Canadian experience shows that a collaborative approach using a virtual network can provide a means to respond rapidly to advisories at a national level. The Sprint Fidelis and Riata experiences have shown that this approach also has the capacity to provide real-world data to facilitate in the related patient management decisions. The Canadian experience also shows the need for ongoing improvements in the management of device and lead advisories.

A key goal is the creation of an international network of active surveillance and reporting not only to facilitate the identification of advisory situations but also to promote a unified approach to management. Advisory devices and leads can be associated with substantial risk of complications, including death, a key consideration in the development of guidelines in this area. To achieve this goal requires rigorous data definitions, a combination of regulator, health policy, manufacturer, and health care delivery team collaboration, and substantial resources to target improvement in outcomes for patients with CIEDs.

REFERENCES

1. Kurtz SM, Ochoa JA, Lau E, et al. Implantation trends and patient profiles for pacemakers and implantable cardioverter defibrillators in the United States: 1993-2006. Pacing Clin Electrophysiol 2010;33(6):705–11.
2. Mond HG, Irwin M, Ector H, et al. The world survey of cardiac pacing and cardioverter-defibrillators: calendar year 2005 an International Cardiac Pacing and Electrophysiology Society (ICPES) project. Pacing Clin Electrophysiol 2008;31(9):1202–12.
3. Uslan DZ, Tleyjeh IM, Baddour LM, et al. Temporal trends in permanent pacemaker implantation: a population-based study. Am Heart J 2008;155(5): 896–903.
4. Ross H, Howlett J, Arnold JM, et al. Treating the right patient at the right time: access to heart failure care. Can J Cardiol 2006;22(9):749–54.
5. Tang AS, Wells GA, Talajic M, et al. Cardiac-resynchronization therapy for mild-to-moderate heart failure. N Engl J Med 2010;363(25):2385–95.
6. Wells G, Parkash R, Healey JS, et al. Cardiac re-synchronization therapy: a meta-analysis of randomized controlled trials. CMAJ 2011;183(4):421–9.
7. Maisel WH, Sweeney MO, Stevenson WG, et al. Recalls and safety alerts involving pacemakers and implantable cardioverter-defibrillator generators. JAMA 2001;286(7):793–9.
8. Krahn AD, Simpson CS, Parkash R, et al. Utilization of a national network for rapid response to the Medronic Fidelis lead advisory: the Canadian Heart Rhythm Society Device Advisory Committee. Heart Rhythm 2009;6:474–7.
9. Kay GN, Brinker JA, Kawanishi DT, et al. Risks of spontaneous injury and extraction of an active fixation pacemaker lead: report of the Accufix Multicenter Clinical Study and Worldwide Registry. Circulation 1999;100:2344–52.
10. Medtronic, Marquis patient management information. Minneapolis (MN): Medtronic; 2005.
11. Guidant advisory update, Contak renewal and Contak Renal 2, models H 135 and H155. Indianapolis (IN): Guidant; 2005.
12. Gould PA, Krahn AD. Complications associated with implantable cardioverter-defibrillator replacement in response to device advisories. JAMA 2006;295: 1907–11.
13. Krahn A, Champagne J, Healey J, et al. Outcome of the Fidelis implantable cardioverter-defibrillator lead advisory: a report from the Canadian Heart Rhythm Society Device Advisory Committee. Heart Rhythm 2008;5:639–42.
14. Cox JL. Optimizing disease management at a health care system level: the rationale and methods of the improving cardiovascular outcomes in Nova Scotia (ICONS) study. Can J Cardiol 1999;15(7):787–96.
15. Parkash R, Crystal E, Bashir J, et al. Complications associated with revision of Sprint Fidelis leads: report from the Canadian Heart Rhythm Device Advisory Committee. Circulation 2010;121:2384–7.

16. Birnie DH, Parkash R, Exner DV, et al. Clinical predictors of Fidelis lead failure: report from the Canadian Heart Rhythm Society Device Committee. Circulation 2012;125:1217–25.

17. Krahn AD, Morissette J, Lahm R. Radiographic predictors of lead fracture: a systematic case control analysis. Heart Rhythm 2013;10(5):S70–1.

18. Parkash R, Exner D, Champagne J, et al. Failure rate of the Riata lead under advisory: a report from the CHRS Device Committee. Heart Rhythm 2013;10: 692–5.

19. Roux JF, Page P, Dubuc M, et al. Laser lead extraction: predictors of success and complications. Pacing Clin Electrophysiol 2007;30(2):214–20.

20. Moss AJ, Zareba W, Hall WJ, et al. Prophylactic implantation of a defibrillator in patients with myocardial infarction and reduced ejection fraction. N Engl J Med 2002;346(12):877–83.

21. A comparison of antiarrhythmic-drug therapy with implantable defibrillators in patients resuscitated from near-fatal ventricular arrhythmias. The Antiarrhythmics versus Implantable Defibrillators (AVID) Investigators. N Engl J Med 1997;337(22):1576–83.

22. Moss AJ, Hall WJ, Cannom DS, et al. Improved survival with an implanted defibrillator in patients with coronary disease at high risk for ventricular arrhythmia. Multicenter Automatic Defibrillator Implantation Trial Investigators. N Engl J Med 1996; 335(26):1933–40.

23. Kadish A, Dyer A, Daubert JP, et al. Prophylactic defibrillator implantation in patients with nonischemic dilated cardiomyopathy. N Engl J Med 2004; 350(21):2151–8.

24. Connolly SJ, Gent M, Roberts RS, et al. Canadian implantable defibrillator study (CIDS): a randomized trial of the implantable cardioverter defibrillator against amiodarone. Circulation 2000;101(11): 1297–302.

25. Hohnloser SH, Kuck KH, Dorian P, et al. Prophylactic use of an implantable cardioverter-defibrillator after acute myocardial infarction. N Engl J Med 2004; 351(24):2481–8.

26. Carlson MD, Wilkoff BL, Maisel WH, et al. Recommendations from the Heart Rhythm Society Task Force on device performance policies and guidelines endorsed by the American College of Cardiology Foundation (ACCF) and the American Heart Association (AHA) and the international Coalition of Pacing and Electrophysiology Organizations (COPE). Heart Rhythm 2006;3(10):1250–73.

27. Canadian Medical Devices Sentinel Network pilot project. Available at: http://www.hc-sc.gc.ca/dhp-mps/medeff/cmdsnet-resscmm-eng.php. Accessed October 1, 2010.

28. Guidance document for mandatory problem reporting for medical devices. Available at: http://www.hc-sc.gc.ca/dhp-mps/pubs/medeff/_guide/2011-devices-materiaux/index-eng.php. Accessed March 10, 2011.

29. Kramer DB, Buxton AE, Zimetbaum PJ. Time for a change–a new approach to ICD replacement. N Engl J Med 2012;366(4):291–3.

30. Hauser RG. Here we go again–failure of postmarketing device surveillance. N Engl J Med 2012;366(10): 873–5.

31. Carlson MD. ICD leads and postmarketing surveillance. N Engl J Med 2012;366(10):967.

32. Nielsen JC. National registry data on implantable cardioverter defibrillator treatment: what are they useful for? Europace 2009;11(4):405–6.

33. Gradaus R, Block M, Brachmann J, et al. Mortality, morbidity, and complications in 3344 patients with implantable cardioverter defibrillators: results from the German ICD Registry EURID. Pacing Clin Electrophysiol 2003;26(7 Pt 1):1511–8.

34. Peinado R, Torrecilla EG, Ormaetxe J, et al. Spanish implantable cardioverter-defibrillator registry. 5th official report of the Spanish Society of Cardiology working group on implantable cardioverter-defibrillators (2008). Rev Esp Cardiol 2009;62(12): 1435–49.

35. Lee DS, Birnie D, Cameron D, et al. Design and implementation of a population-based registry of implantable cardioverter defibrillators (ICDs) in Ontario. Heart Rhythm 2008;5(9):1250–6.

Lead Extraction and Registry Experiences in Europe

Maria Grazia Bongiorni, MD[a],*, Simone L. Romano, MD[a],
Charles Kennergren, MD, PhD, FETCS, FHRS[b], Carina Blomström-Lundqvist, MD, PhD[c]

KEYWORDS

- Infections • Malfunctions • Cardiac implantable electronic device • Lead extraction
- Clinical practice • Registry

KEY POINTS

- With the rise of Pacemakers and implantable cardiac defibrillators (ICDs), implantations, infections, and malfunctions related to these devices have increased.
- Transvenous lead extraction (TLE) is the gold standard treatment in case of cardiac implantable electronic device (CIED) infection or failing leads. This procedure was developed in terms of technology and techniques, improving success rates and showing its safety in experienced centers.
- The number of European hospitals performing TLE has increased in recent years. The European Heart Rhythm Society (EHRA) started to characterize them and published the results of 2 surveys about clinical practice of TLE in Europe. These surveys highlighted the need for a prospective registry for a better analysis of this procedure among European countries.
- ELECTRa (European Lead Extraction Controlled) Registry is the first large, prospective, multicenter registry for TLE in Europe. It will describe the European real world practice on TLE and will improve the quality of patient care.

INTRODUCTION

The number of cardiac implantable electronic device (CIED) implant procedures has grown considerably in recent years. Despite advances in technology, the number of infective and noninfective complications related to these devices has increased.[1,2]

Transvenous lead extraction (TLE) is the gold standard for treatment of CIED-related infective complications and is often required in the management of lead malfunction. TLE is a percutaneous procedure, which consists of extracting leads from the venous system used for CIED implantation. This procedure does not require surgical opening of the chest, and it is performed using appropriate instruments for operating in the veins of implantation.[3–5]

TLE has evolved enormously in the last 30 years since the early attempts, which were done with little expertise and inappropriate tools. Over time, numerous techniques and many instruments have been added to improve the results of TLE.[5–7]

TLE EVOLUTION
Mechanical Techniques

Since the beginning of TLE, traction on leads has played a significant role. The success rate of simple manual traction on leads is dwell time

Disclosures: Charles Kennergren: Presented on behalf of, advised and/or performed scientific studies with: Boston Scientific, Biotronic, ELA/Sorin, Medtronic/Vitatron/TYRX, Mentice, Sim Suite, St Jude.
[a] Second Cardiology Department, Santa Chiara University Hospital, Paradisa Street 2, Pisa 56100, Italy;
[b] Department of Cardiothoracic Surgery, Sahlgrenska University Hospital, Gothenburg, S-413 45, Sweden;
[c] Department of Cardiology, Institution of Medical Science, Uppsala University, Akademiskasjukhuset ing. 35, 2 tr 751 85, Uppsala, Sweden
* Corresponding author. Second Cardiology Department, Santa Chiara University Hospital, Paradisa Street 2, Pisa 56100, Italy.
E-mail address: m.g.bongiorni@med.unipi.it

Card Electrophysiol Clin 6 (2014) 335–344
http://dx.doi.org/10.1016/j.ccep.2014.03.005
1877-9182/14/$ – see front matter © 2014 Elsevier Inc. All rights reserved.

dependent; leads implanted for less than 6 months can often be removed by simple traction, whereas leads with implant times longer than 2 years have a low success rate, and traction has to be considered just one of the steps of a potentially complex extraction procedure.

To improve traction results, attention was focused on developing systems that allow traction energy to be applied at the tip of the lead and/or on a section of the lead, in order to free the lead while avoiding coil disruption or leaving the lead tip behind. Locking stylets engaging the lead tip were an essential part of the original mechanical technique and were used in combination with mechanical dilatation sheaths.[5–8] The use of a stylet makes the lead stiffer, thus helping dilatation or ablation (in case of powered sheaths) of scar tissue, independent of the energy used. One initial drawback of locking stylets was that once the stylet was locked, it was impossible to unlock and withdraw it. This was a significant problem in cases of failed extraction. Later, a new type of locking stylet was developed, allowing the stylet to be locked and unlocked when necessary; traction ability was not affected by this feature.

Other traction devices were developed in subsequent years.[9,10] The lead locking device (LLD) comes with a mechanism that expands a coil in the inner lumen of the lead, providing locking to the tip as well as to the length of the lead. Extraction tension is thus distributed, minimizing the risk of lead damage. Reports on LLD use suggest that the added ability to remove leads using a locking stylet compared with simple traction is limited.[11–13]

Published data also suggest that the success rate of pulling out leads with or without locking stylets not using sheaths can be estimated to be about 30% in the overall population of leads. These results support the opinion of many experienced centers, that the key point of transvenous extraction is freeing the lead tip and body from binding fibrous tissue, more than applying traction to pull out the lead.

At the end of the 1980s, Charles Byrd developed the first effective technique for transvenous extraction of chronic pacing leads.[8] This original technique used locking stylets and mechanical dilatation of fibrotic binding sites by means of dilating sheaths.[14] Later, his technique included a transfemoral approach by means of a transvenous workstation and several different tools (retrieval basket, snares) to approach lead fragments or free-floating leads.[14] The clinical results of mechanical dilatation described by Byrd were published using data from the US database on transvenous extraction.[15] The first report analyzed

data from December 1988 to April 1994, relating the extraction of 2195 intravascular pacing leads from 1299 patients. Extraction was attempted via the implanted vein using locking stylets and dilator sheaths, via the femoral vein using snares, retrieval baskets, and sheaths, or via both approaches. Using this technique, 86.8% of leads were completely removed; 7.5% were partially removed, and 5.7% were not removed.[15] Fatal and near-fatal complications occurred in 2.5% of patients, including 8 (0.6%) deaths. The incidence of serious complications was found to be acceptable, particularly when compared with surgical removal techniques. In 1999, a new set of data from the US database on lead extraction was published.[16] It showed an increase in the number of procedures and also in success rate.

This experience refers to a period when extraction techniques were not undergoing development, and most of the limited numbers of active operators were well trained and experienced. From January 1994 through April 1996, extraction of 3540 leads from 2338 patients (mean age 64 years, range 5 to 96) was attempted at 226 centers. The conventional techniques for mechanical dilatation, including Cook Medical (Bloomington, Indiana) extraction kit tools, were used. Extraction was attempted via the implant vein using locking stylets and dilator sheaths, and/or transfemorally using snares, retrieval baskets, and sheaths. Complete removal was achieved in 93% of leads; partial removal was achieved in 5% of leads, and 2% of leads were not removed. Major complications were reported in 1.4% of patients (<1% at centers with >300 cases); minor complications were reported in 1.7%. The report underlined that the experience of operators played a key role in achieving a high success rate as well as in reducing the occurrence of major complications. Following these initial reports, many single-center experiences were published, but no significant contributions for improved techniques or results were added.

During the second half of the 1990s Maria Grazia Bongiorni and colleagues[17] developed a new transvenous approach using mechanical sheaths through the right internal jugular vein in cases of free-floating leads and leads difficult to expose, providing a significant contribution to developing techniques. Their modification of the technique of mechanical dilatation by polypropylene sheaths and the use of the jugular approach led to a significant improvement in results. In 2008, this group published the results of its single-center experience demonstrating the effectiveness of both the use of a single sheath technique and the use of the transjugular approach in presence of difficult leads. Transvenous extraction was attempted in 2062 leads (1825 pacing and 237 ICD leads, including 73 free-floating leads) in 1193 consecutive patients. The approach of mechanical dilatation from the venous entry site was effective in 1799 leads (90.4%). The use of the transjugular approach in the presence of free-floating leads or after failure of the conventional approach allowed complete removal of 2032 leads (98.4%) and partial removal of 18 leads (0.9%); removal failed in 12 leads (0.6%). Major complications were observed in 8 patients (0.7%), causing 3 deaths (0.3%).

These results suggest that mechanical dilatation techniques are effective and acceptably safe, particularly when different approaches are used by skilled operators.

Powered Techniques

Excimer laser
In the early 1990s, an extraction system using dilating sheaths powered by an excimer laser was developed and introduced in clinical practice by Spectranetics.[18] The system consists of sheaths connected to a laser generator; pulses of laser energy are delivered at the tip of the sheath, causing scar vaporization and binding site disruption. This new technique was well received, particularly in the United States, and its use rapidly expanded in the following years.

Results of the first multicenter experience were released in 2002.[19] From October 1995 to December 1999, 2561 pacing and defibrillator leads were treated in 1684 patients at 89 sites in the United States using laser sheaths. Complete removal was achieved in 90% of the leads, and partial removal was achieved in 3%; failure occurred in 7%. Major perioperative complications (tamponade, hemothorax, pulmonary embolism, lead migration, and death) were observed in 1.9% of patients, with in-hospital death in 13 patients (0.8%). Minor complications were observed in an additional 1.4% of patients.

Similar results were shown by the European multicenter experience.[20] Charles Kennergren published the final report of the PLESSE (Pacing Lead Survelllance Study in Europe) trial in 2007.[20] From August 1996 to March 2001, 383 leads implanted in 292 patients were extracted at 14 European centers. Complete extraction was achieved in 90.9% of the leads, and partial extraction was achieved in 3.4%; extraction failed in 5.7% of the leads. The total complication rate, including 5 minor complications (1.7%), was 5.1%. Cardiac tamponade occurred in 10 cases, but no in-hospital mortality was observed. In this study, contrary to most others, training experience was included.

Results of single-center experiences were published subsequently, in most cases using a second-generation laser sheath model.[21–24] The results of the LExICon Study (Multicenter Observational Retrospective Study of Consecutive Laser Lead Extractions) reported the results of laser-assisted lead removal of 2405 leads in 1449 patients at 13 centers between January 2004 and December 2007. Data showed a 97.7% clinical success rate and a 96.5% complete lead removal success rate. The major adverse event rate was a 1.4%, which was a 26% relative reduction compared with a previous multicenter study evaluating the original laser sheath.[25]

The previously mentioned results demonstrate the high efficacy of the laser technique. However, no significant improvement in success rate was observed in this or previous laser studies in comparison with the best single-center studies using nonpowered tools, although procedural time was reduced. In the LExICon Study, concern was raised by the slightly increased incidence of major complications, mainly due to venous or myocardial wall injury. Mortality was, however, very low.

Electrosurgical dissection
During the 1990s, Cook Medical developed a new powered sheath using electrosurgical dissection (ESD). The depth of the lesion induced by electrosurgical dissection seems to be larger than that of laser-assisted sheaths, but it is delivered only at the cutting dipole and not all over the circumference of the rim of the sheath. After its introduction in clinical practice, its use did not spread in the same way as that of the laser did. Although it is still used in a consistent but limited number of centers, particularly in the United States, only few experiences have been published in the literature, most of which are preliminary reports.[26]

The evolution mechanical dilator sheath
A new tool for extraction was introduced in 2006 by Cook Medical. The Evolution Mechanical Dilator Sheath is a rotationally powered telescoping device powered by a steel inner sheath. The rotation mechanism is manually operated, allowing rotation of small cams fitted near the distal sheath tip. The system provides a technique combining counterpressure, rotation, and action of the threaded end of the sheath, in order to enhance the effectiveness of dilatation at binding sites. The original version provides 1-way rotation with laterally directed dilatation forces. Preliminary experiences using this device have been reported in literature.[27,28] The results suggest effectiveness of the tool in overcoming binding sites similar to other powered sheaths; further data are necessary to understand

possible improvement in outcomes using this technique.[29]

Studies presenting results of different extraction techniques should be compared with caution. Comparing multicenter studies, sometimes including results from learning the techniques, with single-center studies may lead to inaccurate conclusions. Many biases, including patient selection, apply to presently available studies on lead extraction. Unfortunately, no major, prospective, randomized trial comparing techniques is yet available. The experience and training of the operator are probably more important for success and complication rates than the extraction technique. Presently available studies show that first-class results can be achieved with all available sheath methods, provided enough experience has been obtained.

TLE has been developed and has become a specialized procedure. Its different technological possibilities are well known and, as previously mentioned, its use continues to rise in the various centers. Initially, the NASPE (North American Society of Pacing and Electrophysiology)[30] and later Heart Rhythm Society (HRS)[31] published recommendations describing precise indications, settings, facilities, training, and accreditation for the extraction procedures. These recommendations are likely to be developed, and much improvement can be obtained by future multicenter studies.

EVOLUTION OF LEAD EXTRACTION IN EUROPE

In recent years, the CIED implantation rate also has grown in Europe (**Fig. 1**), and an increasing number of centers have started to perform TLE. In the past, not many centers performed TLE in Europe. Every country had a few reference centers; some of them published their results on TLE, and only 2 of these studies were randomized.[5–7,32–35] However, these studies and clinical practice have shown that, in general, the success rate and the safety of TLE have increased over time. This statement is especially true for most reports that share the experience of high-volume centers with experienced operators. For low-volume centers, especially those with limited experience, lower success rates and higher major complication rates can be expected.[34,35]

Unlike the United States, large-scale registries on TLE have been lacking in Europe. The aforementioned PLESSE trial, involving 14 European centers and 292 patients, until now has been the largest multicenter study for TLE specifically on this continent. In 2012, the results of the LEADER (Lead Extraction Device Evaluation and Results) database were presented. Between October 2009 and April 2012, this study collected data on consecutive patients undergoing TLE from approximately 600 centers in North America and Europe, for a total of 2021 cases. The registry only reports data from extractions made with a representative of Cook Medical present. The study, although limited to most procedures using at least 1 Cook instrument and offered by a commercial company, is still one of the largest on TLE. Europe was involved, helping to take a further step toward the description of the real-world practice of TLE; unfortunately, specific data about the old continent are not available.[5,36]

In Europe the majority of currently active centers only recently started to perform TLE; thus objective data on their activity are lacking.[34,35] TLE is partially unexplored in European countries in regard to appropriate indications, techniques, success rates, safety, and follow-up. Therefore, the

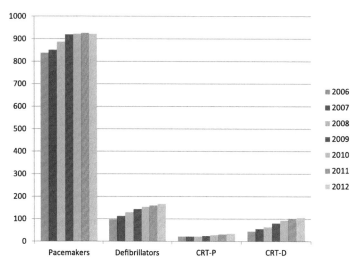

Fig. 1. CIED implantation trends in Europe from 2006 to 2012. (*Data from* Eucomed Medical Technology, Brussels, Belgium. Available at: http://www.eucomed.org/uploads/_medical_technology/facts_figures/Graphs_CRM_2013.pdf.)

European Heart Rhythm Association (EHRA), decided to initiate a process to characterize centers performing TLE.

In 2010, the Scientific Initiative Committee (SIC) of the EHRA administered a questionnaire via the SIC-network (EHRA EP Wire), to learn more about the practice of extraction in Europe, with a special focus on the management of redundant leads.[37] The answers were compared with the recommendations of the 2009 HRS Expert Consensus document[31] to evaluate adherence.

Most extraction procedures were transvenous and performed by cardiologists and/or cardiac surgeons (cardiologists were the primary operators in 63% of centers). Forty-seven percent of responding centers performed TLE in 10 to 40 patients per year, and almost equally, 40% of responding centers performed less than 10 extractions annually, this being below the minimum annual number of extractions recommended for each operator according to the 2009 consensus.[31]

More than 40 extractions annually were performed by 13% of responding centers, fulfilling the definition of being a major extracting center. On average, 10% of patients, especially those with chronic and infected leads, were referred to experienced centers.

In many centers, extraction of redundant leads in the absence of infection, especially with certain clinical characteristics (age, comorbidities) present, was considered with caution. However, 57% of centers claimed to consider replacing a failing ICD lead a better option than adding another lead. Importantly, infection was still, in percentage terms, the main indication for extraction.

Regarding methods, traction alone (34%) and traction in combination with extraction tools (46%) were most often used. Only 14% of centers reported use laser sheaths. Extraction techniques varied slightly depending on the type of lead to be extracted.

After this survey a task force of the EHRA in 2012 published a consensus document on training and accreditation for TLE of chronically implanted pacing and defibrillator leads.[34]

The scope was to integrate the previous consensus documents on indications, facilities, training, and management of TLE published by the HRS and the document of the American Heart Association on infections, into a European setting.[31,38] The resulting paper focused on lead extraction tools, techniques, and training creating a present baseline for TLE. A particular focus of this document was to provide more precise recommendations on training.[34] In order to understand the future need of lead extraction in Europe, the task force calculated the approximate total need

by using the incidence of CIED infections times 1.5 as the denominator. This calculation was approximate, given the difficulty in finding uniform and clear data on infection rates across the European countries and centers.

In fact, the task force considered many databases and national registries to be inaccurate regarding the number of TLEs performed and the incidence of infections. In addition, it noted the lack of standards to define and categorize collected data. To make up for the heterogeneity of these data, the EHRA document recommended improved local registries as well as establishing a European registry, both registry types providing uniform data regarding indications, patients, technologies, approaches, complications, and outcomes, in order to monitor real-world extraction.

As a prelude to a European EHRA-supported registry, another exploratory survey on the experience of TLE across Europe was carried out; it was more extensive and widespread than the previous survey.[35] During 2012, EHRA presented European implanting centers with 2 electronic questionnaires. The first one (30 questions) focused on the technical details of the procedure; the second questionnaire (28 questions) focused on the clinical experience of operators. This was the most extensive survey yet published on TLE, being very representative of the European situation, involving 30 European countries and 164 centers.[35,37,39]

The survey showed an increase in the number of European centers performing TLE. Compared with the previous survey, the number of hospitals treating less than 10 patients per year decreased from 40% to 23%, and the number of hospitals treating more than 40 patients increased from 13% to 31%.

Cardiologists as first operators increased from 63% to 88% (**Fig. 2**). All centers reported having at least 2 experienced and trained operators. Importantly, the majority of centers reported having cardiac surgeons available for treating complications. The responses showed good adherence to recent international recommendations regarding personnel.

As far as the tools for TLE are concerned, answers to the first questionnaire showed a general confidence with all kinds of tools and alternative venous approaches (femoral 65%, jugular 37%). Manual traction was used by 44% of the centers, locking stylets by 88%, and mechanical sheaths by 79%. The laser was used by 28% of the centers, and electrosurgical dissection was by 36% of centers (**Fig. 3**).

These percentages confirm, as in the 2010 survey, a greater familiarity with nonpowered sheaths

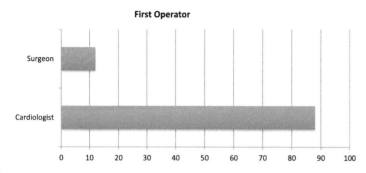

Fig. 2. Centers with a surgeon as the first operator and centers with a cardiologist as first operator for TLE according to the responses to the EHRA questionnaire 2012. (*Data from* Bongiorni MG, Blomström-Lundqvist C, Kennergren C, et al. Current practice in transvenous lead extraction: a European Heart Rhythm Association EP Network Survey. Europace 2012;14(6): 783–6.)

than with powered sheaths. The indication for lead extraction was more often infection (70%) than other conditions (30% of patients).

When systemic infection was suspected, a transesophageal echocardiogram (TEE) was usually performed in 88% of centers. The rates of success and complication were comparable with those of the major single-center experiences as well as results of international surveys, suggesting the reliability of these results as a good snapshot of TLE management in Europe. It should be noted that few surgical centers performing lead extraction in Europe were surveyed. This noted, the survey gave further strong encouragement to the creation of a European registry on TLE.

ELECTRA REGISTRY

In 2012, EHRA initiated the ELECTRa (European Lead Extraction Controlled) Registry: the first large

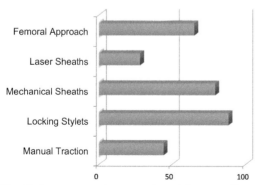

Fig. 3. Percentage of centers that claim to utilize a specific extraction technique and approach according to the responses to the EHRA questionnaire 2012. (*Data from* Bongiorni MG, Blomström-Lundqvist C, Kennergren C, et al. Current practice in transvenous lead extraction: a European Heart Rhythm Association EP Network Survey. Europace 2012;14(6):783–6.)

prospective, multicenter registry for TLE in Europe. Management was given to the ESC (European Society of Cardiology) EURObservational Research Programme (EORP).[40]

The primary objective of the registry was to evaluate the acute and long-term safety of TLE, while the secondary objectives were

- Description of demographic and clinical characteristics of patients undergoing a TLE procedure
- Analysis of characteristics of leads
- Evaluation of indications for TLE procedures
- Definition of the routine diagnostic and therapeutic approaches of physicians performing TLE
- Assessment of the acute and chronic outcome of TLE procedures.

The study started recruitment of patients on Nov. 6, 2012, and is expected to stop inclusion in May 2015. The target is to achieve a statistically relevant sample of at least 3500 patients, the most extensive of all large studies on TLE (**Fig. 4**). All national societies from the EHRA White Book and all other identified European lead extraction centers have been invited to participate. Seventy-five centers enrolled patients on a voluntary basis from most European countries; centers were stratified on the basis of their volume of extraction. Participating centers have to consecutively enroll and follow patients for 1 year.

Indications for performing procedures were left completely to the participating physicians. No specific protocol or recommendations for procedure, materials, extraction technique, or postoperative treatment were mandated during this observational study. Data were collected using a Web-based system in the EORP database (www.eorp.org). The eCRFs (electronic Case Report Form) includes 7 questionnaires, 15 main sections, and 150 questions in total (**Box 1**).

The first part of the questionnaire focuses on preprocedure evaluation: patient characteristics, NYHA (New York Heart Association) class,

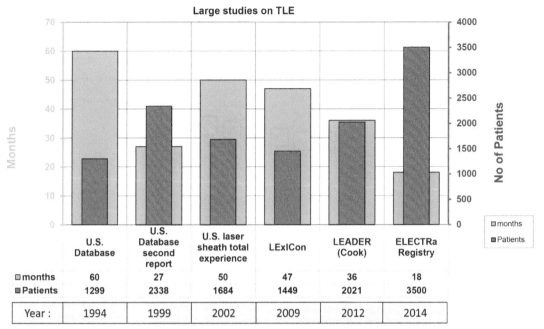

Fig. 4. Main large studies with more than 1000 patients on the TLE. The light blue rectangles show the duration of the studies in the month; the red rectangles show the number of patients. On the bottom of the chart, the years of publication of the studies are shown along a time line. (*Data from* Refs. [6,36,40].)

concomitant cardiovascular diseases, risk factors, and concomitant other diseases. The next part concerns CIED history, preprocedure investigations, pharmacologic treatment, and indications for lead extraction. The central part of the

---

Box 1
Main sections of the eCRF of ELECTRa Registry

1. Patient characteristics
2. Investigations
3. Indications for lead extraction
4. Treatments before procedure
5. Lead extraction preparation
6. Preprocedure lead information
7. Lead extraction procedure
8. Target lead characteristics
9. Lead extraction approaches and tools
10. Lead extraction results
11. Postprocedure lead information
12. Acute and postprocedural complications (prior to discharge)
13. Lead reimplantation procedure
14. Investigations and treatment at discharge
15. Follow-up

---

questionnaire focuses on the lead extraction procedure (personnel, tools, techniques, approaches, procedural room setting, type of anesthesia, procedural time, fluoroscopic exposure) and acute outcome and complications (major, minor). The third section covers postprocedure evaluation, reimplantation, and investigations and treatments at discharge. The final part covers the 1-year follow-up data.

From the start in 2012 to the end of January 2014, 75 centers from 19 countries enrolled 2521 patients (**Fig. 5**). Among the 19 countries involved, 16 are from Europe; the other 3 are Russia, Israel, and Azerbaijan.

The main characteristics of this registry are independence, consecutiveness of enrollment, and monitoring of collected data. Centers have been monitored according to the general rules of EORP; a data manager reviews all data forms for completeness, correctness, and compliance to the protocol. In addition, on-site random audits were carried out in 40% of centers.

Information collected in the survey will provide a description of the European real-world practice on TLE, a comparison of data from centers and countries, with potential evaluation of adherence to guideline recommendations, differences between small- and large-volume centers, experience-based outcomes, need of learning curve, and timing and method of reimplantation after extraction.

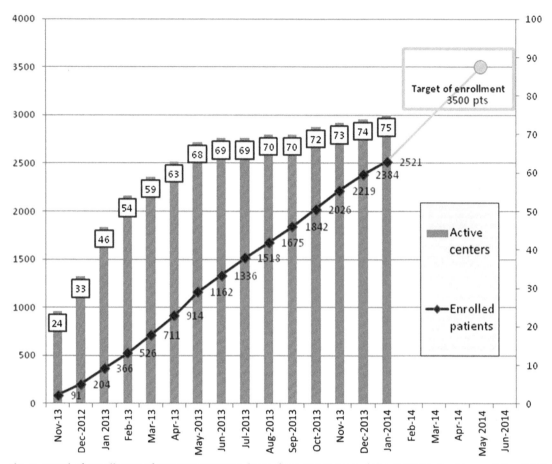

Fig. 5. Trend of enrollment of ELECTRa Registry. (*Data from* Newsletter of the ELECTRa Registry and the EORP EURObservational Research programme Data-base [www.eorp.org.])

The ELECTRa Registry has the potential to increase the quality of care for lead extraction patients, to disseminate more knowledge on lead extraction treatment, and to help verify and potentially adjust standards for lead extraction procedures in Europe.

REFERENCES

1. Greenspon AJ, Patel JD, Lau E, et al. Trends in permanent pacemaker implantation in the United States from 1993 to 2009: increasing complexity of patients and procedures. J Am Coll Cardiol 2012;60:1540–5.
2. Van Veldhuisen DJ, Maass AH, Priori SG, et al. Implementation of device therapy (cardiac resynchronization therapy and implantable cardioverter defibrillator) for patients with heart failure in Europe: changes from 2004 to 2008. Eur J Heart Fail 2009; 11:1143–51.
3. Madigan NP, Curtis JJ, Sanfelippo JF, et al. Difficulty of extraction of chronically implanted tined ventricular endocardial leads. J Am Coll Cardiol 1984;3: 724–31.
4. Rettig G, Doenecke P, Sen S, et al. Complications with retained transvenous pacemaker electrodes. Am Heart J 1979;98:587–94.
5. Maytin M, Epstein LM. The challenges of transvenous lead extraction. Heart 2011;97(5):425–34.
6. Bongiorni MG, editor. Transvenous lead extraction from simple traction to internal transjugular approach. Milan, Dordrecht, Heidelberg, London, New York: Springer; 2011.
7. Diemberger I, Mazzotti A, Giulia MB, et al. From lead management to implanted patient management: systematic review and meta-analysis of the last 15 years of experience in lead extraction. Expert Rev Med Devices 2013;10(4):551–73.
8. Byrd CL, Schwartz SJ, Hedin NB, et al. Intravascular lead extraction using locking stylets and sheaths. Pacing Clin Electrophysiol 1990;13:1871–5.
9. Eckhard A, Neuzner J, Binner L. Three year experience with a stylet for lead extraction: a multicenter study. Pacing Clin Electrophysiol 1996;19: 18–25.
10. Vassilikos VP, Maounis TN, Chiladakis J, et al. Percutaneous extraction of transvenous defibrillator leads

using the VascoExtor pacing lead removal system. J Interv Card Electrophysiol 1999;3(3):247–51.

11. Bracke F, Meijer A, Van Gelder B. Extraction of pacemaker and implantable defibrillator leads: patient and lead characteristics in relation to the requirement of extraction tools. Pacing Clin Electrophysiol 2002;25(7):1037–40.

12. Bracke FA, Meijer A, Van Gelder LM. Lead extraction for device related infections: a single centre experience. Europace 2004;6:243–7.

13. Marijon E, Boveda S, De Guillebon M, et al. Contribution of advanced techniques to the success and safety of transvenous lead extraction. Pacing Clin Electrophysiol 2009;32(Suppl 1):S38–41.

14. Byrd CL, Schwartz SJ, Hedin NB. Intravascular techniques for extraction of permanent pacemakers leads. J Thorac Cardiovasc Surg 1991; 101:989–97.

15. Smith HJ, Fearnot NE, Byrd CL, et al. Five-years experience with intravascular lead extraction. US Lead Extraction Database. Pacing Clin Electrophysiol 1994;17(11 Pt 2):2016–20.

16. Byrd CL, Wilkoff BL, Love CJ, et al. Intravascular extraction of problematic or infected permanent pacemaker leads: 1994-1996. U.S. Extraction Database, MED Institute. Pacing Clin Electrophysiol 1999;22(9):1348–57.

17. Bongiorni MG, Soldati E, Zucchelli G, et al. Transvenous removal of pacing and defibrillating leads using single sheath mechanical dilatation and multiple venous approaches: high success rate and safety in more than 2000 leads. Eur Heart J 2008;29(23):2886–93.

18. Wilkoff BL, Byrd CL, Love CJ, et al. Pacemaker lead extraction with the laser sheath: results of the pacing lead extraction with the excimer sheath (PLEXES) trial. J Am Coll Cardiol 1999;33:1671–6.

19. Byrd CL, Wilkoff BL, Love CJ, et al. Clinical study of the laser sheath for lead extraction: the total experience in the United States. Pacing Clin Electrophysiol 2002;25:804–8.

20. Kennergren C, Bucknall CA, Butter C, et al. PLESSE Investigators Group. Laser assisted lead extraction: the European experience. Europace 2007;9(8): 651–6.

21. Kennergren C, Bjurman C, Wiklund R, et al. A single-centre experience of over one thousand lead extractions. Europace 2009;11(5):612–7.

22. Moon MR, Camillo CJ, Gleva MJ. Laser-assist during extraction of chronically implanted pacemaker and defibrillator leads. Ann Thorac Surg 2002;73: 1893–6.

23. Roux JF, Pagé P, Dubuc M, et al. Laser lead extraction: predictors of success and complications. Pacing Clin Electrophysiol 2007;30(2):214–20.

24. Jones SO, Eckart RE, Albert CM, et al. Large, single-centre, single-operator experience with transvenous lead extraction: outcomes and changing indications. Heart Rhythm 2008;5(4):520–5.

25. Wazni O, Epstein LM, Carrillo RG, et al. Lead extraction in the contemporary setting: the LExICon study: an observational retrospective study of consecutive laser lead extractions. J Am Coll Cardiol 2010;55(6): 579–86.

26. Wilkoff BL. Transvenous leads extraction with electrosurgical dissection sheaths. Initial experience. Pacing Clin Electrophysiol 2000;23:679–84.

27. Dello Russo A, Biddau R, Pelargonio G, et al. Lead extraction: a new effective tool to overcome fibrous binding sites. J Interv Card Electrophysiol 2009;24: 147–50.

28. Hauser RG, Katsiyiannis W, Gornik C, et al. Deaths and cardiovascular injuries due to device-assisted implantable cardioverter–defibrillator and pacemaker lead extraction. Europace 2010;12:395–401.

29. Hussein A, Wilkoff B, Martin D, et al. Initial experience with the Evolution mechanical dilator sheath for lead extraction: safety and efficacy. Heart Rhythm 2010;7(7):870–3.

30. Epstein AE, DiMarco JP, Ellenbogen KA, et al. ACC/AHA/HRS 2008 guidelines for device-based therapy of cardiac rhythm abnormalities: a report of the American College of Cardiology/American Heart Association Task Force on Practice Guidelines (Writing Committee to Revise the ACC/AHA/ NASPE 2002 Guideline Update for Implantation of Cardiac Pacemakers and Antiarrhythmia Devices) developed in collaboration with the American Association for Thoracic Surgery and Society of Thoracic Surgeons. J Am Coll Cardiol 2008;51(21):e1–62.

31. Wilkoff BL, Love CJ, Byrd CL, et al. Transvenous lead extraction: Heart Rhythm Society expert consensus on facilities, training, indications, and patient management. Heart Rhythm 2009;6: 1085–104.

32. Neuzil P, Taborsky M, Rezek Z, et al. Pacemaker and ICD lead extraction with electrosurgical dissection sheaths and standard transvenous extraction systems: results of a randomized trial. Europace 2007; 9:98–104.

33. Bordachar P, Defaye P, Peyrouse E, et al. Extraction of old pacemaker or cardioverter-defibrillator leads by laser sheath versus femoral approach. Circ Arrhythm Electrophysiol 2010;3:319–23.

34. Deharo JC, Bongiorni MG, Rozkovec A, et al. Pathways for training and accreditation for transvenous lead extraction: a European Heart Rhythm Association position paper. Europace 2012;14: 124–34.

35. Bongiorni MG, Blomstrom-Lundqvist C, Kennergren C, et al. Current practice in transvenous lead extraction: a European Heart Rhythm Association EP Network Survey. Europace 2012;14:783–6.

36. Love CJ, Kutalek SP, Starck C, et al. Results of the lead extraction device evaluation and results (leader) database. Journal of Heart Disease 2012; 9(1):78–9.
37. Van Erven L, Morgan JM. Attitude towards redundant leads and the practice of lead extractions: a European survey. Europace 2010;12:275–6.
38. Baddour LM, Epstein AE, Erickson CC, et al. Update on cardiovascular implantable electronic device infections and their management: a scientific statement from the American Heart Association. Circulation 2010;121:458–77.
39. Henrikson CA, Zhang K, Brinker JA. A survey of the practice of lead extraction in the United States. Pacing Clin Electrophysiol 2010;33:721–6.
40. Bongiorni MG, Romano SL, Kennergren C, et al. ELECTRa (European Lead Extraction ConTRolled) Registry—Shedding light on transvenous lead extraction real-world practice in Europe. Herzschrittmacherther Elektrophysiol 2013;24(3):171–5.

Lead Design for Safer Lead Extraction

Melanie Maytin, MD*, Laurence M. Epstein, MD

KEYWORDS

- Lead • Design • Extraction • Implant • Cardiovascular implantable electronic device

KEY POINTS

- A detailed understanding of lead design is critical to making appropriate implant choices and crucial to safely and effectively extracting each unique lead model.
- Safety in lead extraction depends on the ability to apply sufficient traction to the lead and locking stylet, without disruption, to create a rail to allow the sheath to track the lead.
- A desirable lead design for extraction should encompass the following features: (1) adequate tensile strength to allow minimal lead distortion and stretching with the application of significant traction, (2) the effect of traction is applied to all components evenly (lead control), (3) lead delamination and destruction do not occur with marked traction (maintenance of lead integrity), (4) lumen integrity to allow placement of a locking stylet, (5) isodiametric lead design and designs that minimize ingrowth of scar tissue and lead encapsulation, and (6) a reliably retractable active fixation mechanism.

 Video of overcoming an engaged active fixation mechanism accompanies this article at http://www.cardiacep.theclinics.com/

INTRODUCTION

With the advent of subcutaneous implantable cardioverter-defibrillators (ICDs) and the ongoing development of leadless and even biologic pacemakers, the need for transvenous pacing and ICD leads will continue to decrease. However, the future is not here and there are millions of patients currently living with implanted leads. An understanding of lead design and the components of the ideally extractable lead are required to appropriately manage patients with implanted leads and devices. Cardiovascular implantable electronic device (CIED) and lead management starts before implantation and may extend to include the need for lead extraction. A detailed understanding of lead design is critical to making appropriate implant choices and is crucial to safely and effectively extract each unique lead model. CIED use continues to increase rapidly,[1–3] with more than 4.5 million active devices and more than 1 million new leads implanted annually worldwide.[4,5] With expanded indications for device therapy and increased CIED use, observed complications have increased in parallel.[6–14] More frequent device system revisions for complications,[6–8] system upgrade,[15–17] and/or lead malfunction,[9–13] and longer patient life expectancies, have all mandated a paradigm shift toward premeditated lead management strategies, from implantation to removal or replacement. Proactive lead management requires both forethought and conscious decisions at the time of CIED implantation with respect to a variety of factors, including hardware selection.

Lead design and construction are closely connected with the implantability, function, and

Dr M. Maytin has received research grants from Medtronic and Spectranetics and is a consultant for St. Jude Medical. Dr L.M. Epstein has received research grants from and is a consultant for Boston Scientific, Medtronic, Spectranetics, and St. Jude Medical, and has equity in and has served as a board member for Carrot Medical.

Cardiovascular Division, Brigham & Women's Hospital, 75 Francis Street, Boston, MA 02115, USA
* Corresponding author.
E-mail address: mmaytin@partners.org

Card Electrophysiol Clin 6 (2014) 345–354
http://dx.doi.org/10.1016/j.ccep.2014.03.004
1877-9182/14/$ – see front matter © 2014 Elsevier Inc. All rights reserved.

extractability of the lead. The lead must be designed and constructed to withstand several unique applied forces from manipulation at implantation to bending and torqueing with arm and chest movement, to beat-to-beat contraction with each cardiac cycle, to the harsh chemical and oxidative stress of an in vivo environment. In addition, the lead must maintain electrical integrity even in the face of the extremely high voltages seen with ICD leads. Some of the same characteristics required for implant ease and dislodgement prevention may make extraction more challenging. Lead implantation mandates both flexibility and durability to negotiate and withstand these factors. In contrast, extractability depends on the tensile strength and stiffness of the lead. Overcoming areas of fibrotic adhesions necessitates that specific forces be applied to both the lead and sheath; namely counterpressure, traction, and countertraction. Safety in transvenous lead extraction is critically dependent on the ability to apply sufficient traction to the lead and locking stylet, without disruption, to create a rail to allow the sheath to track the lead. A desirable lead design for extraction should encompass the following features: (1) adequate tensile strength to allow minimal lead distortion and stretching with the application of significant traction, (2) the effect of traction is applied to all components evenly (lead control), (3) lead delamination and destruction do not occur with marked traction (maintenance of lead integrity), (4) lumen integrity to allow placement of a locking stylet, (5) isodiametric lead design and designs that minimize ingrowth of scar tissue and lead encapsulation, and (6) a reliably retractable active fixation

mechanism. The ideal lead has the optimal balance of all these features. In choosing a lead for an implant, clinicians should consider all of these characteristics. In addition, when faced with extracting a lead, understanding how that specific lead model fails to meet any of the criteria listed earlier helps the extractor plan for obstacles to a safe and effective procedure.

LEAD CONSTRUCTION

The lead consists of the body, conductors, electrodes, insulation, fixation mechanisms, and connectors. Each component has important features that can affect both implantation and extraction procedures.

Older leads can be unipolar with only 1 conductor. These leads have a smaller external diameter, are more flexible for easier manipulation at implantation, and can be more fragile. Although some older unipolar leads are robust, most modern leads are bipolar with lead body constructions that can be coaxial (brady and cardiac resynchronization therapy [CRT] leads), coradial (brady and CRT leads), multilumen (ICD and CRT leads), or lumenless (brady leads) (**Fig. 1**).

Coaxial lead body design consists of an outer coil to ring electrode that is layered over an inner coil to tip electrode with a central lumen and insulation between the coils, as well as encompassing the lead. This design construction yields a slightly larger diameter and stiffer lead. During traction, the inner and outer coils can begin to delaminate.

Coradial lead assembly features parallel wound insulated coils surrounded by outer insulation and

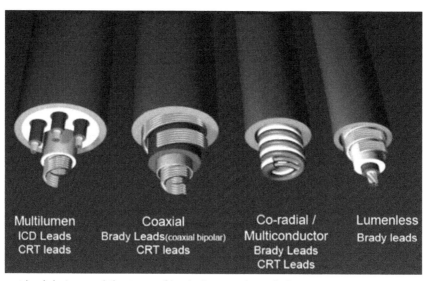

Fig. 1. Different lead designs and the types of leads that use these designs.

allows a smaller diameter lead body than coaxial construction. The result is a highly flexible lead with the potential for less durability and less tensile strength. In addition, the ethyltetrafluoroethylene (ETFE) insulation coating the coils has a low coefficient of friction and can allow slipping of the locking stylet.

Multilumen lead design is the mainstay of current ICD lead technology. Each company has its own design features with respect to number, orientation, and distribution of the internal elements. In general, the multiple lumens contain both cable and coil conductors sheathed in insulation with or without additional compression lumens. The lead body is composed of silicone and an outer protective layer of insulation (in all current ICD models but not some older models). Multilumen design has yielded a thinner and more complex lead with more connection points. These points of attachment are not only sites of potential lead malfunction but also areas vulnerable to lead disruption when traction is applied to the lead at the time of extraction.

Lumenless leads have a coaxial lead body with an outer coil to ring electrode over an inner cable to tip electrode separated by and covered with insulation. Although the inner cable contributes tensile strength to the lead, the absence of a lumen limits the distribution of applied traction forces.

As with any technology, early, solid rudimentary designs are replaced over time by smaller and structurally more complex ones. Early high-voltage leads were large and nonisodiametric, posing specific challenges at both implantation and the time of extraction. Complex lead design resulted in isodiametric leads with downsized lead diameters; however, reliability remains an issue. ICD lead failure rates approach 20% at 10 years after implantation.[10]

LEAD ELEMENTS
Conductors

The specific metallurgic components of pacing and ICD lead conductors are beyond the scope of this article. Conductor types include both coils, unifilar and multifilar, and cables. Unifilar coils consist of a single wire wound spirally around a central axis and are less common than multifilar coils. With multifilar coils, 2 wires are wound together in parallel around a central axis. Multifilar design allows for redundancy in the event of filar fracture and reduces pacing impedance. Cables consist of 2 or more wires wound together into a strand and then twisted with other strands into a rope. With this construction, cables can provide high tensile strength with high flex fatigue resistance.

Insulation

Lead insulation options include silicone, polyurethane, and hybrids. Like all design elements, each material has its advantages and disadvantages. Silicone is a biocompatible substance that is chemically inert and has excellent biostability. It tends to be highly flexible and soft with a lower tear/abrasion strength and a higher coefficient of friction. Although it can withstand the harsh in vivo environment, it is highly susceptible to electrocautery, abrasion, and failure caused by cool flow at sites of prolonged pressure. In contrast, polyurethane has a higher tensile strength and abrasion resistance. It yields a smaller diameter lead with better handling because of a lower coefficient of friction. However, polyurethane may not be as durable in vivo because both environmental stress cracking and metal ion oxidation have been observed with polyurethane insulation. More recently, copolymers have been designed to offer the advantages of both silicone and polyurethane. Although early results seem promising, long-term in vivo performance data remain limited. Other insulating materials, such as polytetrafluoroethylene (pTFE) or ETFE, offer biostability and abrasion resistance but are too stiff to be used as primary insulation. Current ICD leads use a combination of insulation materials. The lead body is composed of silicone, the high-voltage cables are coated with pTFE or ETFE, and the lead is encased in an outer jacket of polyurethane or a hybrid polymer.

The insulation is essential to the tensile strength of the lead. When traction is applied to a lead, the integrity of the lead is maintained so long as the insulation remains intact. Once the insulation disrupts, further traction results in coil deformation and lead disruption.

Lead Fixation

Lead fixation mechanisms can be passive or active. Passive fixation leads are tined, nonisodiametric, and often result in more scar formation at the lead-endocardial surface (**Fig. 2**). Active fixation leads have a screw and are isodiametric. They can have a fixed helix or one that is extendable and retractable. Certain active fixation leads (eg, Guidant Endotak Endurance EZ 0154, 0155, 0156) require specialized stylets to retract the active fixation mechanism. Retracting the helix of chronic active fixation leads can be difficult and sometimes is not possible. The bends that a lead takes throughout its course and scar formation at the fixation site may limit the transmission of torque through the lead body to the helix. Often difficulties in helix retraction can be overcome through

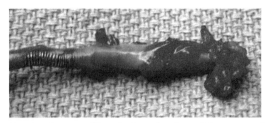

Fig. 2. Vigorous fibrosis that developed in areas of direct contact between the passive fixation mechanism and the myocardium. Extracted ventricular lead with intense fibrosis at the electrode tip–myocardial interface.

patience and withdrawing and readvancing a stylet halfway up the length of the lead. If the inner coils have fractured, the screw mechanism will not be functional. In cases in which the screw does not retract, or for fixed-screw lead models, the fixation mechanism can be overcome by tensile force (Video 1; available online at http://www.interventional.theclinics.com/). In almost every case, traction on the lead results in stretching of the fixation screw with release. In addition to the fixation mechanism (ie, tines) of passive leads their nonisodiametric design makes them more difficult to extract. Isodiametric lead construction lends itself to easier extractability because any variability in the lead serves as substrate for fibrotic adhesion formation. Moreover, animal data have shown that the tensile force necessary for lead removal is 5-fold higher for passive compared with active fixation leads in a chronic pacing model in dogs.[18]

Distal Lead Construction

Lead construction from pin to distal electrode affects tensile strength. Some leads have different design features at the distal portion of the lead. For example, silicone rubber distal tip-ring spacers have been used in lead design to provide a more flexible lead tip. The joint between the lead and the silicone is rubber bonded and can delaminate if the tensile load applied to the lead exceeds the strength of the bond. Lead designs with wide spacing between the proximal and distal electrodes similarly may not withstand the tensile load applied during lead extraction and lead disruption can occur. When extracting leads with these types of distal lead designs, it is important to ensure that the locking stylet is inserted the full length of the lead and to watch the entire lead under fluoroscopy during extraction for early evidence of lead disruption such as changes in electrode spacing. In some lead models, the design that makes them thin and flexible can pose challenges to extraction. The electrodes of

some coradial leads are only attached to a single filar and the outer insulation, which makes them susceptible to lead disruption with separation of the electrodes from the lead body during extraction.

ICD LEADS
ICD Lead Coils

ICD leads have specific design elements that can affect the extractability of the lead. The challenges and risks of transvenous lead extraction are related to the foreign-body response to the device. Robust fibrosis develops in areas of direct contact between the lead and both the vasculature and endocardium. The most common adhesion sites include the venous entry site, the superior vena cava (SVC), and the electrode tip–myocardial interface.[19] Studies have shown equivalent defibrillation efficacy, first shock efficacy, and all-cause mortality in patients with single-coil and dual-coil ICD leads.[20–23] Despite this equivalency, most implanted ICD leads remain dual coil. It is estimated that single-coil lead implantation in the United States has accounted for only 5.4% to 13.2% of device implants[24] but it is hoped that this is changing. Exposed defibrillator coils of ICD leads enable fibrous tissue ingrowth, resulting in more dense vascular and myocardial adhesions (Fig. 3A). Aggressive fibrosis of a SVC coil, which lies in a thin-walled area at high risk for vascular injury, is associated with increased difficulty and risk of transvenous lead extraction.[25] A group of high-volume, experienced operators found transvenous lead extraction of ICD leads with an SVC coil to be associated with a 1.0% major complication rate compared with no major complications during removal of single-coil ICD leads despite longer lead implant durations among the single-coil leads. In addition to a markedly higher observed complication rate, dual-coil ICD leads were 2.57 times more difficult to remove (more frequent use of powered sheaths and longer extraction times) on adjusted analysis. A postmarket extraction surveillance study found that 72% of all major adverse events and 79% of mortality was associated with the removal of dual-coil ICD leads. Therefore, given the lack of clinical benefit of dual-coil ICD leads, their simple elimination may dramatically improve the safety of ICD lead extraction. This possibility is a clear example of how thinking before you choose can have a significant impact on patient outcomes.[26]

In the past, the high-voltage shocking coils of ICD leads have created significant extraction challenges. Early ICD leads were not isodiametric. There was often a step-up in size of the coil

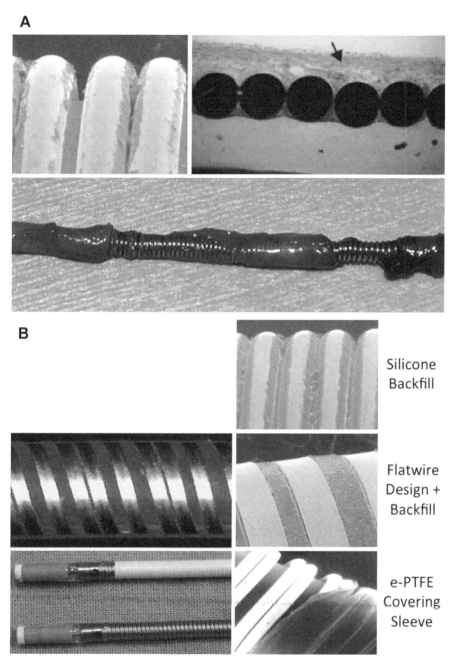

Fig. 3. Tissue ingrowth in ICD coils and treated coil strategies. (*A*) Tissue ingrowth (clockwise from top left). High-powered photomicrograph of standard ICD coil showing spacing that permits tissue ingrowth; cross-section of ICD coil with *arrow* showing tissue ingrowth between high-voltage coils (hematoxylin and eosin staining); extracted ICD lead showing extensive fibrosis and tissue adhesion at the level of the high-voltage coil. (*B*) Treated ICD coils. (*Top*) High-powered photomicrograph showing Medtronic ICD lead treated with silicone backfill. (*Middle*) Gross and photomicrograph images of St. Jude Medical's flatwire ICD lead technology with medical adhesive backfill. (*Bottom*) Gross and photomicrograph images of Boston Scientific's expanded polytetrafluoroethylene ICD lead technology. (*Courtesy of* [*A, Top left*; *B, Top*] Medtronic, Minneapolis, MN; and [*B, Middle*] St. Jude Medical, Little Canada, MN; and [*B, Bottom*] Boston Scientific, Natick, MA.)

compared with the lead body. This step-up can create a site of bunching of insulation and snow-plowing of scar tissue. For this reason, engaging the shocking coil with the extraction sheath can be challenging. In addition, early ICD shocking coil design encouraged the active ingrowth of fibrotic tissue, greatly increasing the difficulty of extraction. Newer design elements have been incorporated to address the aggressive fibrotic ingrowth that occurs at the high-voltage electrode. Electrode coils have been treated (either coated with expanded polytetrafluoroethylene or back-filled with medical adhesive) to limit the fibrotic attachments (**Fig. 3**B). Studies comparing transvenous extraction of conventional versus treated ICD leads have shown fewer adhesion sites.[27,28]

ICD Defibrillation Coil Connections

Defibrillation coil connections affect tensile loading with traction (**Fig. 4**A). Different manufacturers have different defibrillation coil connections.

A proximal connection can unravel the coil electrode with traction. In contrast, a distal connection can compress the coil from distal to proximal causing the coil to bunch and bulge. Dual connection results in forces applied to both ends with maintenance of a stable shape. This has important implications not only for transvenous lead extraction but also for surgical extraction. If the lead has only a distal defibrillation coil connection (ie, St. Jude Medical) and the surgeon cuts the SVC coil within the heart and then removes the remainder of the lead from the pocket, a remnant is likely to be left behind as the coil is no longer attached to the proximal portion of the lead (see **Fig. 4**B).

ICD Lead Connectors

Before industry-wide standardization, lead connector pins were proprietary and compatible only within a manufacturer, which frequently necessitated the use of adaptors at generator change

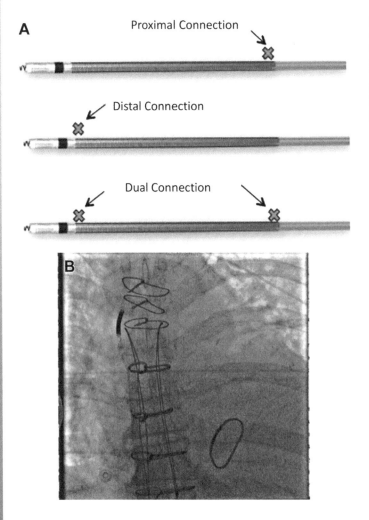

A — Proximal Connection

Distal Connection

Dual Connection

B

Fig. 4. ICD defibrillation coil connectors. (*A*) Defibrillation coil connections affect tensile loading. (*B*) SVC coil remnant following surgical extraction. This coil had a distal connection. The SVC coil was cut and pulled from both directions, leaving the distal portion of the SVC coil behind.

requiring advance planning and introducing another piece of hardware into the system. Standardization led to the advent of IS-1/DF-1 lead connectors with a trifurcated yoke for the pace-sense portion of the lead (IS-1) and the 1 or 2 high-voltage coils (DF-1). The result is a complex, bulky design with multiple connections with the possibility for errors. The bulk in the pocket provides more substrate for scar formation and the yoke connections may be prone to fractures. More recently, IS-4/DF-4 technology has emerged, allowing all the connectors to be merged together into 1 pin. With only 1 pin, the yoke is eliminated, as is the possibility of errors at the time of connection given the single connection. There is also less bulk in the pocket, ICD header size is reduced, and less extensive dissection is required at the time of generator change. This standard has only recently been introduced and only time will tell whether this design will result in improved lead/device performance. Although the advantages of IS-4/DF-4 technology may not apply directly to the ease of extraction, their features may help prevent the need for extraction.

EXTRACTION CONSIDERATIONS ASSOCIATED WITH SPECIFIC LEAD DESIGNS

Each lead design has its own unique extraction characteristics. Reviewing each available lead is not the goal of this article. Before extraction, the physician must know what lead models are present, and, if unfamiliar, research the specifics of that model's design (always readily available from the manufacturer). However, it is useful to address a few specific leads that either have a significantly high incidence of the need for extraction (advisories) or pose particularly difficult challenges.

Sprint Fidelis

The Sprint Fidelis lead (Medtronic, Inc, Minneapolis, MN) was introduced as a small-diameter ICD lead with reduced insulation and stiffness yielding a lead that was easier to implant but at the expense of more stress on the coils and cables. On October 15, 2007, Medtronic voluntarily suspended distribution of the Sprint Fidelis lead because of growing concerns regarding an abnormally high fracture rate.[29] Despite its propensity to failure, the Sprint Fidelis lead is an isodiametric lead with backfilled coils that can be safely extracted by experienced operators. We reported on a multicenter experience of 557 lead extractions removed with 100% complete procedural success, no major complications, and no procedural deaths.[30] A tensilock cable provides additional tensile strength. However, with increasing implant durations, the Fidelis lead is becoming more difficult to extract, almost always requiring the use of powered sheaths.

Attain StarFix

Active fixation coronary sinus leads limit lead dislodgement, may allow avoidance of phrenic nerve stimulation, and represent an attractive option to the implanter. The Attain StarFix 4195 lead (Medtronic, Inc, Minneapolis, MN) is a 5-Fr unipolar pacing lead with an active fixation mechanism that consists of 3 polyurethane lobes that are deployed by advancing the push tubing around the lead. As the push tubing is advanced, it compresses a slotted area of the tubing, forming lobes. Chronic in vivo studies of the long-term adhesions formed between the polyurethane lobes and coronary sinus (CS) endothelium are not available and raise concerns regarding the potential for vigorous fibrotic attachments to occur. Although extraction of passive fixation CS leads is a common and frequently uncomplicated procedure,[31–33] our group of high-volume operators found transvenous lead extraction of the Attain StarFix 4195 lead extremely challenging and it frequently required unconventional techniques.[34] We found removal of the Attain StarFix 4195 lead to be difficult despite short lead implant durations. Complete lobe retraction was unsuccessful in most cases, likely contributing to the challenge of lead removal. The need for unconventional and aggressive approaches with extraction sheath use within the coronary sinus and branch vessels significantly increases the risk of the procedure. Moreover, should a complication such as a tear of the coronary sinus occur, surgical repair would require cardiopulmonary bypass support; a difficult and tenuous undertaking in the CRT patient population. We suggest that this lead should not be used routinely given the concerns noted earlier.

Fineline

The Fineline lead (Boston Scientific, St Paul, MN) was designed to be a thinner, more flexible pacing lead. It is a 5.7-Fr lead with coradial design and with 16 mm between electrodes. Lead extraction without disruption is challenging. Traction on the lead, with or without a locking stylet, results in stretching and distortion of the coils. Further traction frequently results in lead disruption, often at the wide spacing between the proximal and distal electrodes. As noted earlier, the distal electrode of the earlier versions of this model is only attached to a single filar and the out insulation. Even after the lead is freed from the myocardium the distal electrode can become hung up in fibrous tissue as the lead is withdrawn. Because the lead is free from the heat, there is a tendency just to apply additional traction at this point. There is a significant risk of the distal electrode getting stuck and disrupting the lead. It is difficult to retrieve the electrode at this point because it is often embedded in the fibrous sheath. In addition, it may not be stably embedded and may dislodge and migrate. We have adopted a practice of advancing the locking stylet down the central lumen without cutting the lead in an attempt to maintain its limited tensile strength. In addition, we never attempt Fineline lead removal with traction alone and we tend to apply less traction to this lead given its fragile construction. We always try to encompass the distal electrode within the extraction sheath to avoid entrapment in the fibrous sheath.

Riata

The Riata/ST leads (St. Jude Medical, St Paul, MN) are susceptible to a unique problem of insulation abrasion thought to occur as a result of repetitive motion of the ethylenetetrafluoroethylene-coated cables within the silicone-walled lumens exerting disruptive forces that yield inside-out insulation failure, which is frequently manifest by externalized cables.[35] Moreover, it seems that there is an incidence of electrical failure that is discrete from insulation failure.[36–40] In our multicenter experience of transvenous extraction of 577 Riata/ST leads, we observed complete procedural success in 99.1% of cases with a 0.87% major complication rate and 1 procedure-related death.[41] As is the case with extraction of other leads,[25,30] lead implant duration was associated with a significant increase in the need for extraction sheath assistance, thereby increasing the complexity of the extraction procedure. Among leads in which cable externalization was noted, laser sheaths were similarly used more frequently. This lead design poses some unique challenges. As with all ICD leads, an attempt should be made to control all lead elements, particularly for Riata leads. Maintaining traction on all cables sometimes allows extruded cables to be pulled back into the lead, and at a minimum prevents further extrusion. Some clinicians have suggested that there can be difficulty passing the locking stylet to the most distal portion of this lead. Patience and lead manipulation are required in some cases. As mentioned earlier, the shocking coils of Riata leads are only attached distally. Therefore traction placed on the lead can result in bunching of the coil, increasing its diameter and making it more difficult to engage with the extraction sheath. The shocking coils of 1500 series, as opposed to

Table 1
Ease of implantation and extraction of various ICD design elements

Design Element	Implantation Ease	Extraction Ease
Unipolar lead design	↑	–
Silicone	↑	–/↓
Polyurethane	–/↓	↑
SVC coil	–	↓↓
Treated ICD coils	–	↑
DF-4 connector	–	?
Active fixation	–/↑	↑
Isodiametric	↑	↑
Coradial design	–/↑	↓

7000 series, Riata leads are not back filled. They are therefore more subject to fibrous ingrowth. The extruded cables pose their own issues. Significant extrusion can prevent the passage of the extraction sheath. In addition, the extruded cables can be a nidus for thrombus formation and fibrosis. Given all these issues, we always use the largest extraction sheath available from the start and consider the need for an outer sheath as well.

SUMMARY

Lead management mandates premeditated hardware selection with design features that balance implantability and extractability (**Table 1**). The implanter should consider the hardware choices that might result in decreased need for extraction and, if extraction is needed, the hardware choices that will make it safer and easier, keeping in mind the concepts of lead control and tensile strength. The future may mitigate or even obviate these considerations as leadless systems and systems that avoid the vasculature entirely are developed.

VIDEO

Video related to this article can be found online at http://dx.doi.org/10.1016/j.ccep.2014.03.004.

REFERENCES

1. Hammill SC, Kremers MS, Kadish AH, et al. Review of the ICD Registry's third year, expansion to include lead data and pediatric ICD procedures, and role for measuring performance. Heart Rhythm 2009;6: 1397–401.
2. Maisel WH, Moynahan M, Zuckerman BD, et al. Pacemaker and ICD generator malfunctions: analysis of

Food and Drug Administration annual reports. JAMA 2006;295:1901–6.

3. DeFrances CJ, Lucas CA, Buie VC, et al. 2006 National Hospital Discharge Survey. Natl Health Stat Report 2008;(5):1–20.

4. Borek PP, Wilkoff BL. Pacemaker and ICD leads: strategies for long-term management. J Interv Card Electrophysiol 2008;23:59–72.

5. Agarwal SK, Kamireddy S, Nemec J, et al. Predictors of complications of endovascular chronic lead extractions from pacemakers and defibrillators: a single-operator experience. J Cardiovasc Electrophysiol 2009;20:171–5.

6. Eckstein J, Koller MT, Zabel M, et al. Necessity for surgical revision of defibrillator leads implanted long-term: causes and management. Circulation 2008;117:2727–33.

7. Voigt A, Shalaby A, Saba S. Continued rise in rates of cardiovascular implantable electronic device infections in the United States: temporal trends and causative insights. Pacing Clin Electrophysiol 2010;33:414–9.

8. Cabell CH, Heidenreich PA, Chu VH, et al. Increasing rates of cardiac device infections among Medicare beneficiaries: 1990-1999. Am Heart J 2004;147:582–6.

9. Haqqani HM, Mond HG. The implantable cardioverter-defibrillator lead: principles, progress, and promises. Pacing Clin Electrophysiol 2009;32:1336–53.

10. Kleemann T, Becker T, Doenges K, et al. Annual rate of transvenous defibrillation lead defects in implantable cardioverter-defibrillators over a period of >10 years. Circulation 2007;115:2474–80.

11. Dorwarth U, Frey B, Dugas M, et al. Transvenous defibrillation leads: high incidence of failure during long-term follow-up. J Cardiovasc Electrophysiol 2003;14:38–43.

12. Ellenbogen KA, Wood MA, Shepard RK, et al. Detection and management of an implantable cardioverter defibrillator lead failure: Incidence and clinical implications. J Am Coll Cardiol 2003;41:73–80.

13. Luria D, Glikson M, Brady PA, et al. Predictors and mode of detection of transvenous lead malfunction in implantable defibrillators. Am J Cardiol 2001;87:901–4.

14. Pakarinen S, Oikarinen L, Toivonen L. Short-term implantation-related complications of cardiac rhythm management device therapy: a retrospective single-centre 1-year survey. Europace 2010;12:103–8.

15. Vatankulu MA, Goktekin O, Kaya MG, et al. Effect of long-term resynchronization therapy on left ventricular remodeling in pacemaker patients upgraded to biventricular devices. Am J Cardiol 2009;103:1280–4.

16. Sweeney MO, Shea JB, Ellison KE. Upgrade of permanent pacemakers and single chamber implantable cardioverter defibrillators to pectoral dual chamber implantable cardioverter defibrillators: indications, surgical approach, and long-term clinical results. Pacing Clin Electrophysiol 2002;25:1715–23.

17. Foley PW, Muhyaldeen SA, Chalil S, et al. Long-term effects of upgrading from right ventricular pacing to cardiac resynchronization therapy in patients with heart failure. Europace 2009;11:495–501.

18. Amitani S, Sohara H, Kurose M, et al. Tensile force of pacing lead extraction. A comparison between tined type and screw-in type. Jpn Heart J 1996;37:495–501.

19. Smith HJ, Fearnot NE, Byrd CL, et al. Five-years experience with intravascular lead extraction. U.S. Lead Extraction Database. Pacing Clin Electrophysiol 1994;17:2016–20.

20. Rinaldi CA, Simon RD, Geelen P, et al. A randomized prospective study of single coil versus dual coil defibrillation in patients with ventricular arrhythmias undergoing implantable cardioverter defibrillator therapy. Pacing Clin Electrophysiol 2003;26:1684–90.

21. Schulte B, Sperzel J, Carlsson J, et al. Dual-coil vs single-coil active pectoral implantable defibrillator lead systems: defibrillation energy requirements and probability of defibrillation success at multiples of the defibrillation energy requirements. Europace 2001;3:177–80.

22. Aoukar PS, Poole JE, Johnson GW, et al. No benefit of a dual coil over a single coil ICD lead: evidence from SCD-HeFT. Circulation 2010;122:A13672.

23. Mokabberi R, Haftbaradaran A, Pranesh S, et al. Defibrillation thresholds in single versus dual coil ICD lead systems: is there any difference? Circulation 2011;124:A17919.

24. Neuzner J, Carlsson J. Dual- versus single-coil implantable defibrillator leads: review of the literature. Clin Res Cardiol 2012;101:239–45.

25. Epstein LM, Love CJ, Wilkoff BL, et al. Superior vena cava defibrillator coils make transvenous lead extraction more challenging and riskier. J Am Coll Cardiol 2013;61:987–9.

26. Epstein LM. Think before you choose: the case against the routine use of dual coil ICD leads. EP Lab Digest 2013;13:2.

27. Di Cori A, Bongiorni MG, Zucchelli G, et al. Transvenous extraction performance of expanded polytetrafluoroethylene covered ICD leads in comparison to traditional ICD leads in humans. Pacing Clin Electrophysiol 2010;33:1376–81.

28. Hackler JW, Sun Z, Lindsay BD, et al. Effectiveness of implantable cardioverter-defibrillator lead coil treatments in facilitating ease of extraction. Heart Rhythm 2010;7:890–7.

29. Sprint Fidelis Model 6949 lead performance physician letter - dated October 15, 2007. Available

at: http://www.medtronic.com/product-advisories/physician/sprint-fidelis/PROD-ADV-PHYS-OCT.htm.

30. Maytin M, Love CJ, Fischer A, et al. Multicenter experience with extraction of the Sprint Fidelis implantable cardioverter-defibrillator lead. J Am Coll Cardiol 2010;56:646–50.

31. Dic A, Bongiorni MG, Zucchelli G, et al. Large, single-center experience in transvenous coronary sinus lead extraction: procedural outcomes and predictors for mechanical dilatation. Pacing Clin Electrophysiol 2012;35(2):215–22.

32. Williams SE, Arujuna A, Whitaker J, et al. Percutaneous lead and system extraction in patients with Cardiac Resynchronization Therapy (CRT) devices and coronary sinus leads. Pacing Clin Electrophysiol 2011;34:1209–22.

33. Hamid S, Arujuna A, Khan S, et al. Extraction of chronic pacemaker and defibrillator leads from the coronary sinus: laser infrequently used but required. Europace 2009;11:213–5.

34. Maytin M, Carrillo RG, Baltodano P, et al. Multicenter experience with transvenous lead extraction of active fixation coronary sinus leads. Pacing Clin Electrophysiol 2012;35(2):215–22.

35. Hauser RG, McGriff D, Retel LK. Riata implantable cardioverter-defibrillator lead failure: analysis of explanted leads with a unique insulation defect. Heart Rhythm 2012;9:742–9.

36. Schmutz M, Delacretaz E, Schwick N, et al. Prevalence of asymptomatic and electrically undetectable intracardiac inside-out abrasion in silicon-coated Riata and Riata ST implantable cardioverter-defibrillator leads. Int J Cardiol 2013;167(1):254–7.

37. Kodoth V, Cromie N, Lau E, et al. Riata lead failure; a report from Northern Ireland Riata lead screening programme. Eur Heart J 2011;32:1838. Abstract.

38. Parkash R, Exner D, Champagne J, et al. Failure rate of the Riata lead under advisory: a report from the CHRS Device Committee. Heart Rhythm 2013;10: 692–5.

39. Larsen JM, Riahi S, Nielsen JC, et al. Nationwide fluoroscopic screening of recalled Riata defibrillator leads in Denmark. Heart Rhythm 2013;10(6):821–7.

40. Parvathaneni SV, Ellis CR, Rottman JN. High prevalence of insulation failure with externalized cables in St. Jude Medical Riata family ICD leads: fluoroscopic grading scale and correlation to extracted leads. Heart Rhythm 2012;9:1218–24.

41. Maytin M, Love CJ, Bongiorni MG, et al. Multicenter experience with extraction of the Riata/Riata ST ICD lead. Heart Rhythm 2013;10:1.

Complications and Errors Made in Lead Extraction

Charles J. Love, MD, FHRS, CCDS[a],*, Charles Kennergren, MD, PhD, FETCS, FHRS[b]

KEYWORDS

- Lead extraction • Implantable cardioverter-defibrillator • Complications • Pericardiocentesis
- Lead management • Pacemaker

KEY POINTS

- Evaluate the patient carefully and make sure you have reviewed every facet of the patient's medical and device history.
- Have a low threshold to look for and diagnose a complication.
- Have a low threshold to treat a complication.
- Remember the Boy Scout motto, "be prepared"; when doing this procedure it is important that proper planning has taken place. Have the appropriate people and the proper tools present.

PERFORMING A PROCEDURE THAT IS NOT NECESSARY

Each lead extraction must be performed by evaluating the risk to the individual patient given the total circumstances present, and includes evaluation of the number of leads implanted, duration of implant of the targeted lead(s), age of the patient, comorbidities present, indication for the extraction, and the degree of skill and experience of the operator and personnel. There is broad consensus that leads falling into the Class I indications for extraction should be removed in nearly all patients.[1] However, leads falling into Class II indications require somewhat more consideration. For example, extracting a normally functioning lead in an elderly patient because of a lead "recall" may expose the patient to a significantly higher risk from the extraction procedure relative to the risk of continuing to use the lead, or that of simply placing another lead while abandoning the targeted lead. It would be difficult to justify the addition of any surgical risk in such a patient.

Unfortunately, many of these decisions are not simple, requiring consideration of several issues specific to the individual patient. One of the main axioms of performing this procedure safely is to carefully review all aspects of the device history, all dictated implant notes, and the patient's medical history.

PERFORMING A PROCEDURE WITHOUT ENOUGH EXPERIENCE

Lead extraction is not the same procedure with regard to success and risk for every patient. Many issues such as the duration of implant will have an effect on the risk to the patient. Whereas a physician with minimal experience would be capable of removing a lead that had been implanted a few years previously, a lead that is 20 years old with calcification present would pose an entirely different risk. It is important that physicians undertaking lead extraction start with leads that potentially are easier to remove. As experience is gained, more challenging leads may be attempted. This aspect is

Disclosures: **Dr Love:** Medical Advisory Board or Consultant: Medtronic, Spectranetics, WL Gore, Leadexx, Eximo, St Jude Medical. **Dr Kennergren:** Performed studies in cooperation with, advised, and/or presented on behalf of: Biotronic, Boston Scientific, Ela/Sorin, Medtronic/Vitatron, Mentice, Spectranetics, St Jude, TYRX.
[a] Division of Cardiology, The New York University Langone Medical Center, 403 East 34th Street, RIV-4th Floor, New York, NY 10016, USA; [b] Department of Cardiothoracic Surgery, Sahlgrenska University Hospital, Goteborg S-413 45, Sweden
* Corresponding author.
E-mail address: charles.love@nyumc.org

Card Electrophysiol Clin 6 (2014) 355–360
http://dx.doi.org/10.1016/j.ccep.2014.03.003

especially important when considering the risks and benefits of removing leads considered for Class II indications. Until such experience is gained, additional mentoring or referral of the patient to a physician with more experience is appropriate.

PERFORMING A PROCEDURE WITHOUT THE CORRECT TOOLS

One of the more common issues that can result in failure to extract a lead or in a complication resulting from working too hard with a certain tool is the failure to recognize that all leads cannot be extracted with a single type of extraction system. The highly successful physician, who is able to change techniques as needed given the circumstances present during the extraction process, has access to and training with multiple types of extraction tools. This armamentarium includes different types of locking stylets, lead stabilization devices, nonpowered sheaths, LASER sheaths, rotationally powered sheaths, femoral access systems, and multiple types of snares. Knowing when to use which tool, and when to change from one tool or technique to another, requires knowledge and experience. Failure to change technique, pushing and/or pulling harder, or continuing to apply energy at the same site without advancing can lead to complications.

PERFORMING A PROCEDURE WITHOUT THE APPROPRIATE TEAM(S)

Lead extraction obviously requires a trained operator. However, failure to have a trained and experienced team can result in complications, failure to recognize a complication, or failure to rescue a patient when a complication occurs. The staff must be familiar with all of the equipment being used, including the theory of traction/countertraction, and calibration and safety regarding the laser. Staff must be knowledgable about the types of complications that can occur, at which points during the procedure they are likely to occur, and the anatomic sites that are vulnerable to damage. Staff must be fully focused on the procedure at all times, but especially during sheath application. Emergency procedures need to be known and practiced, with specific roles assigned to individual members of the team. If the primary extractor is not a cardiac surgeon, the surgeon and his or her team must be fully aware of the types of injuries that can occur, and must be prepared to provide the procedures required to rescue the patient. It is strongly advised that a checklist be developed and reviewed before each procedure, with the extraction team present, to assure that all personnel, equipment, and supplies are readily available and prepared.

NOT RECOGNIZING THAT A COMPLICATION HAS OCCURRED

It is not uncommon for the blood pressure to drop during the performance of a lead extraction. This event can be due to vasodilation from anesthetic agents, vagal responses to traction on the lead, vagal response to pain, or inversion of the right ventricle. These causes are usually quickly reversible. However, it is imperative that the first consideration regarding the cause of a drop in blood pressure be the possibility of a tear in the myocardium or venous system. Likewise, failure of a finger pulse oximeter to register is often due to the probe falling off the patient's finger. However, this can also be attributable to the lack of blood pressure from an intravascular complication. Failure to consider one of the serious complications as the cause of loss of blood pressure or oximeter readings may delay the diagnosis of a major complication and, thus, the efforts to begin the needed rescue procedure. Delays of even several minutes to diagnose a complication requiring surgical rescue can lead to a poor outcome for the patient. Having transesophageal echo or portable transthoracic echo available in the operating room is very helpful in assisting in the differential diagnosis relating to hypotension. Most operators consider this essential equipment in the room. In some laboratories, intracardiac echo is placed to allow online simultaneous monitoring of the right and left ventricle for an effusion. The bottom line is that ideally some form of echo should be in the room, or at least immediately available.

NOT RESPONDING IMMEDIATELY TO A POSSIBLE COMPLICATION

Just as failure to recognize that a complication has occurred delays the surgical rescue required, it is not uncommon for the extraction team to believe that they can manage the situation with conservative measures, and thus delay the involvement of the surgical rescue team. In the case of a small venous or myocardial tear within the pericardium, it is not uncommon that pericardiocentesis is effective in relieving tamponade. In many of these cases the small leak is sealed by a thrombus, and the chest does not need to be opened. However, it would be a mistake to believe that all cases can be managed in this manner, or that all patients will respond well to pericardiocentesis. When a complication has occurred, the extraction attempt should be halted (if the lead is not removed already), and all attention and resources should be focused on resuscitation and management of the patient. If the cardiac surgery team is not already present, they should be summoned immediately, even while attempts to further define the nature of the complication and intervene to manage the complication are in process. It is far better to have the extra support present and not needed than to need them and not have them available. In these situations, hesitating for a period of time as short as 5 to 10 minutes may make the difference between a good and a poor outcome.

SHEATH BECOMES STUCK ON THE LEAD

Many extractors prefer to size the inner diameter of the extraction sheath closely to the size of the lead. Unfortunately, fibrous tissue, calcification, loose insulation, and deformable shock coils can become wedged or jammed inside the sheath. In some cases, a sheath may become kinked and lock on to the lead. When either of these events occur, it is possible for the sheath to become stuck in such a way that it can no longer be advanced or withdrawn. If the inner sheath is stuck and an outer sheath is present, it may be possible to advance the outer sheath over the inner sheath and complete the extraction. If the outer sheath has kinked, the inner sheath may be able to be advanced through the outer sheath to relieve the kink and remove the sheath system. It is possible to minimize the risk of these events occurring by using properly sized sheaths, and using the sheaths in a telescoping manner. However, many operators often use the more flexible laser sheaths without an outer sheath. Therefore, upsizing these sheaths from the recommended sizes provided on the reference sheet is a strategy often used.

TEAR OF THE SUPERIOR VENA CAVA

Tear of the superior vena cava (SVC) has become one of the most significant and feared complications of lead extraction, as there can be rapid and massive blood loss, and repair of the damage can be difficult or impossible. It has been noted that more than 70% of these types of injuries are associated with the extraction of dual-coil implantable cardioverter-defibrillator (ICD) leads, because the proximal coil sits against the SVC and innominate veins. The leads often become integrated with the vein owing to fibrosis. Leads without adhesive backfill in the coils or a Gore-tex covering over the coils seem to be more likely to adhere aggressively to the vein. As the extraction sheath passes over the coil the vein can be torn or cut, leading to a major complication. This type of injury must be addressed by surgical intervention without delay. Use of extracorporeal membrane oxygenation rapidly instituted through previously placed femoral arterial and venous sheaths can buy some time, but should not delay sternotomy and cardiopulmonary bypass. The surgeon charged with rescue of the patient should be prepared for and able to manage this type of severe injury; this requires knowledge of the types and locations of the injuries common to lead extraction, and the experience to be able to quickly and expertly stabilize the patient and repair the injury.

TEAR OF THE MYOCARDIUM

Tear of the atrial or ventricular myocardium resulting in pericardial tamponade is one of the more common complications. As noted earlier, it may be possible to relieve the tamponade by performing a pericardiocentesis. While these efforts are proceeding the surgical team should be summoned, if not already present. Sternotomy should be performed if the bleeding does not stop rapidly, or if the tamponade is not able to be relieved by simple drainage.

AIR EMBOLISM

Air embolism is uncommon, but does occur. The sheaths used to extract leads are large, ranging from 7F to 20F internal diameter. If the lead is removed with the sheath still in the vessel to maintain access, it is possible for a significant amount of air to be sucked into the central circulation. The resulting drop in cardiac output may be significant, resulting in hemodynamic instability. Supportive measures may be needed, and even using a catheter placed into the right ventricular outflow area or main pulmonary vein to aspirate some of the air can be attempted. Prevention of air embolism requires attention to occlusion of the sheath opening by placing a finger over the sheath or clamping the sheath.

EMBOLISM OF A VEGETATION

One of the more common questions posed to experts is "What size of vegetation should cause one to not perform a transvenous extraction procedure?" There are no absolute limits in this regard, but most experts agree that when the vegetation or thrombus is the size of the main pulmonary artery or larger, there should be serious consideration of using an alternative technique. The risk of embolization seems to be related not only to the size of the vegetation but also to its shape and consistency. A pedunculated or massive vegetation seems to have a higher risk of causing symptomatic pulmonary embolization. Alternatives to standard sheath-based extraction techniques include using a suction device from the femoral approach to remove all or part of the mass,[2] or proceeding to a sternotomy or limited atriotomy approach to remove the mass and or lead(s). Smaller embolic events are usually tolerated, although they may cause transient hemodynamic changes. If the vegetation contains a large bacterial load or is full of necrotic or pyogenic material, the patient may require significant support with fluids and/or pressors for a period of time.[3] However, nearly all of these events appear to be reversible. It is important to keep in mind that removal of leads in the presence of infection is a Class I indication,[1] and that most patients will not be able to clear the infection until the leads are removed. Thus, the risk of complication is almost always lower than the risk of not operating.

PULMONARY EMBOLISM (THROMBUS)

Another type of pulmonary embolism (PE) is that of a thrombus which was not originally present before the extraction. This event may occur because of trauma to the venous system arising from the extraction sheaths. PE may occur when either the superior or femoral approach is used. The femoral approach usually uses a 16F sheath, with inner sheaths and snares being manipulated in the central circulation. Thrombus may occur at the insertion site of the sheath, or on areas of the venous system that sustain trauma from the sheaths and snares. Even when the superior approach is used, there is trauma to the endothelial surface of the veins and there is disruption of fibrous tissues that may expose thrombogenic surfaces to the blood, resulting in clot formation. If the clot is large enough and it embolizes, it is possible for a hemodynamically significant event to occur. This event may happen during the procedure or even days following the operation.

TRICUSPID VALVE DAMAGE

Once thought to be rare, tricuspid valve damage has been found to be a relatively common occurrence.[4] However, it is rarely of clinical significance.[5] The lead can perforate the valve during implant, or become highly adherent and scarred to the valve over time. In either case, extraction can avulse a portion of the valve, or create a significant defect in a valve leaflet from sheath application. As tricuspid insufficiency is not an uncommon normal variant, small and even moderate disruptions of the valve are usually well tolerated, as evidenced by the lack of need for subsequent valve repair. However, on rare occasions damage to the valve can be significant, requiring reconstruction or replacement of the valve.

ARTERIOVENOUS FISTULA

An uncommon and unforeseeable complication is that of an arteriovenous (AV) fistula.[6] This event can be caused by improper implant technique, or result from erosion of the lead through a vein into an artery or direct damage to the artery from the extraction process. When the venous system is accessed at the time of implant, it is possible to for the introducer needle (and thus subsequently the lead) to go through an artery and into the target vein. There is often no immediate symptom associated with this; however, it is not uncommon to have excessive bleeding at the extraction site or to have bright red (arterial) blood flow back through the extraction sheath. Postoperatively one may notice a bruit over the site of the fistula, or even a palpable thrill over the site. If the fistula is large enough, the patient may have symptoms of fatigue or high-output heart failure. Therapy for this type of injury in the past has involved open surgical repair, which may be difficult if the vessels are underneath the clavicle. However, the development of covered stents and embolic therapy has made open repairs of AV fistulas largely unnecessary.

INFECTION OF NONTARGETED LEAD

Occasionally when a new device is placed following removal of an infected device, it or the new lead system becomes infected. Although this can occur with proper timing and therapy, there are several scenarios whereby infection of the new system is far more likely to occur. First, some patients are referred for extraction of an infected system by a physician who has already placed a new system on the contralateral side. In the case of a pocket infection, the bacteremia that may occur from the extraction process as sheaths are placed into the vasculature through the infected site results in contamination of the new device and/or leads. This approach is clearly wrong and should never be allowed to occur. The second way that contamination of a new system can occur is when a new system is placed into the same area where a recently extracted and infected system had been located. Despite good debridement and irrigation, contamination is likely to remain. Even if placing the new device in a different tissue plane, it is difficult to maintain a completely sterile and uncontaminated new implant. The third and most common reason for contamination of a new system is placement of new transvenous leads in a patient who is still bacteremic or who still has infected vegetations within the heart. It is very important to ensure that the patient is cleared of the infection and that blood cultures are negative for at least several days before the new implant.

DISLODGMENT OF NONTARGETED LEAD

A common situation involves targeting only 1 of 2 or more leads for extraction, with the intent of preserving the other lead or leads. This scenario occurs when a malfunctioning lead is targeted or an upgrade from a pacemaker to an ICD is attempted. As the extraction sheath is advanced or withdrawn, the interaction between the sheath and the other lead(s) in the vessel pushes, pulls, or twists the lead(s), resulting in displacement; this is not uncommon, frustrating, and frequently unavoidable. The risk of affecting a nontargeted lead can be minimized through stabilizing the lead by placing a standard stylet into its lumen. One must be cautious about placing the stylet too far into the lead, thus dislodging it. During the extraction process, the operator is usually fixated on the targeted lead and the venous and cardiac structures. It may be useful to assign 1 member of the team to observe the nontargeted lead(s) so that the physician can stop and possibly modify the sheath position to avoid dislodgment. This point is important when one evaluates a patient for lead extraction. For example, it would be a poor outcome to remove a nonfunctional right atrial or right ventricular lead and in the process dislodge a left ventricular lead, and then not be able to find a satisfactory branch in a cardiac vein to replace the left ventricular lead.

INABILITY TO PLACE A LOCKING STYLET INTO A SECONDARY TARGETED LEAD

When more than 1 lead is targeted for extraction, it is essential that all targeted leads have locking stylets placed into them before extraction of the first lead. Just as a nontargeted lead can be twisted and moved about by the extraction process, the same can happen to other targeted leads. However, if the subsequent lead is twisted or damaged during the extraction of the first lead, it may be impossible to pass the locking stylet into it, making extraction much more challenging. A good technique (and highly recommended by the authors) is to place locking stylets into all leads that are targeted for extraction before applying a sheath to a lead. Even if traction alone is applied to the first lead, the other lead may be dragged back and looped or twisted, such that stylet application is difficult or impossible. Occasionally it is not possible to place a locking stylet into a lead because of damage to the inner coil, lead fracture,

or severe tortuosity. Such cases provide greater challenges for the extracting physician, and may require careful use of sheaths without the support of a stylet, or consideration of an alternative approach such as from the femoral vein.

LOSS OF VENOUS ACCESS

One of the most critical mistakes made during extraction is loss of venous access after a targeted lead is removed. A common reason for this is that the lead pulls free and out of the vessel before the extraction sheath is placed into the vessel. To avoid this, great care must be taken to ensure that the lead is not pulling back while the locking stylet is placed or the sheath is being applied to the lead. If the lead does seem to be pulling out too easily, or it is pulling out as the sheath is being advanced (and there is a desire to maintain access via the current site, especially in the setting of an occluded vessel), one should stop pulling on the lead immediately. At this time a snare can be placed via the femoral route, and the free end of the lead grasped.[7] By having an assistant maintain traction on the lead from below, the extraction sheath may be advanced over the lead through the occluded vessel. The lead is removed through the sheath while keeping the sheath in the vessel in a position beyond the occlusion. A guide wire is then placed through the sheath, thus providing venous access. A variation on this technique involves placing a 0.014-inch (0.356 mm) guide wire into the lead as far as it will go. The lead is then snared from below and pulled out of the femoral vein, leaving the guide wire through the occlusion. Balloon venoplasty may then be performed or, using an exchange catheter, a wire of larger diameter can be placed into the central circulation.

If a lead pulls through a sheath while the sheath is partially through an occluded vessel, it is often still possible to place a hydrophilic guide wire or a 0.014-inch guide wire into the lumen left by the lead that was removed. It is critical that the sheath be left in place if the lead pulls out; this will keep it aligned with the lumen left by the extracted lead. The guide wire is then placed into the sheath, and with probing and manipulation it is often possible to thread into and through the tubular lumen left by the lead.

Sometimes one simply forgets about the need to maintain access and pulls the sheath out with the lead. In this case, as with the previous scenario, it is often possible to regain access. If it is possible to perform a venipuncture into a patent area of the vein peripheral to the occlusion, an angulated hydrophilic guide wire is placed into the vein.

Using patience and probing, the lumen left by the extraction sheath may be regained and the lead passed through the occluded vessel. If the occlusion is very localized in the subclavian vein, it may be possible to access the venous system more centrally (eg, a "medial subclavian stick"), and thus regain access. It should be noted that using the latter technique may result in early lead failure owing to "subclavian crush."

Finally, the process of lead extraction may cause a thrombus to develop in the subclavian or innominate vein, which may make passage of a guide wire difficult or impossible. Although the vessel may have appeared patent before the extraction, there is now a problem in passing a new lead. To avoid this, the authors recommend that a guide wire (or guide wires if more than 1 lead is to be placed after the extraction) be placed from the implant site into the inferior vena cava so that there are no issues with access or loss of access after the extraction. Obviously this technique does not apply if the central circulation is occluded.

ENDING UP IN A FALSE LUMEN

One potentially serious complication that occurs is placement of a guide wire or new lead into a false lumen of the vessel. As leads are removed, it is not uncommon for small dissection in the venous vessel wall to occur. As a guide wire is passed into the vessel, it follows what initially seems to be a normal course. However, the guide wire seems to "hang" at some point, often in the superior vena cava. It will often loop back on itself, or resistance will be met. If there is any problem passing the guide wire or if it seems to be taking an unusual course, one should stop and assess the situation. Contrast venography can be used to evaluate the course of the true lumen, after which the guide wire can be steered into the appropriate vessel. Failure to recognize this problem can result in a lead ending up in the mediastinum or even the pericardium. This complication can be avoided by leaving the extraction sheath tip in the inferior vena cava or low right atrium, then using a long guide wire and introducer to maintain access to the true lumen of the vessel. Another cogent point is that the tip of the guide wire should have free access to the inferior vena cava. If the guide wire can be maneuvered to below the diaphragm, it essentially rules out that the guide wire is in a false lumen.

STENTING LEADS INTO PLACE

If stenting of a vessel is being planned, extraction of any leads within that vessel before the stenting

is essential. Failure to do so will result in "incarceration" or "jailing" of the leads between the vessel wall and the stent. Attempting to extract a chronic lead that has been pinned into place could result in a vascular catastrophe. Failing to recognize that a lead was stented into a vessel wall and attempting an extraction could result in this undesired outcome. It should be noted that some stents are very radiolucent and may not be visible on fluoroscopic examination. For this reason, obtaining historical information regarding any history of stenting is essential.

SUMMARY

Lead extraction is a complex procedure that is relatively safe and highly successful when performed by competent physicians, in an appropriate venue, with the appropriate team and tools. Proper planning for each operation, and careful consideration of each patient's individual situation and needs, can prevent several of these complications and errors.

REFERENCES

1. Wilkoff BL, Love CJ, Byrd CL, et al. Transvenous lead extraction: heart rhythm society expert consensus on facilities, training, indications, and patient management. Heart Rhythm 2009;6: 1085–104.
2. Epstein LM, Love CJ, Wilkoff BL, et al. Superior vena cava defibrillator coils make transvenous lead extraction more challenging and riskier. J Am Coll Cardiol 2013;61(9):987–9.
3. Patel N, Azemi T, Zaeem F, et al. Vacuum assisted vegetation extraction for the management of large lead vegetations. Journal of Cardiac Surgery 2013; 28(3):321–4.
4. Coffey JO, Sager SJ, Gangireddy S, et al. The impact of transvenous lead extraction on tricuspid valve function. Pacing and Clinical Electrophysiology 2014;37(1):19–24.
5. Rodriguez Y, Mesa J, Arguelles E, et al. Tricuspid insufficiency after laser lead extraction. Pacing and Clinical Electrophysiology 2013;36(8):939–44.
6. Cronin EM, Brunner MP, Tan CD, et al. Incidence, management, and outcomes of the arteriovenous fistula complicating transvenous lead extraction. Heart Rhythm 2014;11(3):404–11.
7. Fischer A, Love B, Hansalia R, et al. Transfemoral snaring and stabilization of pacemaker and defibrillator leads to maintain vascular access during lead extraction. Pacing and Clinical Electrophysiology 2009;32(3):336–9.

New Advances in Left Ventricular Lead Technology

George H. Crossley, MD, FACC, FHRS, CCDS

KEYWORDS

• Lead technology • Cardiac resynchronization therapy • Congestive heart failure

KEY POINTS

- Cardiac resynchronization therapy (CRT) has been demonstrated highly efficacious in the treatment of congestive heart failure in patients with a wide QRS.
- Achieving successful left ventricular (LV) lead placement is the key step in achieving successful CRT.
- Leads have been developed that reduce the possibility of lead dislodgement after implantation.
- Lead technology has been developed that allows for the reprogramming of the stimulation vector so that phrenic nerve stimulation can be avoided while maintaining successful resynchronization therapy.
- Implantation tools have been developed that help achieve successful CRT implantation.

INTRODUCTION

CRT has been demonstrated to improve outcomes and mortality in patients with moderate to severe congestive heart failure and a wide QRS complex.[1–5] The LV lead position is critical to the success of CRT.[6–8] The limiting factor in the implementation of successful CRT is usually the anatomy of the coronary veins and the association of the cardiac veins with the phrenic nerve.[9–13] Challenges include the unavailability of a good vein position, the possibility of lead movement after implantation, and the problem of patient posture causing a change in the relationship of the LV stimulation site and the phrenic nerve. In one study, there was a 12% rate of CRT failure postoperatively related to either loss of LV capture or phrenic nerve stimulation.[14]

In response to this challenge, manufacturers of leads for CRT devices have developed an array of leads. In addition to the original unipolar LV leads, bipolar leads and quadripolar leads are now available.

The initial studies of leads developed specifically for CRT showed promising results. For example, the Medtronic 4193 lead was studied in more than 1000 patients. The mean chronic stimulation threshold was approximately 2 V. The overall complication rate was approximately 10%.[15] Another comparative study of several different Medtronic LV leads showed phrenic nerve stimulation in 13% of patients. Of these, 1.6% required either reoperation or discontinuation of LV pacing. Unipolar leads were more likely to have phrenic stimulation, and leads positioned in a midventricular site and an apical site were more likely to have phrenic nerve stimulation.[16]

ADDRESSING THE VENOUS POSITION ISSUE

In an attempt to address the problem of the variety of venous anatomy, manufacturers have

Disclosures: Dr Crossley receives significant income from consulting and speaking for both Boston Scientific and Medtronic.
Vanderbilt Heart Institute, Vanderbilt University, 1215 21st Avenue North, Nashville, TN 37232-8802, USA
E-mail address: george.crossley@vanderbilt.edu

Card Electrophysiol Clin 6 (2014) 361–369
http://dx.doi.org/10.1016/j.ccep.2014.03.002
1877-9182/14/$ – see front matter © 2014 Elsevier Inc. All rights reserved.

developed an array of leads to help fit and engage the veins and an array of additional tools to help place the leads into position. There is huge variation in the anatomy of the coronary sinus venous branches. **Fig. 1** displays examples of the variety in coronary venous anatomy.

One of the challenges in LV pacing is that the phrenic nerve lies adjacent to the lateral LV, a common site for LV pacing. The original LV leads were all unipolar and the anode was typically the right ventricular (RV) coil. Later, widely spaced bipolar leads were developed. In both of these designs, the virtual electrode size is often large enough to capture the phrenic nerve.[10,13,16,17]

It has been demonstrated that reducing the interelectrode spacing reduces the size of the virtual electrode and thus the incidence of phrenic nerve stimulation.[18] As discussed later, programmability of the vector of LV leads has undoubtedly helped avoid phrenic nerve stimulation. Leads with narrow interelectrode spacing are now available throughout most of the world. **Fig. 2** displays the choices in these LV leads. In the Medtronic leads, the interelectrode spacing

is identical on the 3 leads but the shapes are different. The Medtronic 4298 lead is a canted shape and the force of the cant is intended to provide stability. The S shape is intended for smaller veins and the straight lead, with tines, is intended to provide stability in small, short veins. There is a great deal of variability in the preference of implanters. Boston Scientific leads have varying interelectrode spacing between poles 1 and 2. This is intended to keep the short-spaced bipole away from the tip and allow for distal lodging, allowing electrical stimulation distance from the phrenic nerve. **Table 1** displays the characteristics of LV leads that are currently available.

Another concept in LV pacing is that the presence of LV stimulation at a high output may not prevent achievement of good long-term lead performance. In one study, the presence of phrenic nerve capture at 4 times the LV stimulation threshold was considered acceptable.[19] Using this approach, only 2 of 174 patients had phrenic nerve stimulation that was not remedied by reprogramming.

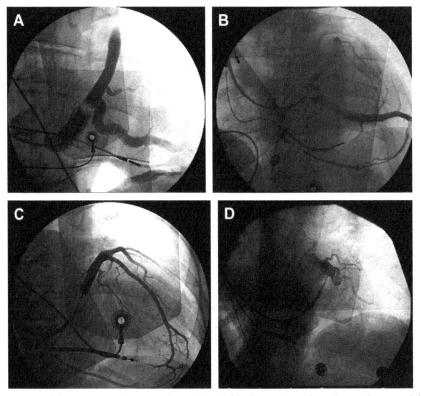

Fig. 1. The anatomy of the coronary sinus vasculature is variable. Sometimes the veins are large and there may be difficulty lodging a lead in place (*A, B*). Sometimes the veins are smaller (*C*), and sometimes the veins are small and tortuous, presenting great difficulty engaging the lumen (*D*).

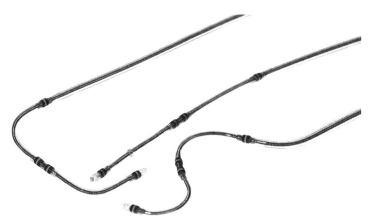

Fig. 2. Medtronic 4298, 4398, and 4598 leads have interelectrode spacing that is wide, narrow, and wide. The purpose of the narrow spacing is to reduce the risk of phrenic nerve stimulation. The shapes are intended to give physicians choices based on venous anatomy. In general, the straight lead is intended for small veins and the canted and S-shaped leads are intended for larger veins.

ADDRESSING THE POSITION STABILITY ISSUE

The long-term stability of leads in the coronary sinus has been problematic. Lead movement in the first few months after implantation is common. Physicians often have to balance the need for lead stability against the desire for the best electrical parameters. In general, once the leads have scarred into place (6 months), dislodgement is unusual.

Leads of various shapes have been developed to enhance the long-term stability of the lead. Some are straight (**Fig. 3**A), some are canted (see **Fig. 3**B), and recently several S-shaped or helical-shaped leads (see **Fig. 3**C) have been developed.[20] These shaped leads have been designed to exert lateral force, holding the lead in place as a result, even if the tip of the lead is not wedged in position. The utilization of these leads has helped to achieve lead stability.

An active fixation lead was developed by Medtronic (StarFix, model 4195). This lead has an outer push tubing that deploys 3 sets of lobes that provide radial force against the vein wall (**Fig. 4**). This fixation mechanism affords 2 benefits. First, it becomes possible to lock the lead into positions in large veins and to position proximal positions of veins that might be otherwise inaccessible. Second, the mechanism likely improves the dislodgement rate. The results with this lead have been reported and show impressive avoidance of dislodgement compared with historic controls.[21–23]

Concern has been raised by some investigators regarding the long-term ability to extract

this lead.[24,25] Results of a large clinical trial of LV lead extraction reveal that when standard extraction techniques are used, this lead is extractable, occasionally with a bit of difficulty.[26] The technique that was most successfully involved passage of the extraction sheath to the lobes for application of counter-traction at that point.

One of the problems in LV lead use is that the association of the phrenic nerve (fixed on the parietal pericardium) with lead (attached to the heart) changes when a patient's posture is different from the supine posture on the operating table. This can easily create phrenic nerve stimulation in a patient's daily life that is not observed at the time of lead implantation. If a patient has a unipolar lead, then the only nonoperative option is to decrease the output and to create a window where cardiac stimulation occurs and phrenic nerve capture does not occur.[27] Otherwise, a lead repositioning is needed. In an attempt to remedy this situation, multipolar leads were developed. These leads allow for what has often been euphemistically called *electronic repositioning*. This technique has been used successfully with bipolar leads.[27] Recently, several manufacturers developed quadripolar leads that have been successful in allowing physicians to reprogram the pacing vector and to lessen phrenic nerve stimulation.[27–30] Occasionally, however, a vein is found that lies entirely along the phrenic nerve. In this case, electronic repositioning fails.[31] Alternatively, by using quadripolar leads, there can be up to 16 vectors chosen using the 4-electrode on the lead, the RV coil, and the pulse generator can.

Table 1
Characteristics of currently available LV leads

	Medtronic							
	Attain OTW	Starfix	Attain Ability	Attain Ability Plus	Attain Ability Straight	Attain Performa	Attain Performa	Attain Performa
	4194	4195	4196	4296	4396	4298	4398	4598
Compatibility	IS-1	IS-1	IS-1	IS-1	IS-1	IS-4	IS-4	IS-4
OTW delivery	Yes	Yes	Yes	Yes	Yes	Yes	Yes	Yes
Stylet delivery	Yes	Yes	Yes	Yes	Yes	Yes	Yes	Yes
Distal lead diameter	5.4 Fr	5.3 Fr	4.6 Fr	4.6 Fr	4.6 Fr	5.1 Fr	5.1 Fr	5.1 Fr
Proximal lead diameter	6.0 Fr	5.0 Fr	4.0 Fr	5.3 Fr	4.0 Fr	5.3 Fr	5.3 Fr	5.3 Fr
Distal shape	Angled	Canted	Angled	Angled	Straight	Canted	Straight	S Shaped
Fixation	Angled body	Deployable lobes	Dual canted	Dual canted	Tined fixation	Dual canted	Tines	S Shaped
Polarity	Bipolar	Unipolar	Bipolar	Bipolar	Bipolar	Quadri-polar	Quadri-polar	Quadri-polar
Distal ESA (mm^2)	5.8	5.8	5.8	5.8	5.8	5.8	5.8	5.8
Proximal ESA (mm^2)	38.0 mm^2	NA	5.8 mm^2	5.8 mm^2	5.8 mm^2	5.8 mm^2	5.8 mm^2	5.8 mm^2
Electrode separation	11.0 mm	NA	21.0 mm	21.0 mm	21.0 mm	22.5 mm, 2.7 mm, 22.5 mm	22.5 mm, 2.7 mm, 22.5 mm	22.5 mm, 2.7 mm, 22.5 mm
Lead lengths	78, 88 cm	78, 88, 103 cm	78, 88 cm	78, 88 cm	78, 88 cm	78, 88 cm	78, 88 cm	78, 88 cm
Electrodes	2	1	2	2	2	4	4	4
Outer insulation	Polyure-thane	Polyure-thane	Polyure-thane	Polyure-thane	Polyure-thane	Polyure-thane	Polyure-thane	Polyure-thane

Abbreviations: ESA, electrode surface area; Fr, French; IS-1, International Standard 1; IS-4, International Standard 4; OTW, over the wire.

The decision of which electrode is best is made by considering electrode position, threshold, and the presence of phrenic nerve stimulation (see **Fig. 5**). To make quadripolar leads feasible, a new connector standard had to be developed (as displayed in **Fig. 6**).

These leads are designed to give physicians an opportunity to choose from many possible vectors. They also present a prospect of pacing from more than 1 LV site. There may be an additive hemodynamic effect from multisite pacing.[32] Although theoretically appealing, this approach would have a significant adverse effect on the longevity of the power source.

The use of these quadripolar leads has been demonstrated to achieve excellent results.[9,30,33] They have also been demonstrated to allow for successful electronic repositioning when phrenic nerve stimulation occurs after implantation.[34]

	Boston Scientific							St. Jude		
	Easy-track 2	Easy-track 3	Acuity Steerable	Acuity Spiral	Acuity X4 Spiral	Acuity X4 Spiral L	Acuity X4 Straight	Quartet	Quickflex	Quicksite
	4514, 4518, 4520, 4542, 4543, 4544	4524, 4525, 4527, 4548, 4549, 4550	4554, 4555	4591, 4592, 4593	4674, 4675	4671, 4672	4677, 4678	1458Q	1258T	1056K
	IS-1	IS-1	IS-1	IS-1	IS-4	IS-4	IS-4	IS-4	IS-1	IS-1
	Yes	Yes	Yes	Yes	Yes	Yes	Yes	Yes	Yes	Yes
	No	No	Yes	No	No	No	No	Yes	Yes	Yes
	5.2	5.3	5.3	4.1	3.9	3.9	3.9	4.0 Fr	3.8 Fr	5.6 Fr
	5.3	6.3	6	4.5	5.3	5.3	5.3	4.7 Fr	4.3	0
	Straight	Helix	Curve	Helix	Variable	Variable	Variable	S Shaped	S Shaped	S Shaped
	Tines	Helix	Curve	Helix	Helix/Tines	Helix/Tines	Tines	S Shaped	S Shaped	S Shaped
	Bipolar	Bipolar	Bipolar	Unipolar	Quadri-polar	Quadri-polar	Quadri-polar	Quadri-polar	Bipolar	Unipolar
	4	8.5	7.8	5.2	4.1	4.1	4.1	4.9	5	4.8
	4.2	9	9	No	8.3	8.3	8.3	7.4	7.35	NA
	11	11	8	NA	20.5, 7.5, 7.5	35.5, 7.5, 7.5	12, 12, 12	20, 10, 17	20	NA
	80, 90, 100	80, 90, 100	80, 90	80, 90, 100	86, 95	86, 95	86, 95	76, 86, 92	76, 86, 92	76, 86
	2	2	2	1	4	4	4	4	2	1
	Polyure-thane	Polyure-thane	Polyure-thane	Polyure-thane	Silicone	Silicone	Silicone	Optimum	Optimum	Optimum

IMPLANTATION TOOLS

When CRT was first used, there were no tools to help with lead implantation. Stylets were manually shaped to guide the leads into the branches of the coronary sinus. Soon thereafter, peel-away sheaths were developed. Now, all manufacturers have an array of sheaths to help with lead deployment. Some manufacturers use a steerable sheath within a sheath to allow for engagement of venous branches that veer off at an angle greater than 90°. These technologies have been exceptionally well reviewed elsewhere.[35] A hybrid guide wire has been developed that has the back-end characteristics of a stylet and the front-end characteristics of a guide wire. In a clinical trial, the use of this tool reduced the procedure duration and enhanced the accessibility to venous branches.[36]

Other pulse generator–based advances have augmented the efficacy of LV leads. One example is the use of automated threshold detection that has allowed physicians to operate the LV leads

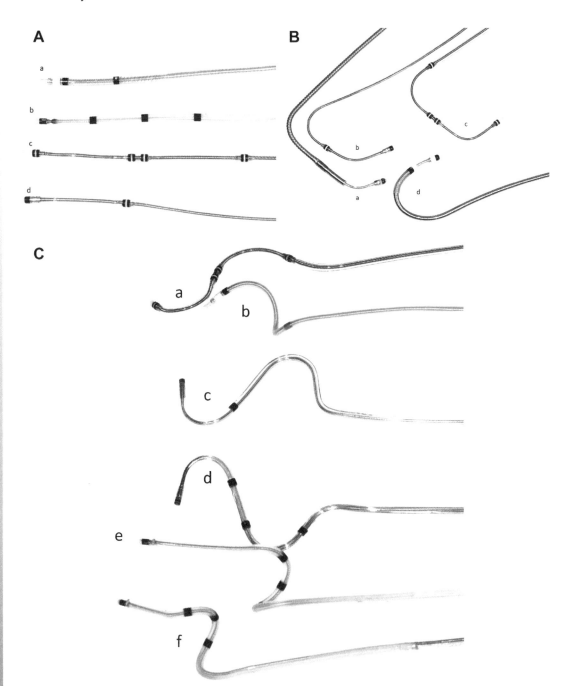

Fig. 3. (*A*) Examples of the available straight LV leads are displayed. The Boston Scientific 4543 lead is a bipolar lead (a). The Boston Scientific 4672 is a quadripolar lead with evenly spaced electrodes (b). The Medtronic 4398 is a quad-ripolar lead has asymmetrically spaced electrodes (c). The Medtronic 4396 lead is bipolar (d). (*B*) Examples of the available canted or curved LV leads are displayed. The Medtronic 4194 lead is a larger diameter bipolar lead (a). The Medtronic 4396 lead is a smaller diameter bipolar lead (b). The Medtronic 4298 is a quadripolar lead with asym-metric interelectrode spacing (c). The Boston Scientific 4554 lead is a curved, narrowly spaced electrode lead (d). (*C*) The newest designs in LV leads are the S-Shaped or spiral-shaped leads. The Medtronic 4598 lead is a quadripolar lead with asymmetrically spaced electrodes (a). The Boston Scientific 4591 is a spiral shaped lead that has a widely spaced bipole (b). St. Jude has the model 1258T (c), which is a bipolar lead, and the 1458T, which is a quadripolar lead with evenly spaced electrodes (d). Boston Scientific has 2 quadripolar leads. The model 4678 (e) has wider spacing between electrodes 1 and 2 and the model 4675 (f) has narrower spacing between electrodes 1 and 2. Quartet, Quickflex and St. Jude Medical are trademarks of St. Jude Medical, Inc., or its related companies. Used with permission of St. Jude Medical, © 2014. All rights reserved. Medtronic leads used with permission of Med-tronic, Inc. Boston Scientific leads used with permission of Boston Scientific Corporation.

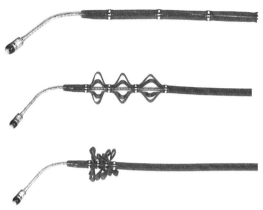

Fig. 4. The Medtronic 4195 lead is an active fixation lead. The push tubing is moved forward, forcing the lobes to deploy. The lead is slightly canted and is deployed either over a guide wire or with the use of a stylet.

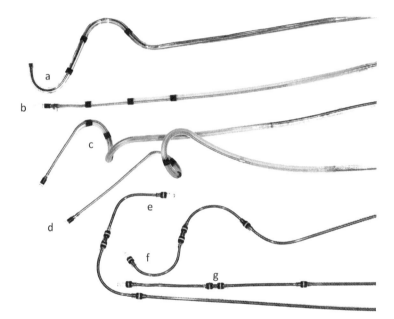

Fig. 5. Examples of available quadripolar leads are displayed. The St. Jude Medical 1458Q lead is an S-shaped lead with evenly spaced electrodes (a). The Boston Scientific leads include the straight model 4677 lead (b) in addition to the model 4674 lead (c) and model 4671 (d) leads, which are spiral shaped with different spacing between electrodes 1 and 2. The Medtronic leads include the model 4298 with a canted shape (e), the model 4598 (f), which is S-shaped, and the model 4398 (g), which is straight. All leads are intended to be deployed in an over-the-wire method. At the time of publication, the Boston Scientific and Medtronic leads are not available in the United States. Quartet, Quickflex and St. Jude Medical are trademarks of St. Jude Medical, Inc., or its related companies. Used with permission of St. Jude Medical, © 2014. All rights reserved. Medtronic leads used with permission of Medtronic, Inc. Boston Scientific leads used with permission of Boston Scientific Corporation.

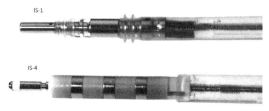

Fig. 6. IS-1 and IS-4 pin configurations are displayed.

safely with a lower output.[37] This improves longevity while maintaining safety. Advances now allow for LV pacing alone, where that is appropriate, and permits the automatic measurement of thresholds in patients with quadripolar leads with many vectors.

REFERENCES

1. Abraham WT, Fisher WG, Smith AL, et al. Cardiac resynchronization in chronic heart failure. N Engl J Med 2002;346(24):1845–53.
2. Cazeau S, Leclercq C, Lavergne T, et al. Effects of multisite biventricular pacing in patients with heart failure and intraventricular conduction delay [see comments]. N Engl J Med 2001;344(12):873–80.
3. Salukhe TV, Dimopoulos K, Francis D. Cardiac resynchronisation may reduce all-cause mortality: meta-analysis of preliminary COMPANION data with CONTAK-CD, InSync ICD, MIRACLE and MUSTIC. Int J Cardiol 2004;93(2–3):101–3.
4. Stellbrink C, Breithardt OA, Franke A, et al. Impact of cardiac resynchronization therapy using hemodynamically optimized pacing on left ventricular remodeling in patients with congestive heart failure and ventricular conduction disturbances [see comments]. J Am Coll Cardiol 2001;38(7):1957–65.
5. Young JB, Abraham WT, Smith AL, et al. Combined cardiac resynchronization and implantable cardioversion defibrillation in advanced chronic heart failure: the MIRACLE ICD trial. JAMA 2003;289(20):2685–94.
6. Ypenburg C, van Bommel RJ, Delgado V, et al. Optimal left ventricular lead position predicts reverse remodeling and survival after cardiac resynchronization therapy. J Am Coll Cardiol 2008;52(17):1402–9.
7. Khan FZ, Virdee MS, Fynn SP, et al. Left ventricular lead placement in cardiac resynchronization therapy: where and how? [review] [58 refs]. Europace 2009;11(5):554–61.
8. European Heart Rhythm Association, European Society of Cardiology (ESC), Heart Rhythm Society, et al. 2012 EHRA/HRS expert consensus statement on cardiac resynchronization therapy in heart failure: implant and follow-up recommendations and management. Europace 2012;14(9):1236–86.
9. Mehta PA, Shetty AK, Squirrel M, et al. Elimination of phrenic nerve stimulation occurring during CRT: follow-up in patients implanted with a novel quadripolar pacing lead. J Interv Card Electrophysiol 2012;33(1):43–9.
10. Biffi M, Boriani G. Phrenic stimulation management in CRT patients: are we there yet? [review]. Curr Opin Cardiol 2011;26(1):12–6.
11. Seifert M, Schau T, Moeller V, et al. Influence of pacing configurations, body mass index, and position of coronary sinus lead on frequency of phrenic nerve stimulation and pacing thresholds under cardiac resynchronization therapy. Europace 2010;12(7):961–7.
12. Thibault B, Karst E, Ryu K, et al. Pacing electrode selection in a quadripolar left heart lead determines presence or absence of phrenic nerve stimulation. Europace 2010;12(5):751–3.
13. Biffi M, Bertini M, Ziacchi M, et al. Management of phrenic stimulation in CRT patients over the long term: still an unmet need. Pacing Clin Electrophysiol 2011;34(10):1201–8.
14. Knight BP, Desai A, Coman J, et al. Long-term retention of cardiac resynchronization therapy. J Am Coll Cardiol 2004;44(1):72–7.
15. Johnson WB, Abraham WT, Young JB, et al. Long-term performance of the attain model 4193 left ventricular lead. Pacing Clin Electrophysiol 2009;32(9):1111–6.
16. Biffi M, Exner DV, Crossley GH, et al. Occurrence of phrenic nerve stimulation in cardiac resynchronization therapy patients: the role of left ventricular lead type and placement site. Europace 2013;15(1):77–82.
17. Biffi M, Zanon F, Bertaglia E, et al. Short-spaced dipole for managing phrenic nerve stimulation in patients with CRT: the "phrenic nerve mapping and stimulation EP" catheter study. Heart Rhythm 2013;10(1):39–45.
18. Biffi M, Foerster L, Eastman W, et al. Effect of bipolar electrode spacing on phrenic nerve stimulation and left ventricular pacing thresholds: an acute canine study. Circ Arrhythm Electrophysiol 2012;5(4):815–20.
19. Jastrzebski M, Bacior B, Wojciechowska W, et al. Left ventricular lead implantation at a phrenic stimulation site is safe and effective. Europace 2011;13(4):520–5.
20. Fatemi M, Etienne Y, Gilard M, et al. Short and long-term single-centre experience with an S-shaped unipolar lead for left ventricular pacing. Europace 2003;5(2):207–11.
21. Crossley GH, Exner D, Mead RH, et al. Chronic performance of an active fixation coronary sinus lead. Heart Rhythm 2010;7(4):472–8.
22. Nagele H, Azizi M, Hashagen S, et al. First experience with a new active fixation coronary sinus lead. Europace 2007;9(6):437–41.
23. Luedorff G, Kranig W, Grove R, et al. Improved success rate of cardiac resynchronization therapy implant by employing an active fixation coronary sinus lead. Europace 2010;12(6):825–9.
24. Moynahan M, Duggirala H, Dwyer D, et al. FDA approved the Medtronic model 4195 attain starfix coronary sinus lead. Heart Rhythm 2010;7(8):e3–4.
25. Maytin M, Carrillo RG, Baltodano P, et al. Multicenter experience with transvenous lead extraction of active fixation coronary sinus leads. Pacing Clin Electrophysiol 2012;35(6):641–7.
26. Sorrentino RA, Adler S, Exner DV, et al. Multicenter extraction experience with chronic medtronic LV leads. Heart Rhythm 2013;10(5):S229 [ref type: abstract].

27. Klein N, Klein M, Weglage H, et al. Clinical efficacy of left ventricular pacing vector programmability in cardiac resynchronization therapy defibrillator patients for management of phrenic nerve stimulation and/or elevated left ventricular pacing thresholds: insights from the efface phrenic stim study. Europace 2012;14(6):826–32.

28. Shetty AK, Duckett SG, Bostock J, et al. Initial single-center experience of a quadripolar pacing lead for cardiac resynchronization therapy. Pacing Clin Electrophysiol 2011;34(4):484–9.

29. Sperzel J, Danschel W, Gutleben KJ, et al. First prospective, multi-centre clinical experience with a novel left ventricular quadripolar lead. Europace 2012;14(3):365–72.

30. Forleo GB, Della Rocca DG, Papavasileiou LP, et al. Left ventricular pacing with a new quadripolar transvenous lead for CRT: early results of a prospective comparison with conventional implant outcomes. Heart Rhythm 2011;8(1):31–7.

31. Kirubakaran S, Rinaldi CA. Phrenic nerve stimulation with the quadripolar left ventricular lead not overcome by 'electronic repositioning'. Europace 2012; 14(4):608–9.

32. Thibault B, Dubuc M, Khairy P, et al. Acute haemodynamic comparison of multisite and biventricular pacing with a quadripolar left ventricular lead. Europace 2013;15(7):984–91.

33. Shetty AK, Duckett SG, Bostock J, et al. Use of a quadripolar left ventricular lead to achieve successful implantation in patients with previous failed attempts at cardiac resynchronization therapy. Europace 2011;13(7):992–6.

34. Champagne J, Simpson CS, Thibault B, et al. The effect of electronic repositioning on left ventricular pacing and phrenic nerve stimulation. Europace 2011;13(3):409–15.

35. Worley S. Left ventricular lead implantation. In: Ellenbogen KA, Kay GN, Lau CP, et al, editors. Clinical cardiac pacing, defibrillation, and resynchonization. 3rd edition. Philadelphia: Saunders; 2007. p. 653–825.

36. Giannola G, Iacopino S, Lombardo E, et al. Efficacy of a tool combining guide-wire and stylet for the left ventricular lead positioning. Europace 2011;13(2):244–50 [ref type: abstract].

37. Crossley GH, Mead H, Kleckner K, et al. Automated left ventricular capture management. Pacing Clin Electrophysiol 2007;30(10):1190–200.

Index

Note: Page numbers of article titles are in **boldface** type.

Card Electrophysiol Clin 6 (2014) 371–376
http://dx.doi.org/10.1016/S1877-9182(14)00034-3
1877-9182/14/$ – see front matter © 2014 Elsevier Inc. All rights reserved.

Moving?

Printed and bound by CPI Group (UK) Ltd, Croydon, CR0 4YY

03/10/2024

01040376-0020

.